'An understanding of Human Growth and Development is ess[...] social work practice. This book is a friendly, comprehensive guide to human growth and development suitable for social work students and more experienced practitioners alike.'
— Dr Anna Harvey, Senior Clinical Lecturer in Social
Work and Social Care, Tavistock and Portman Clinic

'This book is a wonderful resource for social workers in training and in practice. It is very accessible, with materials arranged to allow the reader to tailor the depth of their learning according to their needs. Theory and research are explained with care and there are practice examples throughout the book to help the reader engage with these frameworks as tools to guide and develop understanding of service users' lived experiences.'
— Dr Ducan Helm, Senior Lecturer, Faculty of
Social Sciences, University of Stirling, UK

'In this 2nd edition of John Sudbury's book, now with Andrew Whittaker, the psychodynamic orientation of the original text has been retained whilst content and form have been updated and refreshed. Developments refer to: the influence on young lives of social media; work with refugees fleeing war and conflict; gender variant and transgender identities; and recent data on culturally sensitive work with older adults.'
— Clare Parkinson, Clinical Lecturer, Senior Social Worker,
SFHEA, The Tavistock Centre, London, UK

Human Growth and Development

Social workers work with people at all stages of life, tackling a multitude of personal, social, health, welfare, legal and educational issues. As a result, all social work students need to understand human growth and development throughout the lifespan.

This fully revised and expanded second edition of this introductory text for social workers provides a knowledge base about human development from conception to death. It is designed to encourage understanding of a wide range of experiences: from the developmental trajectories of children in care, to adult mental distress and the experiences of people with dementia, to bereavement. Using engaging narratives to illustrate each topic, the authors clearly introduce and analyse different theoretical approaches, and link them to real-life situations faced by social workers.

Packed with case studies, this student-friendly book includes overviews, summaries, questions and further reading in each chapter, as well as a 'Taking it further' section providing greater depth on key theoretical issues. A reference section contains a glossary and overviews of the principal theories discussed throughout the book. It is an essential read for all social work students.

John Sudbery is Senior Research Fellow in Social Work at the University of Salford, UK. He has been teaching Human Growth and Development for the past ten years and is on the editorial board of *The Journal of Social Work Practice*.

Andrew Whittaker is Associate Professor and Head of Social Work at London South Bank University, UK, where he teaches Human Growth and Development. He was a Research Fellow at the Centre for Social Work Research at the Tavistock Clinic, an area director for the mental health charity Mind and a senior social worker in child protection and child and adolescent mental health teams.

STUDENT SOCIAL WORK

www.routledge.com/Student-Social-Work/book-series/SSW

This exciting new textbook series is ideal for all students studying to be qualified social workers, whether at undergraduate or masters level. Covering key elements of the social work curriculum, the books are accessible, interactive and thought-provoking.

New titles

Social Work Placements
Mark Doel

Social Work
A Reader
Viviene E. Cree

Sociology for Social Workers and Probation Officers
Viviene E. Cree

Integrating Social Work Theory and Practice
A Practical Skills Guide
Pam Green Lister

Social Work, Law and Ethics
Jonathan Dickens

Becoming a Social Worker, 2nd edn
Global Narratives
Viviene E. Cree

Social Work and Social Policy, 2nd edn
An Introduction
Jonathan Dickens

Mental Health Social Work in Context, 2nd edn
Nick Gould

Social Work in a Changing Scotland
Edited by Viviene E. Cree and Mark Smith

Social Theory for Social Work
Ideas and Applications
Christopher Thorpe

Human Growth and Development, 2nd edn
An Introduction for Social Workers
John Sudbery and Andrew Whittaker

Human Growth and Development

An Introduction for Social Workers

Second Edition

John Sudbery and Andrew Whittaker

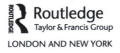

Routledge
Taylor & Francis Group

LONDON AND NEW YORK

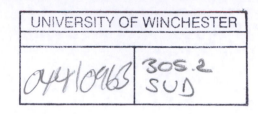

Second edition published 2019
by Routledge
2 Park Square, Milton Park, Abingdon, Oxon OX14 4RN

and by Routledge
711 Third Avenue, New York, NY 10017

Routledge is an imprint of the Taylor & Francis Group, an informa business

First edition published by Routledge 2010

British Library Cataloguing-in-Publication Data
A catalogue record for this book is available from the British Library

Library of Congress Cataloging-in-Publication Data
Names: Sudbery, John, author. | Whittaker, Andrew, 1966- author.
Title: Human growth and development : an introduction for social workers / John Sudbery and Andrew Whittaker.
Description: 2nd edition. | Abingdon, Oxon ; New York, NY: Routledge, 2018. | Series: Student social work | Includes bibliographical references and index.
Identifiers: LCCN 2018005610| ISBN 9781138071278 (hardback : alk. paper) |
ISBN 9781138304093 (pbk. : alk. paper) | ISBN 9780203730386 (ebook : alk. paper)
Subjects: LCSH: Developmental psychobiology. | Life cycle, Human. | Human growth. | Social service.
Classification: LCC BF713 .S83 2018 | DDC 305.2—dc23
LC record available at https://lccn.loc.gov/2018005610

ISBN: 978-1-138-07127-8 (hbk)
ISBN: 978-1-138-30409-3 (pbk)
ISBN: 978-0-203-73038-6 (ebk)

Typeset in Akzidenz Grotesk
by Keystroke, Neville Lodge, Tettenhall, Wolverhampton

Visit the companion website of the First Edition: http://cw.routledge.com/ textbooks/hgdsudbery/

Contents

Figures

Tables

Acknowledgements

Many people have contributed to the completion of this book. The support and commitment of Claire Jarvis and Georgia Priestley at Routledge were essential, together with others involved in the editing and production processes. Our thanks are due to the anonymous academic reviewers for their time and care.

John Sudbery would like to acknowledge the following people. He owes a particular debt of gratitude to the late Colin Woodmansey, and to Joan Meredith, from whom he learnt so much of what he has tried to communicate in this book. The text would not have been possible without the wide-ranging theoretical and practical knowledge which Jeff Edwards, a colleague at the University of Salford, shared with him.

Andrew Whittaker would like to thank his colleagues at London South Bank University for their support, including Martyn Higgins, Alison Leary, Jane Wills, Tirion Havard, Andrea Colquhoun, Jo Rawles, Jill Yates, Darlene Lamont, Iain Campbell-King, Michelle Evans, Claire Felix-Baptiste, James Ganpatsingh and John Macdonough. He would also like to thank current and former colleagues at the Tavistock Clinic, including Stephen Briggs, Anna Harvey, Hannah Linford and Andrew Cooper. Finally, he would like to thank his mother, father, sister Sally, Joe, Lauren-Kate and Ben for their support and encouragement. He would like to thank Rebecca, Samantha and Lily and, most of all, he would like to thank his wife, Christina, for all of her love and support.

Finally, thanks must go to the service users, parents and children to whom we provided a service, to the staff we have supervised, and students, all of whom over the years have taught us about human development.

Introduction

This book is an introduction to human growth and development for social workers. Although designed for a first-year undergraduate course, it contains sufficient depth to be a resource which remains useful afterwards.

FOR THE STUDENT

It is written so as to capture the interest which you will inevitably find in your work with people. You will become involved in their lives and development, and at times will have a significant responsibility as to the direction this takes. The subject is endlessly fascinating, as much for experienced and expert workers as for the new student. By making this human and professional interest the focus of the text, it has been possible to create a textbook for all students – suitable for readers who have already studied some psychology and sociology and for those who are tackling these academic subjects for the first time.

For the student who has already studied some child development, psychology or sociology, the book uses this academic knowledge, as well as additional descriptive research material, to help you to see how varied human life is, to see the world imaginatively through other people's eyes, and to think about the impact of 'welfare' interventions on people's lives and development. It will prompt you to think more deeply about whether you understand the theories and whether they describe life adequately. Information you need about the theories is summarised in the chapters, and provided at more length in the technical reference section. Because this is much more of an applied practical study, you may find that the perspective and emphasis given to theories in this book is different from that you acquired in previous purely academic study. In this course, you are learning to study life, using different theories as appropriate, which may be a subtle contrast to academic study which equips you with knowledge about research findings and theories.

For the student who has not studied 'social sciences' before, the chapters are designed to provide you with understanding, knowledge and theories about human development. The main chapter text takes you on an imaginative journey into the experience of life, its variety, complexity and its challenges, and shows how different theories and research help us to understand the world. To include the detail of the theories or research would make the chapters too long and complex, and you will need to study also the 'Essential background' sections, which we think you will find as interesting as the main chapters, so that you are properly informed.

Areas considered in greater depth. Textbooks at this level always give an overview of the basics required by students. By remaining at this introductory level, however, many texts fail to reflect the different levels at which even first-year students in this subject must operate. Each student has (and is required to demonstrate) areas in which they make use of more complete knowledge. These areas are different for every student – about pregnancy for one, attachment theory for another, learning disability, older age, and so on. They may arise from placement work, previous experience, special interest, or academic choices made during a study course. In such a broad field, the options for more detailed study are endless. In this book, six chapters end with a section which examines an aspect of growth and development in more depth. They provide examples of how basic knowledge is taken further and can be written about in more detail.

When you have finished the book, if you return and re-read it, you will probably understand the text very differently. Casual references which you glossed over on first reading actually hint at a host of additional understanding which will be evident by the end of the book. This is how it is in real life too – your experience of someone else's life (or your own) changes when you have had cause to reflect and explore some of the complexities of the life cycle. This is also true in this book because you will know far more about the people in the examples after you have read the book – just like in real life and in social work practice, an incident at a point in time will have a different significance after you have had a chance to understand more about the person and their life.

HOW TO USE THIS BOOK

There are three different sorts of learning material in this book:

Main text of
each chapter

- Intended to deepen insight into human life and its processes of change and development.

- Puts lived experience in the foreground – theoretical approaches and factual research evidence are presented as tools for exploration. The language is not technical, but makes demands on the reader to use imagination and empathy as well as intellect.

- Within this, the coverage of key theoretical ideas should be appropriate for both students already familiar with the theories and those for whom they are new. For the former it recapitulates the ideas as a preliminary to showing how they integrate (or not) with each other and how they illuminate developmental experience; for the latter, key ideas are introduced without going into technical detail or specific evidence.

■ The aim of the text is to equip the student both to see life more clearly from the inside, and to become confident in examining it as a subject of study.

Essential background

Concise accounts of commonly used developmental theories. They focus on 'understanding theories' as distinct from 'understanding life', but we hope students will nevertheless find them stimulating and thought-provoking. They give a picture of each theory covered, largely from within that theory's point of view. They give space to evidence and conceptual frameworks. Obviously, they are relevant to imaginatively understanding life and development, but they are written as reference material. By clearly presenting them as introductory summaries, it is hoped that they forestall inappropriate attempts to use elementary presentations as a basis for critical evaluation. They are written in standard language accessible to first-year university students.

Taking it further

These sections explore a selected topic in greater depth. In general, these are more demanding intellectually, and we do not expect every student will read them all. They are written in the appropriate academic style for the subject – more detached when they are more scientifically oriented, but more flexible in language when considering emotions and personal explorations. Some give a flavour of current research knowledge (the interaction between genes and environment, for example); some explore a theory in more detail (attachment theory, or Bronfenbrenner's ecological model); and others pick a facet of life to explore (for example, guilt and conscience).

FOR THE TEACHER

In this subject, a student is challenged to:

■ assimilate a range of factual information, often research findings whose validity can only be understood in conjunction with an appraisal of the research methods which generated them.
■ understand various theories and models of development which attempt to unify a range of observations and give them a coherent narrative, often supporting a particular **paradigm** about the processes that occur.
■ engage emotionally and socially with the material, integrating this with their cognitive efforts.

The module materials, from lectures to discussions and textbooks, therefore provide information, offer an explanation of theories and models, and nurture the ability to enter imaginatively into someone else's life. In relation to the latter, the course equips students to be open to the diversity of life, to avoid ignorant prejudgements, to refrain from interpreting life purely through the filter of theory, and yet to be equipped with the categories, concepts, attitudes and empathy which form the basis of accurate rapport and critical thinking.

In this book, the chapter text (including 'Taking it further') is essentially about exploration — exploring life, its development, and its complexities. It helps with the student's task of exploring the value of different theories and approaches, attempting to integrate their implications and application. Although the ten technical resources in the 'Essential background' section include discussion, we regard their purpose as primarily informational.

First-year social work students need a general overview of human growth and development as well as knowledge beyond the elementary in some areas (not least because within the year they will be 'practising' on real people with complex and urgent needs). In this subject and at this level, students appropriately will choose some areas which they explore in more depth than others, perhaps linked to previous work experience, elective seminar presentations, or special topics for course work and assessment. In addition, realistically, some complete their programme with a much more sophisticated grasp of the subject than others. We are conscious that not all teachers may welcome a book which states from the outset that not all students will master all the material. Nevertheless, if we are to meet the legitimate learning needs of the students, we must be aware that some will study material which others avoid. To include both a basic survey and all the necessary advanced material would require a far larger book than this and one not well suited to first-year students. On the other hand, keeping all the material at a basic level results in the typical problems of first-year social work textbooks in this subject — a 'middle of the road' or introductory approach which lacks depth and gives no real guidance to the student about where their studies should take them. In this textbook we have tried to create a resource which avoids the dangers of superficiality and blandness. As scholars, practitioners and educators we find our own solutions to this conundrum in the lecture room, in the seminar room and in the structures we create for student research and learning. The text is intended to provide a written resource to match the creativity we put into this task.

In physics, as with plumbing, more basic concepts and procedures are practised first and the more complex knowledge builds on these foundations. In our subject, students (whether they recognise it or not) are already operating at an extremely sophisticated level in their own lives, and the basics of analysis have to be learnt simultaneously with the refinement of already complex skills.

The book does not include any formal introduction to research methods or critical appraisal. However, it is simply not possible for professional workers in training to acquire all the information they need from a single textbook and classroom learning, and we have assumed throughout that seminar and assessed written work require the student to integrate these sources with additional material from their own investigations.

OTHER LEARNING FEATURES

Other features additional to the main chapter text are:

Glossary	The glossary explains the meaning of terms which may be unfamiliar. Most are technical terms whose use is explained when the word is first used. The first time they occur within a chapter, glossary words are printed in **bold**. This is not done for every occurrence because the use of bold distorts the rhythm and visual emphasis of a sentence.
Reflective questions	These are interactive sections which use open-ended activities to direct the readers' attention to themselves and their development. Their purpose is varied – sometimes to bring home the particular aspect of development which has been described more academically, sometimes to provide an alternative learning experience to reading; sometimes as a small contribution to helping students avoid the trap of treating 'clients', 'service users', as if they were a different category from themselves; and sometimes to underscore that in social work, self-understanding is essential.
Questions to the student in the text	Sometimes as a variant to continuous prose, questions are asked, to prompt an active engagement with the academic material. Sometimes they highlight that a suggested research approach in the text is not the only one possible; sometimes they check understanding or illustrate how an apparently simple statement may have complex ramifications.
'Links'	There are a number of marked 'links', directing the reader's attention to a different part of the book where a related topic is covered.
Further reading	At the end of each chapter, indications are given for sources of further information and discussion. Several of these include further reading appropriate also for the use of service users (for example, information designed for children in care, information about mental health issues provided by the charity Mind).
'For you to research'	From the numerous further avenues of exploration, a few topics related to the subject matter of each chapter are singled out as suggestions for independent research by the student. These may well be worked on by small groups of students collaboratively for seminar presentation or portfolio work. In our experience, students produce excellent work from these investigations, and remember the material well.

The chapters follow a roughly chronological sequence. Pauses along the route to consider particular theories or perspectives do not have an entirely logical place in this scheme – the influence of genes and environment, for example, or poverty, are relevant to all stages of life. A compromise has to be made to keep the chapters to a manageable size.

The narratives and examples

A measure of continuity is provided by a number of narratives. Although the stories are coherent and reflect changing social, economic and cultural factors in development over the last eighty years, chapters and examples are always self-contained and do not require knowledge of the earlier narrative. For those who do follow the narratives there are occasional questions or discussion points which encourage thought about the differences made by knowing an individual's personal or social history.

The majority of additional vignettes are based on real-life accounts. Except where published references are provided, names and some details have been changed. We are grateful to those represented here for the permission they gave for us to quote from their lives.

Finally, a reiteration to the student that, frustrating though it may possibly seem, in this subject a textbook does not replace the need for other exploratory reading and research, attention to television programmes and discussion. We hope the technical summaries in particular are useful when you need an instant summary (for an assignment, perhaps), but the subject requires you to read more in depth, to assemble, collate and critically compare your own resources. The website which accompanies the book gives links to an extensive range of additional material – more detailed information, original research reports and relevant policy and guidance. The subject is endlessly fascinating but, as explained in Chapter 10, does require creative intellectual and emotional engagement.

CHAPTER 1

Beginnings

In this chapter you will find:

■ **Introductory reading**

■ **Making sense of development requires biological, psychological and sociological knowledge**

■ **Bio-psychosocial knowledge: an overview of the approaches which will be used in the book**

■ **Genes, environment and behaviour: a section written in a more formal academic style**

INTRODUCTORY READING

'I'm pregnant,' she said, 'I've not told anyone else yet.'

These words point to the different ways in which a social worker needs to be able to understand human development.

In the first three months after conception the baby can be said to be 'taking shape' – developing the basic plan of a human body, including a head, arms, legs, hands and feet. In the next three months, the organs and limbs will be developing in size, complexity and functionality; the mother can feel her baby moving, and the baby responds to stimuli. Continuing to simplify this finely tuned and intricate process, in the next three months each interlinked part of the tiny body will continue to grow in size, efficiency and complexity until birth, and the baby in this period becomes increasingly able to survive outside the womb. In keeping with this simplified account, if drugs interfere with the process in the first three months, parts of the baby may be malformed or missing; and malnutrition is more likely to cause small size if it occurs in the final three months rather than in the earlier phases.

During pregnancy, a special enzyme in the placenta acts to block the stress hormone cortisol from reaching the foetus (DiPietro et al., 2006). However, if a mother experiences intense or chronically stressful situations where she feels out of control, such as domestic abuse or severe poverty, this can over time affect the enzyme, leading to it being less effective (Gerhardt, 2015). The result is that the baby can be flooded with stress hormones, which can lead to later difficulties. For example, they are likely to be born more irritable and prone to crying (van der Waal et al., 2007). This is because of the effects that stress hormones have on the baby's amygdala (involved in emotions) and the hypothalamus (involved in memory). An amygdala that has had to cope with considerable stress in early life tends to react more, working harder and growing larger. Unfortunately, this means the person is more sensitive to stress and the mechanisms for managing the stress response are weakened. This is an important finding, but there is a danger that it can be used as a form of 'victim blaming', in which mothers who experience considerable stress (such as being victims of domestic abuse) are viewed as being responsible for their child's difficulties. It is important to bear in mind that there are positive aspects of later caregiving that can have a positive effect. For example, secure attachment and positive bonding during the first year can enable a small hippocampus affected by stress to be restored to normal volume (Buss et al., 2012; Gerhardt, 2015).

We have no words that can accurately describe the unborn baby's experience. We know that it hears sound, as after birth it will respond differently to pieces of music which have been played repeatedly during pregnancy – presumably most of these sounds are the internal noises of its mother's body and the muffled penetration of her voice, talking, singing, shouting. In a fascinating series of observations, Piontelli (2002) found that at the age of 5, twins were still using routines for mutual comforting which had been observed by ultrasound when they were in the womb. And then at some point the baby will be gripped harder than it is ever likely to be gripped again, so hard that the bones of its skull fold over each other. Over a period between seven and fourteen hours on average, it will be propelled in repeated shoves down a narrow tube until it bursts into a noisy, bright, colourful environment totally different from the world it has experienced previously. This shocking experience will usually have the effect you might predict – having been massively stimulated the baby will be awake for an initial period and then fall into a deep exhausted sleep.

You will be able to find many sources of further information about pregnancy, including websites which you can locate for yourself. Detail appropriate to this level of study can be found in Chapter 2 of Boyd and Bee (2014).

We could tell a related story for the mother's own bodily development during pregnancy, but instead, let us think about a different perspective: the developmental meaning of the pregnancy in a woman's life, its significance and implications, which are different for every mother.

Nicola

Perhaps the young woman is Nicola, pregnant with her second child, anticipating that she will leave paid work for at least the next five or six years.

She is a 26-year-old Black British woman who has made a good start to her career. She and her partner have planned – to the degree that these things can be planned – that his income and some state benefit will support the family until she goes back to work when both children are at school. She is not very clothes-conscious, but usually looks smart in her business suit when she goes to work. She's very busy day-to-day with her first child – let us say a boy – but her partner, a neighbour with whom she's close, her mother whom she sees once or twice a week and some friends who had babies at the same time as her, are all involved in the planning for when she has her new baby. During her first pregnancy, she had many thoughts and daydreams about how the life of her child would turn out; she has similar thoughts now, but when asked about the future she says, 'Oh, I just hope everything's going to be OK, I'm really quite stretched this time, what with work, my son Matthew, Steve's job and the pregnancy as well. I just hope the baby will be healthy, have ten fingers and ten toes, and we'll get everything sorted in time.' What she says, of course, depends on whom she is talking to; she has a friend at work with whom she particularly chats about her toddler and the pregnancy.

Naoko

But every pregnancy, every woman, is different. Maybe the young woman is Naoko and this is her first baby. She was born and brought up 6,000 miles away in Japan, and is now living in the UK with Paul, whom she met as a student. She sees her mother only once a year. Her partner's parents are supportive, but although they are geographically closer, their routines, expectations, standards of healthcare, religious beliefs and daily language are all a second culture for her. English people find her rather quiet and reserved, and she still occasionally struggles to find the word she wants. She is sometimes surprised by the behaviour of boys and girls and by the attitudes of women where she lives.

Tia

And a social worker must be prepared to understand a myriad of different developmental stages. The mother-to-be may be Tia, aged 16 and having just left a children's home. She's talking on the phone to Claire, the only person she trusts. Claire is 15 and also in care. The children's home, known as 'Number 24', has been Tia's third placement in two years, before which she lived in six foster homes. Her keyworker sometimes listens, alarmed, as she jabs her finger into her belly and says, 'I hate *it*', deliberately emphasising the word 'it', and continuing, 'I hope it's gone when I wake up.' She doesn't say much at all to this worker, whom she has known for only four months, since she left the children's home. However, she does speak about the time she thinks she got pregnant, which was when she stayed out all night at a friend's squat, and felt pressurised into sex, almost without caring what she did. The significance of the pregnancy in her life? Her ferocious displays of independence and wilfulness had always been partly a reaction to her pervasive sense of helplessness before fate; defiant strivings to carve out some control for herself in the midst of major events which usually seemed just to happen to her. The pregnancy was little different. She is defiantly independent, proclaiming her competence to do whatever is required; she also has the sneaking hope, daydream, that the baby might be the one person in the world who will really love her, who will be *hers*; sometimes she is terrified of the responsibility and tasks that she hardly dares think about. At the same time, a young woman with a ferocious temper, a short fuse, intolerance born of frustration, she is bitterly angry towards the latest interference in her life. Underlying this is the overwhelming sense of helplessness and lack of control over events. As earlier in her life, she feels that things are done to her, they happen without her permission, and her attempts at effective influence repeatedly seem to dissolve into a position of impotence.

Social support

One feature common to each story is that however independent and competent each pregnant woman is (and all have demonstrated great strength and resourcefulness in their lives to date), each needs emotional and practical support, and this will have particular significance at the birth and afterwards. This support may come from many different directions – a partner; a circle of female friends; the woman's mother; a religious grouping; various official, medical or social staff, for example. As a social worker, you could potentially be involved in any of these situations, and it would be a routine part of your professional assessment to understand the nature of the woman's needs, how what you have to offer fits in with all the other sources of support available (or missing), and the potential outcome of offering support.

Toddlers to grandparents

There are of course other people involved in this scenario, each at a different stage of life. It is typical of social work that these all have to be kept in mind. Unlike doctors, psychologists, counsellors or many other human service professionals, as a social worker, it is usual for you to have professional responsibility for several different life stages at the same time.

For Matthew, Nicola's first child, this pregnancy, and more importantly the birth, may represent a big milestone. Until now, he has been the sole focus of parental attention, love, annoyance and preoccupation. In this attention, the adults who keep him safe are concerned about his welfare, ensure they are there for him, focus all their parental love solely on him. His experience is that they are captivated by him when he offers a single smile or takes a first few tottering steps. One utterance that sounds as if it might be a word evokes doting admiration. This is shortly to change for ever, a dramatic change as he is supplanted by a rival for his mother's love and attention – 'Can't we just put her in the bin?' as one boy said of his young sister.

It may be, too, that the partner is facing some of the most stressful periods in his life as he juggles new responsibilities at work, financial responsibilities at home – and he too may have troubles about the direction of Nicola's affections, the time she has for him, changes in her sexual impulses – he turns over choices, perhaps dilemmas, as to how to satisfy his sexual needs; with her he will be finding his way, managing and relating to an increasingly independent toddler, and later a schoolchild. Then there are Nicola's parents, in whose development grandchildren are likely to be extremely significant. They were older than many – 64 when Nicola became pregnant again – and they are a major part of their grandchildren's lives. Nicola's first child has experienced much of his daytime care at their house.

On the other hand, think of the world from the point of view of Naoko's parents. They see their daughter and grandchild for only one week in the year. They will perhaps have questions, worries, about the starkly contrasting gender attitudes and child-rearing practices compared with those they have believed to be 'correct' and 'necessary' in the provincial Japanese village which is their home.

The mother of 16-year-old Tia is Bella – perhaps she hasn't seen her daughter for twelve years. If she is like many mothers in such a situation, she will describe the loss of her daughter into care as 'like a death, only worse'. Birth parents of adopted children say that long after the event, they still think of their lost child 'every day, or two or three times a week'; decades later, they describe themselves as 'still screaming'. Her sense of loneliness, hurt and loss may be intensified if she hears by a circuitous route that her daughter has had a baby. Or perhaps Tia's mother is still in touch with her, and alongside her fury with social workers for what they did in the past, desperately hopes they will be able to help her daughter so her grandchild is competently cared for.

From time to time in the coming chapters, you will read more of the world through the eyes of Nicola, Tia, Naoko and their friends and families. We can't simply describe their babies' lives through to old age and death – if we did, we'd have to start in the early 1920s, at the time when 'Tia' might be a girl in a workhouse and might have been locked up for the rest of her life in a mental asylum because she was pregnant; and in a number of occupations Nicola's employment would have been ended because she married. We want to start from pregnancies in circumstances you can relate to. But the book does emphasise the whole sweep of a life, how you have to understand earlier incidents in order to understand the person before you. So in order to understand the development of Tia's grandfather Bob, who dies before the book is finished, you will read snippets about his infancy and earlier adulthood, how he got on with Tia's mother Bella, and how a social worker became involved just before his death.

MAKING SENSE OF DEVELOPMENT AND CHANGE

As we go through life, we all have to make sense of our development – women perhaps more than men are forced to understand their body and its changes; we try to make sense of how we form and manage relationships, our behaviour towards others, and what we may call 'phases' in life. This book is about making a rigorous study of this – study that can be used reliably, not just so we can go about our own private lives, but so we can responsibly be involved in crucial decisions about the lives of others. Generalising from the introductory snapshots at the beginning of the chapter, you can see the areas about which you need to become knowledgeable:

- Biological knowledge about the body, its development, and its influences on emotion and behaviour.
- Psychological knowledge about feelings, behaviour and relationships.
- Social knowledge about how societies and cultures function and influence the individual.
- And, most importantly, the overlap areas between each of these.

However, there is a further complication to which we will return: you will need to understand the view that the word 'knowledge' in the above information box (we could have used the word 'understanding') has to be viewed with caution. It seems to indicate something absolute, to point to 'facts' which exist independently of the researchers who discover or codify them, independent of the language they use and where they publish their findings. But **social constructionists** argue that 'facts' presented by social research are always shaped politically by the cultures of the researchers and the reader. They always represent a 'point of view' and would be different if understood from a different perspective. The categories used are always social creations, and taking them for granted significantly conceals some of what is going on in the activity and publication of such research.

BIO-PSYCHOSOCIAL KNOWLEDGE

One of the most straightforward descriptions of social work is that it is a **psychosocial** activity (Ruch et al., 2010; Wilson et al., 2011), concerned with the 'person-in-the-situation': not just the person on their own, nor just the social arrangements around them, but the two together. In providing a knowledge base about individual development, this book draws attention to biological factors as well as the psychological and sociological – a bio-psychosocial perspective.

Bodies and health

Social workers acquire much of their specific information about the body and brain not in their initial training courses but in particular social work contexts. For example, a social worker working with autistic children will acquire specific information as they work – because of particular children and parents, through continuing professional training, and because of specific multidisciplinary discussions. The same will be true of social workers in a hospice, or social workers in a team that meets the needs of people with dementia and their carers.

This book provides frameworks and examples to prepare you for seeking such specific expertise. This chapter concludes with a discussion about the nature of genetic influence – an introduction to aspects of the nature/ nurture debate. Other chapters contain brief sections about: the influence of emotional relationships on brain development in infants (Chapter 2), physical changes in adolescence (Chapter 4), organic dimensions to mental health problems (Chapter 6), physical aspects of the stress response (Chapter 6) and the ageing process (Chapter 8). There are also shorter references such as that about prenatal development at the beginning of this chapter. 'Essential background', section 1 provides a summary of what is meant by '**genetics**'.

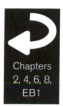

Chapters 2, 4, 6, 8, EB1

Psychological understanding

The core purpose of this book is to promote your understanding of development in people's feelings, behaviour and relationships. Different researchers and practitioners have created different schemes for making sense of these subjects. Sometimes, these different perspectives illuminate different aspects of life, but researchers also sometimes claim that their findings show that another theory is simply mistaken. This book will discuss many of these disagreements.

Using the examples earlier in the chapter for reference, here is a summary of some of the theories which will be used in the course of the book:

■ Stage theories of development, particularly **Erikson's psychosocial model** – in which it is claimed that life can be understood as a series of stages (including infancy, adolescence, older age, for example). This is introduced in Chapter 2 and summarised in 'Essential background', section 6.

What 'stage(s)' of life would you say 16-year-old Tia is in? What about Nicola's mother and father?

This question highlights some of the ambiguity of thinking about universal 'stages'. Tia is an adolescent, a first-time mother, a young adult living in her first independent home. Some would regard becoming a grandparent as the start of a new stage in life – perhaps part of old age; some grandparents would definitely not think so! Different stages can be present at the same time, and different people may follow them in a different sequence. Dividing life into 'stages' can cause as much confusion as clarity.

■ **Attachment theory**, which interprets observational studies as showing that infants are born with a drive to form attachments and parents are programmed to respond with care and protection. The 'attachment style' of an individual develops throughout life in response to external relationships and events, but early attachments are very influential in shaping later attitudes and behaviour. This is introduced in Chapter 2 and summarised in 'Essential background', section 2.

■ **Psychodynamic** theories, which take for granted the existence of conflicting motivations and interests, and view some of them as being unconscious. This is also introduced in Chapter 2, and summarised in 'Essential background', section 4.

What might be some of the conflicting impulses which motivate Nicola's partner Steve? What about her son Matthew, or Nicola herself? What influences how they resolve these conflicts?

■ **Humanistic** models, such as Rogers' person-centred approach, which points out that people from childhood onwards have a drive to achieve something in life, and also a need for unconditional acceptance; it examines achievements and difficulties in life in the light of this. This is introduced in Chapter 4 and summarised in 'Essential background', section 7.

■ Learning theories, including **cognitive behavioural** and **'social learning'** perspectives, which emphasise that behaviour is shaped by rewards and punishments that have been applied in the past, and also by the perception of what is thought to be advantageous or problematic. This is introduced in Chapter 3 and summarised in 'Essential background', section 8.

Think about Matthew when he was 20 months old. In simplified, cognitive behavioural terms, what accounts for how Matthew's behaviour is developing? How might that perspective account for the difference between what Naoko's parents think are good qualities in a woman and what Nicola thinks?

The answer in each case is that the behaviour shown depends on what behaviour has been rewarded and encouraged in the past, and which behaviours punished or discouraged.

■ Models of the experience of 'spoiled identities' – growth to positive self-identity in the face of widespread social attitudes indicating the individual is part of a 'problem group'. Examples are black people brought up in a society with racist attitudes, gay, lesbian and transgendered people brought up in a society in which their sexual identity is seen as 'unnatural' or immoral, or people with disabilities facing attitudes which confuse speech difficulty with cognitive impairment. This is discussed in a number of chapters, but particularly in relation to adolescence in Chapter 5, and adulthood in Chapter 7.

■ Theories of ageing, including the '**social disengagement**' model, '**activity theory**', and '**political economy theory**'. The first of these, for example, builds on research findings to theorise that there is a mutual advantage for the individual and for society if the older generation gradually withdraws from social interaction and responsibility. See Chapter 8 and 'Essential background', section 9.

After the main chapters, the 'Essential background' contains a ready reference summary of these and other theories, as well as an outline of the criticisms that have been directed at them.

Sociological thinking

The life course of mother and baby will be profoundly affected by social factors. If the mother is from a Gypsy Traveller community, the Department of Health's report suggests that the baby is more than twelve times as likely to die from sudden infant death syndrome, and ten times as likely to die from all causes before the age of 2; a third will die before reaching the age of 25 and more than seven out of ten will die before reaching the age of 59 (Parry et al., 2004, explaining they used statistics from Ireland – see McKittrick, 2007). The life course of Naoko's mother in rural Japan may have been profoundly different from that of a woman of comparable age brought up in the UK. A child growing up as part of a stigmatised group which is seen as 'problematic' or 'immoral' by wide sections of the population faces distinctive developmental issues. Whatever genetic differences are at work, there are differences in the experience and expectations of males and females throughout the course of life which are heavily influenced by societal attitudes and expectations.

In general, this book will not focus on sociological theory and debate. It will, however, refer frequently to ways in which social factors and perspectives are areas to explore in relation to individual change and development. It assumes a 'cosmopolitan' view of society – in brief, that people's inner worlds (their identity, values, fears, memories, pleasures) may or may not be primarily embedded in the geographical area in which they live.

One account which sets out systematically the different interpersonal and sociological influences on development is **Bronfenbrenner's ecological model**. This is presented in Chapter 5 and summarised in 'Essential background', section 3.

The '**life course**' approach to development emphasises that there is no universal 'natural cycle' of life. Lives are always located in specific historical, geographical and cultural contexts, and the search for 'normal development' or universal stages may do violence to the diversity of human experience.

Objectivity and subjectivity: facts, theories and viewpoints

This chapter has offered some snapshots, and then referred to the range of ways it is possible to analyse individual development and change. There is no single developmental framework which captures what is happening in life, and if, as a worker in training (and subsequently as a practitioner), you are competent, you will find that you understand development differently as you go through life. Your views about relationships, aggression, culture, people's needs, infantile experience and sexuality are understood differently when you are 15, 20, 35, or 55. As a professional person, this change will be influenced by events in your own life, by what you learn from people to whom you provide service, by scientific research and by informed discussion about challenging situations in which you will be asked to intervene.

ABOUT YOURSELF

Chapter 10

As you follow a course about human growth and development, it is likely that it sets off many thoughts and feelings about yourself. For reasons that are touched on particularly in Chapter 10, self-understanding is important in social work. This book contains a series of activities that allow you to look at aspects of yourself, your attitudes and your development.

The activities can be taken at different levels of sensitivity, but all can touch on painful aspects of life. Ideally, perhaps, they are activities you would undertake with a person whom you know to be kind, competent and understanding in taking care of your feelings. There are no right or wrong answers.

For this first activity, draw a lifeline to represent your life to where you are now (see Figure 1.1 below). Mark some important milestones or transitions you have experienced – for example, being born; birth of siblings; parents' relationship – separation, divorce, remarriage; starting school; getting a job; friendships; marriage, and so on.

There are many different ways this could prompt reflection about your development. For example, the section of this chapter 'Making sense of development and change' stated that you need biological, psychological and sociological knowledge. Discuss how this applies to one of the periods you have identified – why were biological, psychological and sociological factors all involved in the development that was taking place?

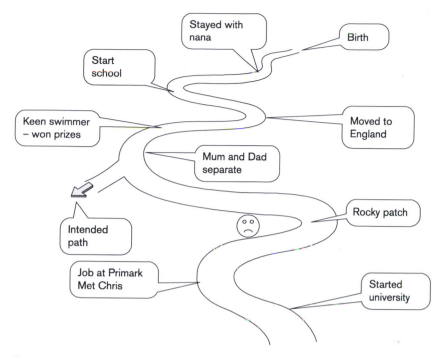

Figure 1.1 An example lifeline

USING THIS BOOK

This is an introductory chapter. It has an explicit and an implicit message. The explicit message is to introduce the range of material that will be covered in the book, to set you thinking about its scope and what knowledge will be involved. The implicit message is that to understand human growth and development you have to engage your social and emotional imagination and to think clearly. In the type of material presented you must be prepared to enter imaginatively into someone else's world even when you have few of the actual details of their lives. As you enter their world, you need to be prepared to find features that are common to everyone, and features that have arisen only because of specific experiences. And you should sometimes be puzzled by which is which.

Furthermore, you only understand an individual's development when you understand the development of other people which is interlocked with it – the baby's experience is interlocked with the mother's, which in turn is interlocked with (for example) the father's and the mother's mother's. As a competent social worker, you have in nearly all situations to understand the developmental experience of several people, often of different ages, at once.

If you just wish to scan for intellectual content we have tried to set this out so it is readily available. The 'Essential background' sections should do this efficiently at the basic level, and the 'Taking it further' essays offer more depth. The main chapter text requires a different kind of attention – a more reflective, personal engagement. The narratives may prompt questions such as, 'I wonder how they got to this stage in their life?' or, 'How easy is it for me to understand their experiences?' In the words of David Howe (2008), it is important that you develop as an 'emotionally intelligent social worker'. You might think about whether you would be interested to meet them, and what your feelings would be in their company – would you know how to set them at ease and so on. In the healthiest possible way, social work is founded on a curiosity about people and a wish that things should be well for them, and this sometimes requires a slower pace of thought as you reflect on an imaginary encounter.

GENETICS AND ENVIRONMENT

Each chapter in this book concludes with a more formal essay, sometimes with more detail, sometimes with greater complexity. In this particular chapter, the theme of the essay is taken from thoughts that will go through many minds as they think about the life that lies ahead of each baby in the womb. As they reflect on this, and naturally consider the differences between a mother in a secure environment living in the suburbs, a 16-year-old care leaver who is pregnant, and the personality and achievements of a young musician living 6,000 miles away from where she was brought up, they are prompted to wonder whether differences are caused by inherited differences or differences in upbringing and environment.

Everyone is different, and all the theories that are used to make sense of the differing paths to people's lives acknowledge that both genetic makeup and different environments play their part in shaping the course of a person's life. There are many areas in which social workers will hear assertions about the relative influences of 'nature' and 'nurture'. They may hear questions asking whether men are by nature more aggressive, or more promiscuous, than women, for example. They will hear psychologists refer to the hereditable nature of intelligence, or the supposed identification of a genetic basis for schizophrenia. In every case, the context may be a discussion about whether the converse is true – that these features are a result of environment – family history, culture, peer influences and so on. On later occasions, this book will refer to some of these topics. This section presents some considerations which are necessary to make sense of particular instances of the 'nature–nurture debate'.

Chapter
EB1

To prepare for this essay, you must check that you understand the information in 'Essential background', section 1. Key ideas that are used in the following 'Taking it further' section are:

- The 'instruction set' that tells your body how to build itself – your eye colour, whether you are male or female, your brain's ability to learn languages, whether you are likely to develop breast cancer – is contained in biological structures called **genes**. There is a complete set of genes in every tiny component cell of your body. It is important to understand that, by and large, you are a conduit for this instruction set and it is passed on faithfully through the generations – you do not change it by becoming a champion weightlifter or a highly qualified academic or a brutal dictator, or by eating well or poorly.
- When a new baby is started, it contains one set of genes from the mother and one from the father. When this baby grows up and has a baby, it may pass on either of these genes. For example, a girl, Tia (whose own eggs were formed inside her when she was in her mother's womb) will have genes from both her father and her mother and may pass either of these on in a particular egg her body releases each month after puberty, as shown in Figure 1.2.

So Tia may pass on characteristics such as straight or curly hair, from her mother or her father. And similarly, her partner's sperm may be passing on details from his mother or his father. For each parent, this selection occurs randomly and more or less independently for every gene in their 'instruction set'.

Figure 1.2 illustrates another feature of genetic reproduction. All the cells in the body contain two sets of genes, one from each parent, except the male sperm and the female egg which only contain one set each. When the egg and the sperm combine to form the start of a new person, the fertilised egg now contains the usual double set.

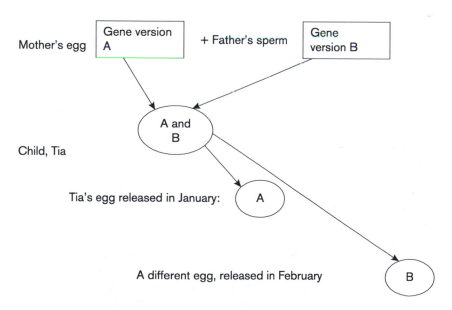

Figure 1.2 Generational transmission of genes

Approximately 25,000–30,000 genes are grouped together into structures called **chromosomes**. The chromosomes come in pairs, one containing the instructions from the father and one from the mother. Although the detail of what they code for may be different (one for blue eyes, one for brown eyes), the genes on each of a matched pair are for the same function (eye colour in this case). The pair of chromosomes determining sex are different from this general pattern. They come in two different forms, called because of their shape X and Y. If the fertilised egg has the pair X-Y, the child will be a boy. If the pair is X-X, the child will be a girl.

Additional basic resources are given on the website which accompanies this book.

?

Lead-up questions

A man has a gene (call it G1) on his Y chromosome. Will that gene ever have been operating in a female?
Answer: No, because women never have a Y chromosome in their body – they are X-X.

A woman has a gene (call it G2) on her X chromosome. Has this ever been operating in a male?
Answer: Yes, because female bodies have X-X and men have X-Y. A daughter will always have one X chromosome from her father.

Of all the Y chromosomes in the population (say, a country), how many are in male bodies?
Answer: All of them.

Of all the X chromosomes in a population, how many are in female bodies at any given time?
Answer: Two out of three. Women have X-X and men have X-Y chromosomes.

What else affects your development and who you are other than your genes?
Answer: Well, we hope you found the answer to that fairly obvious! – How you're brought up, whether you have always eaten well, what illnesses you have suffered, your choices about which school to go to and what career to follow . . . The list is endless. The essay is particularly concerned with the question: what are some of the factors that affect how genes and environment interact?

Some other words and phrases used in the essay:

- *discrete category*: a grouping which contains items which definitely do not belong in a contrasting group – there's a yes/no answer to whether they belong – for example, someone is pregnant or they are not.
- *continuous variable*: a quality which does not fall into discrete categories, but varies by infinitesimally small progressions, progressions so small that whenever you choose two items which differ, you can always specify a third item which is in between (such as height).
- *constitutional*: this is used in the essay as an 'ordinary language' description, not a technical term. It describes how someone's body seems to be in itself, often implying that it's without special treatment or training. Someone might be described as having a 'strong constitution' because they seldom become ill and usually resist infections, or they might be constitutionally suited to being a weightlifter because they have a powerful, compact body.
- *pathways*: a term used to describe the route by which someone's personal qualities come into existence. The pathway to having blue eyes is a genetic makeup which sets off certain chemical and biological processes. The pathway to becoming a good social worker is . . .?
- *correlations*: some factors which have an effect on an outcome can be changed separately from each other. To find what layout of magazine the readers prefer, a publisher can vary the size of print and the colour of print separately, and find whether one has more effect than the other, and what colour, size, and combination of colour and size have a good effect. If for some reason the factors are interlinked, so that changing one changes the other – they are *correlated* in some way. If changing the size would for some strange reason change the colour, then it's a different question to disentangle the effects. When the publishers thought they had measured the effect of size, they might without realising it be measuring the effect of colour. We have chosen this example because it will seem strange. The essay explains that genes and environment have often been understood to vary independently, but in fact there may be complicated ways in which they are linked.

TAKING IT FURTHER

GENES, ENVIRONMENT AND BEHAVIOUR: CORRELATIONS AND INTERACTIONS

Presentations of 'the nature–nurture debate' usually conclude by emphasising that both are involved in human behaviour (for an introductory account, see Holt et al., 2015 – more detail is given in Ridley, 1999; Rutter, 2006). Further analysis explores the particular mechanisms and routes which operate for specific outcomes. These are usually infinitely complicated. Geneticists (Sudbery and Sudbery, 2009; Bateson, 2001) point out that a very large number of genes are required to cooperate to produce behaviour, and the same version of a gene can produce different results in a different 'team' of genes or in different environments. A multitude of environmental differences are relevant in different episodes of development. Given this introduction, the elements highlighted here are:

- ■ 'Biological variation' is not the same as 'genetic variation'.
- ■ Genes can conflict.
- ■ The distinction between behaviours that form a separate category and those that are continuous with the behavioural range in the general population.
- ■ There can be different pathways to the same behavioural characteristics.
- ■ The interdependence of genes and environment – environments are not always independent of genes, and genetic effects are affected by environment.
- ■ The reasons for variability between individuals (the relative importance of heredity and environment) might be different from the reasons for variability between average scores of groups of people.

Running through this are various issues about the meaning and operation of 'cause' in this context. The discussion is illustrated by reference to children's behaviour, gender and mental health issues.

Biological variation is not genetic variation

'Constitutional' conditions may be biological but not necessarily genetic in origin. Even when present at birth, they may be caused by nutrition, prenatal environment in the womb, viruses or complex interactions between genetic factors and environment. For example, Tourette's syndrome is a neurological condition in which people constantly mix little verbal explosions, sometimes swear words, into their speech (National Institutes of Health, 2005). One suggested cause of Tourette's syndrome is that it is manifest after an individual with a particular genetic makeup is exposed to a particular balance of hormones in the womb (Eapen et al., 1997).

There are physiological signs that high-achieving athletes often received higher than average amounts of testosterone in the womb (Paul et al., 2006). If so, this would be a factor which is constitutional, but not in itself genetic.

Genes can be in conflict

Darwin's formulation of evolution was based on the realisation that each individual varies from its parents; and that just as farmers, racehorse owners and pigeon fanciers selectively breed for particular qualities – thereby producing dogs, from pugs to Great Danes; horses, from Shetland ponies to thoroughbred racers – so over much greater periods of time will there be selection and shaping in nature according to which changes survive better and breed more.

This does not, however, imply that the changes that take place in evolution are best for the survival of all the species. For example (see Ridley, 1999: 107–121), some genes are carried only by men, so, in theory, variants which occur are differentially selected if they assist the male body, even if they have indirect consequences harmful to women (as long as these aren't sufficiently harmful to impair breeding success). These are rare, as the genes specific to men are comparatively small in number. They are on a relatively small grouping of genes described because of its shape as the Y-chromosome, and only carried by men. Women, on the other hand, have the chromosome pair X-X. This means that on average over the generations X-chromosomes spend more time (two-thirds of their existence) in females. Variations which make their continuance more likely will preferentially survive. Since they are more often in a female body, these variations are on average those which make the female more likely to survive, even if the consequences are unfortunate for the male of the species (as long as these unpleasant consequences don't lessen breeding success for the female). The conflicts in this example are of course primarily about biological processes in the body, brain and reproductive systems – not in the first instance about psychosocial behaviour.

Separate categories or continuous variables?

A mother may wonder whether her son's aggressiveness (or intellectual level) is a result of his genes or how he was brought up. In an example earlier in this chapter, carers of a teenager in local authority care may wonder whether her seeming lack of maternal feeling towards her unborn baby is because of genes or experience. Social workers, if only to give educated replies to their service users and colleagues, have an interest in the relative importance of genes and environment in 'psychosocial' qualities such as aggression, intelligence and mental confusion.

Rutter (2006: 24) points out that research into behavioural genetics requires clarity (and can create clarity) about whether the quality (or behaviour) forms a separate category from the behaviour of the general population or represents a particularly low (or high) value of something that varies throughout the population.

For example, schizophrenia is listed, with its symptoms, in the authoritative diagnostic manuals of psychiatry (American Psychiatric Association, 2013) as a classification – the individual 'has' it or not. But the nature of the increasing evidence of its heritability indicates that it varies continuously through the population – like intelligence, say – and the 'categorisation' must be understood as a convention, an agreed cut-off point. The reference to intelligence highlights how clarity about this may be important for an accurate understanding. Intelligence varies continuously throughout the population, with increasingly smaller numbers at either extreme – very high or very low. This will have one set of environment–gene interactions. But the

most common forms of mild learning difficulties are not part of this continuous variation. They arise from specific conditions such as Down's syndrome.
This is a category diagnosis (yes/no) and is caused by a specific genetic
condition – the person has an extra chromosome 21. Obviously, people in
the lower third of ability (that is, scoring below two-thirds of the population
on measures of intelligence) may be thus because of the normal variation of
multifactorial determinants of intelligence, or because they come into the
category of Down's syndrome, having the additional copy of chromosome 21.

Multiple pathways

This illustrates another feature of gene–environment antecedents of behaviour. In many cases, the same psychosocial behavioural outcome can arise
from different gene–environment pathways. For example (Rutter, 2006: 29),
depression in adulthood may be caused by a genetic predisposition combined with early negative upbringing (including sexual abuse). But it may also
be the outcome for people without the negative upbringing but with particular
current social stressors. It is likely that some genetic component is implicated
in a propensity to antisocial aggressive behaviour in boys or in men. But some
boys with this genetic makeup will not commit antisocial acts, and others
without the propensity will do so in particular social circumstances.

Gene–environment correlations

The simplicity of the question as to whether genes or environment are
responsible for a particular trait (such as musicality, sportiness or physical
aggressiveness) becomes complicated initially by recognising that both are
always involved. This is shown in line 1 of Figure 1.3 below, which shows
diagrammatically how a person's qualities in the present are the product
of a particular genetic makeup and experiences in life. This diagram, which
is an analysis by Scarr and McCartney (Scarr and McCartney, 1983; Scarr,
1996), goes on to show the ways in which genes and environment do not
vary independently. As explained in the following paragraphs, the environment is affected by a person's genes, so environmental effects may also be
a result of genes.

Line 2 in Figure 1.3 draws attention to correlations in which the child
is *passive*: important features of the child's environment are shaped by the
actions of parents, but since biological parents are formed by the same
genes as the child, a sporty, musical, or violent environment may itself be
part of a genetic influence. Next (line 3), Scarr and McCartney suggest
that differences in environments may be *evoked by* the genetic makeup
of the children. Active, muscular babies evoke active, playful interactive
responses and entertainment choices from those around them; children
with a disposition to musicality may lead their carers into providing musical
environments.

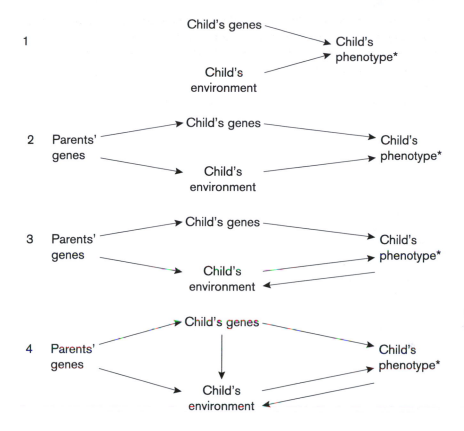

*Phenotype: the observed characteristics of an individual resulting from the interaction of genes and environment

Figure 1.3 The increasingly complex nature of gene–environment correlations as analysed by Scarr and McCartney (Scarr and McCartney, 1983; Scarr, 1996)

Finally (line 4), they point out that children shape environmental characteristics for themselves – choosing those that are compatible with their genetic predisposition. In this, the child is active in selecting environments, and they call this *active gene influences* or niche picking. This links with Eysenck's view (1968) that because their nervous system is underaroused, extroverts seek out stimulation.

So in summary, even studies (say, about aggressiveness) which identify genuine environmental influences may also be picking up intertwined genetic influences – the two are constantly interlinked.

EVOCATIVE GENE INFLUENCES – CHILDREN'S GENETIC MAKEUP EVOKES PARTICULAR ENVIRONMENTS FROM ADULTS

When the Olympic champion Lynford Christie explored the origins of his athletic ability in a television programme, the interviewer suggested he telephone his friends who were also champions and ask for their birth dates. Over three-quarters of them had birthdays between October and March, and Christie revealed that his birthday also fell in this range. Why is this?

This is an effect known as the 'relative age effect', which is discussed later also in relation to academic attainment. Adults do choose children for football teams and special coaching based on 'natural' ability, but in school this often reflects the more advanced development – greater height, weight, motor development – of children whose birthdays make them up to a year older than other children in the class.

This is an environmental effect (special coaching and attention) which is an evocative gene effect, modified itself by a 'random' environmental effect of when the school year begins.

Gene–environment influences

Conversely, the way the genotype (the information in the genes) is expressed is itself shaped by the environment – often through what are now called *epigenetic* effects. **Epigenetics** examines the way in which genetic material controls which genes are switched on or off (resulting for example in the same instruction set producing brain cells in one place and blood cells in another, or determining the changes in function at puberty or old age). The appalling circumstances of Dutch pregnant women under German occupation in the famine of 1942 affected genetically determined factors in their granddaughters' lives (Ceci and Williams, 1999: 13). The genetic information itself was unchanged – there had been no mutation or miscopying of genes – but the eggs within the Dutchwomen's unborn daughters contained instructions for expression that took account of the conditions of scarcity. When these eggs were fertilised decades later in the mature daughters, they grew into offspring (grandchildren of the starved women) with particular characteristics following the epigenetic instructions laid down at the time of their creation (which took account of shortage of nutrition). They were genetically more resistant to diabetes and heart attack. Equivalent effects had been discovered independently for males, in a study of Swedish family records. In this case, the relevant period in the grandfathers' lives was just before puberty, producing seed that reflected the food conditions obtaining at that time (Kaati et al., 2002). The genes were unchanged, but genetic vulnerability to particular illnesses was changed by the environments affecting the grandparents.

This comparatively new branch of study (earlier research concentrated on genetic effects which are irreversible) has according to Rutter (2006: 147) produced few findings specific to psychiatric disorder. Nevertheless, it is recognised as a major set of mechanisms for understanding any genetically transmitted effects, and Schore's work (Schore, 1994, 2003) on the continuing construction of the infant brain after birth has drawn attention to the way this *genetic* process is affected by emotional interaction (see also Corr, 2006: 60). Gerhardt (2015) provides an eminently readable account suitable for people with responsibilities for parents and children, but relevant to all workers concerned with troubled emotions and relationships.

Causal factors, risk and protective processes

'Causation' is a notoriously slippery concept in relation to human behaviour (Ridley, 1999: 98–125). Using the examples quoted earlier in the chapter, this is evident in thinking about the many answers that could be given to the questions: 'What caused the young woman in care to become pregnant at the age of 16?'; or, 'What caused a young woman to settle and start a family 6,000 miles away from where she was brought up?' Plausible answers have to include an account of consciousness and intentionality, but here we are concerned with the complexity of the gene–environment pathways involved. Rutter (quoting Rothman and Greenland) uses the analogy of a light switch. The flick of the switch appears to 'cause' the light to come on, but this is also dependent on the wiring being intact, the power supply working, a bulb being in the socket and so on. There are various 'causes' of different types, and a failure of illumination may be traced to any of these. Furthermore, in relation to genetic/environmental effects, what is known about the causality gives us probabilities, not categorical knowledge. This, as Rutter analyses (2006: 18–39) and illustrates in relation to a range of problems, has relevance to risk and protection factors. Some protective factors may be understood as simply a reduction in the risk factor (consuming less cholesterol reduces the risk of heart disease; caring parenting is a protective factor for antisocial behaviour). In other situations, it makes no sense to refer to this symmetry: 'Adoption is a protective factor for a number of adverse outcomes of abuse and neglect, but it makes no sense to talk of "not being an adopted child" as a risk factor.'

Problems with genetic origins may be entirely remedied by 'environmental' interventions. The learning disability caused by phenylketonurea (PKU – a genetic condition which leaves the child unable to absorb a particular amino acid) will simply not occur if the diagnosis is made at birth and the baby is fed the correct diet. Rutter uses examples of adult depression and antisocial behaviour to summarise how genetic makeup, earlier environment and contemporary situation may interact as risk and protective factors.

Group and individual differences

Statistical investigations into the amount of variation caused respectively by heredity and environment apply only to the group in which the measurement is made. A thought experiment will make this clear. If the environment is optimal and uniform, none of the variation in that study is caused by the environment, so if environment and genes are the two variables under study, the differences in the population (say in respect of IQ score) will be totally attributable to heredity. On the other hand, if relevant features of the environment vary enormously, most of the variation may be caused by the environment. In a population in which people smoke, the influence of heredity relative to environment in causing cancer will be different from that in a population in which no one smokes.

Furthermore, the amount of difference that environment may cause in highly **hereditable** traits can be much larger than intuitively may be expected. Ceci and Williams (1999: 3–5) provide both a qualitative explanation and a mathematically worked example. In this example, a group of adopted children have average IQ measures of 107 in a population with high hereditability. Even if the average IQ of their mothers is 85, a full 22 points lower, this is still consistent with intelligence (as measured by the IQ scores) being 70 per cent hereditable.

This draws attention to a final important point: for groups who typically are subject to different environmental variables (say, European Americans and African Americans), differences in average scores between the two groups will not arise from the same allocation of genetic/environmental influence as do individual differences. The differences in height among a group of friends may be highly genetic in origin, but the differences between their average height and that of another group (say, their parents) may be largely environmental – as a result of changes in nutrition and healthcare.

Conclusion

Social workers sometimes need to understand references to the relative influence of heredity and environment in troublesome aspects of human development. This section has been written with the non-specialist reader in mind, but it builds on rather than explains some of the basics of gene–environment interactions. The basic account concludes that both genes and environment are involved in the creation of a person's psychosocial qualities – her character, the age at which she may have a baby, her behaviour, intelligence, emotional characteristics, vulnerability to illness, and so on. This essay has analysed some factors to be borne in mind when considering this subject: biological features are not necessarily hereditary features; continuously varying features should be distinguished from 'categorical' conditions; the same behavioural outcome can arise from different gene–environment interactions; genes and environment are not two separate independent variables (an environmental effect may be the effect of genes, and a genetic effect may be the result of environmental conditions); the relative contribution of genes and environment to different population averages may not be the same as that applying to differences between individuals. Social workers are not specialists and should not claim to have technical expertise in this field; nevertheless, they will encounter the issue – from antenatal work with people who have had genetic counselling, to questions from parents about the origins of difficult behaviour or emotional difficulties. Historically, social workers were involved both for and against the social management of individuals within **eugenics** philosophies (Payne, 2005: 130; Kennedy, 2008), and with approaches to mental health which underestimated the contribution of genetic factors. It is important for them as laypeople in this field to be sufficiently well-informed so as to avoid oversimplification.

Selected reading for taking it further

Ceci, S. and Williams, W. (1999) *The Nature–Nurture Debate*. Oxford: Blackwell.
Gerhardt, S. (2015) *Why Love Matters*. Second edition. London: Routledge.
Holt, N., Bremner, A. J., Sutherland, E., Vliek, M. and Passer, M. (2015) *Psychology: The Science of Mind and Behaviour*. Third edition. New York: McGraw-Hill Education.
Ridley, M. (1999) *Genome: The Autobiography of a Species in 23 Chapters*. London: Fourth Estate.
Rutter, M. (2006) *Genes and Behaviour: Nature–Nurture Interplay Explained*. Oxford: Blackwell.
Schore, A. (1994) *Affect Regulation and the Origin of the Self*. Hillsdale, NJ: Lawrence Erlbaum.

SUMMARY

This is an introductory chapter, starting with narratives which involved pregnancy. These highlighted some of the ways in which individual development can be considered.

Biological knowledge, psychological understanding and social perspectives are all relevant to social work. Often social workers need to understand the overlap between these aspects, and the mutual influence of body, mind, emotions and society. Social constructionists emphasise that knowledge is not absolute – it is created using specific language, and in specific social contexts.

To promote understanding of feelings, behaviour and relationships, this book will make reference to theories which are summarised in the 'Essential background' section. These include stage theories of development such as Erikson's stage model, psychodynamic theories, attachment theory, humanistic models, learning theories, and various theories of ageing. A number of the perspectives used (such as Bronfenbrenner's and the lifespan perspective) make particular reference to social and historical features.

The chapter concluded with a section written in a more formal academic style. It requires further reading of 'Essential background', section 1, and presented six general factors to bear in mind when studying the relative effects of genes and environment on any specific dimension of behaviour. These include: 'biological variation' is not the same as 'genetic variation'; there can be different gene–environment pathways to the same behavioural characteristic; genes and environment are not independent of each other; and the gene–environment contribution causing population differences (averages) may be different from that at work in individual variations.

FURTHER READING

Further resources are provided on the website which accompanies this book. They include pictures and diagrams, health guidance, a glossary of terms and a summary of research about sensory experience before birth.

About the classic psychosocial formulation of social work:

Ruch, G., Turney, D. and Ward, A. (eds) (2010) *Relationship-Based Social Work: Getting to the Heart of Practice*. London: Jessica Kingsley.

About the experience of pregnancy:

Rayner, E. et al. (2005) *Human Development: An Introduction to the Psychodynamics of Growth, Maturity and Ageing*. London and New York: Routledge. Chapter 2, 'Being pregnant', written by Angela Joyce, is an excellent amplification of the early parts of this chapter, about the experience of pregnancy.

Raphael-Leff, J. (2005) *Psychological Processes of Childbearing*. London: Anna Freud Centre. Although primarily a psychodynamic account, this is written for people who work with parents and parents-to-be, and makes excellent further reading.

Prenatal development:

Boyd, D. and Bee, H. (2015) *Lifespan Development*. Seventh edition. Boston: Pearson/Allyn and Bacon. A readable and engaging textbook set out to take the general student systematically through the subjects.

Reading about each of the theoretical approaches mentioned in the chapter will be given as the topics are covered in more detail. Typical textbooks giving overviews or easy summaries:

Boyd, D. and Bee, H. (2015) *Lifespan Development*. Seventh edition. Boston: Pearson/Allyn and Bacon.

Holt, N., Bremner, A. J., Sutherland, E., Vliek, M. and Passer, M. (2015) *Psychology: The Science of Mind and Behaviour*. Third edition. New York: McGraw-Hill Education.

Giddens, A. and Sutton, P. W. (2017) *Sociology*. Cambridge: Polity Press. Various chapters present a sociological view of the impact of society on the individual.

Genetics:

Further introductory material is available through the website which accompanies this book.

RESOURCES FOR PARENTS

About health and illnesses of all kinds, for children, adults, parents and grandparents:

www.nhs.uk/Conditions/Pages/bodymap.aspx.

Questions

1. Choose a situation in which social work/social care have some responsibilities to illustrate how effective practice may require knowledge of biology, psychology and social factors.
2. What theory of human development considers that human infants are born not only with innate instincts to feed, etc., but also with a drive to form attachments?
3. How many Y-chromosomes does a man normally have? What do you think the genetic conditions 'XYY syndrome' or 'triple X syndrome' may be? Use a reference source to check your answer.

For you to research

Prepare a poster or a short report about one of the following:

- The nine months' development from conception to birth
- The experience of being a grandparent, and the place of grandparents in family life
- Miscarriage – does society understand?
- Three approaches to human psychology

CHAPTER 2

A secure base

In this chapter you will find:

- **Development in early childhood**
- **How early brain development is shaped by affection and attachment**
- **Three models about the relationships between childhood and adulthood:**
  - **Erikson and the first stage of development**
  - **Melanie Klein and 'states of mind'**
  - **Understanding attachment theory**

INTRODUCTION

Sixteen-year-old Tia was frightened. Sitting up in bed on the maternity ward, she just wished it would be over, and the pains would stop. It reminded her of school, when she came in for the tests after she'd missed all the lessons. The other women were all older than her; she was sure they all had husbands who had driven them to the hospital. They probably all had expensive televisions, semi-detached houses and bank accounts. She found it hard to imagine wanting a man with you in the delivery room. As she tried to get comfortable, she hadn't realised she had spoken to herself: 'I want mummy', she had said out loud, and was immediately shocked, looking round to see if anyone had heard, not knowing how loud she had spoken. 'Why did I say that?' she thought, and retraced her train of consciousness. Ah yes, it was because she was thinking about having someone with you in the delivery room. The last person she wanted was Bella, her mum. It was more like she was trying out the words, to see what they sounded like. She rested her hand on her tummy and hoped she hadn't hurt the baby with all that stuff she had done. It was weird to think the baby might say, 'I want my mummy', if he was tired, or hurt, or alone.

Immediately after birth, the baby's experience is undifferentiated in ways that it is difficult for adults to imagine – a busy, technicolour, noisy set of stimuli which makes none of the sense it makes to adults. There are no objects which exist beyond this, let alone other people with feelings. There are sights, colours, warmth, cold, wet, light, dark, hunger and satiation.

As Joyce (2005: 22) puts it, the dramatic discontinuity of birth for the infant must bring about a fundamental psychological reorganisation. Our adult words gesture towards pre-verbal experience but cannot capture it – our words are devised to describe or express a world which is very different from the infant's. However, we should not think of the baby as a 'blank slate' upon which nurture and environment write their message, a body initially equipped only with 'reflexes', as autonomy and identity are integral to an infant's activities at and even before birth (Smitsman, 2001: 72). The sensory experiences may be startlingly and overwhelmingly unfamiliar, but the infant is using aware and constantly active systems day and night.

In this chapter, we will look at some aspects of behaviour in the first two or three years of life, taking your thoughts and feelings through the experience of the early years. At the same time, since a child's life is inextricably linked to that of the adults around it, we will look at the experience of adults, particularly parents, in interacting with the young child – 'there is no such thing as a baby', wrote Donald Winnicott (1952/2007), 'always a baby-and-someone'; and as the saying has it, 'when a child is born, a mother is born'.

There are a number of theories which link later adult development to early experiences. This chapter will refer to three: Erikson's stage model of development; Melanie Klein's idea that later 'states of mind' emerge out of earlier ones; and attachment theory. So although the first part of the chapter is about babies and young children, the later sections build on this to examine adult experience.

Observational research shows the many ways in which a baby is finely tuned to social factors from the earliest days. For a few moments, think of the world through the experiences of Nicola's new baby, Jamie: immediately after birth, he cries less if placed on his mother's belly than if tucked up elsewhere. A first-born baby at four months is more likely to relate equally to both parents if the mother has integrated during pregnancy the transition from being a couple to being a triad (Von Klitzing et al., 1999). Babies mimic bodily movements of parents, specifically facial expressions, soon after birth (interestingly, they later lose this capacity for a while). The schematic pattern of a face (two dots and a line appropriately placed inside a circle) is among the earliest visual stimuli to which babies show preferential recognition. After a few weeks, babies stop crying at the sight of their mothers' faces, but not faces of others (Joyce, 2005). As we shall discuss shortly, babies and their parents (particularly mothers) regulate each other's **hormones** and behaviour.

As the first year progresses, we as adults would describe the child as behaving in a more purposeful, organised way. The baby develops expectations of what happens externally when he or she has certain experiences or responds in certain ways. The presence of different people evokes different patterns of behaviour.

If all goes well, the child comes to *explore* the world in a more coherent, purposeful way, using established relationships with adults as a secure base. Become Jamie again, now aged 11 months in a strange house with his mother, Nicola. At one point he crawls out of the front room door into the hallway. Having had a look round, he scampers back to hook an arm round his mother's leg, hauls himself up to rest his head on her knee and puts his thumb in his mouth. Her presence, her relationship with him, provides the secure base from which he can explore the world.

Reflective thinking

To understand this best, you should pause and think yourself into the body of Jamie – if you are on all fours in this way, what do you see, experience physically and feel emotionally?

Sometimes, the behaviour of the young child will challenge the parents. Babies and toddlers evoke fury and all-consuming anger, as well as the fiercest of protective and love instincts in parents. Faced with a toddler's obstinacy when they need to get out of the house or meet a deadline, parents will feel angry and thwarted. If they want to comfort the child but find it inconsolable, they may feel worn out. Finding that the child erupts into a paroxysm of contorted screaming when crossed, they may feel furious and wonder whether they should be firm or accommodating. Their dilemma may be worsened by advice or by the expectations of others.

EARLY BRAIN DEVELOPMENT AND EMOTIONAL INTERACTION

Almost all of the 100 billion neurons that form the adult brain are formed at the embryo stage (Abbott and Burkitt, 2015). Although human babies are born with a brain that is only a quarter of the size of its final adult size, the baby's brain more than doubles in weight in the first year. The creation of the brain is driven by genes, but the expression of the genes (how they produce an outcome) depends on the environment. Nearly all the brain cells are present at birth, but the increased mass and structure of the brain is made by the connections between the cells ('synapses'). In particular, the brain develops by 'cell death' – many connections are constantly made in the brain, but only those that are repeatedly used become part of the surviving structure. Neuroscientists express this as 'neurons which fire together, wire together', while connections which are not used disappear. This 'pruning' occurs at different times in different parts of the brain. In the second six months when pleasurable interactions between a baby and parents are often at their most frequent and intense, and reaching a climax in early toddlerhood, there is massive growth in connections formed in the part of the brain (the prefrontal cortex) which links the sensory areas with emotional and survival-oriented areas. At this twelve-month stage, the baby's brain is only just reaching the stage of physical development reached by other mammals' brains at birth (we have evolved larger, more complex brains, but this has been possible only by being born at an earlier stage of maturation). So human brain development is much more affected by the specific quality of the parent–child interaction. As Boyd and Bee put it (2014), the human organism comes with a kind of 'programmed plasticity' – 'plasticity' because the outcome of development is flexible according to the environment, but 'programmed' because it is the nature of human development to need the environment in order to take shape.

Researchers are at the very early stages of penetrating the intricacies of links between brain development and human experience and behaviour. One leading authority is Allan Schore, who provided a short, accessible summary of his views in a foreword to a classic work by John Bowlby (Schore, 1999). A quiet revolution has been going on in our understanding of early child development, supported by development in the research technology within neuroscience that enables us to understanding more about our mental processes. It is partly a quiet revolution because the research evidence is contained in a large number of separate studies scattered in academic journals. As mentioned earlier, an excellent book by Sue Gerhardt (2015) brings both the work of Schore and this evidence together and explains it in clear and accessible terms.

Both Schore and Gerhardt examine the way in which a baby 'is an interactive project, not a self-propelled one'. The interaction occurs constantly – in the 'milk, poo, and dribble', in the numerous occasions of mutual physical coordination, and also in the quieter times when the baby's mother sits daydreaming with the baby in her arms. It occurs in tears, anger and laughter, and in talking and singing. What happens in this 'interactive project'? Within your body, hormones regulate **affect** (expression of feelings) and behaviour. The converse is also true – as the neuroscientist Antonio Damasio (1997: sec. 1.1) puts it, 'emotions are the highest order **bioregulation** in complex organisms'. The baby's affect is initially unregulated, but in its interaction with its significant carer, patterns emerge. Schore writes about the finding that the minute-by-minute levels of cortisol (a stress/arousal hormone) and noradrenalin vary in tandem between mother and infant, each influencing the other. He calls this '**co-regulation**' between infant and caregiver. The 'relational context', Schore (2001a) explains, affects the development of the emotions, hormones and brain of both mother and baby. Breastfeeding (as well as childbirth, physical stroking and sexual stimulation) causes major increases in the hormone oxytocin in the mother's body, a hormone which results in a certain detachment from external stressors, an 'inward' orientation and a direction towards relaxation. It promotes daydreaming, a feeling of contentment, and bonding. The hormone is also produced in the baby during breastfeeding. It not only produces an emotional effect at the time and influences the developing structure of the brain, it also provides the developing brain with chemical receptors which enable these same hormones to be better used later in life (Pinker, 2008; Corr, 2006: 180; Gerhardt, 2015). As will be discussed in Chapter 6, this period is immensely developmental for mother as well as child.

Schore (2001a) goes on to discuss how in 'good enough' parenting, the inevitable episodes of misalignment between the child and the caregiver are remedied in a timely fashion. Schore (2001b) outlines how attachment failures which leave the infant emotionally overwhelmed and unregulated prevent the development of resilience. They leave the regulatory systems of the brain inadequate to the emotional challenges which will be faced later in life. As Howe (2005) discusses in more detail, the process of developmental co-regulation of feelings has a direct link with sensitive and insensitive caregiving, and therefore with social work responsibilities for children.

Being a parent is discussed in Chapter 6; brain development and attachment are referred to again in the concluding section of this chapter; neglect and abuse are mentioned in the next section of this chapter, and in Chapters 3 and 7.

WHAT IS A PERSON, WHAT IS A 'MIND'?

The baby's feelings, then, are initially unregulated, but over the first years of life become more amenable to self-regulation through the responsiveness and attunement of a caregiver. The previous paragraphs have pointed towards the biological features of this attunement, the first type of knowledge identified in Chapter 1. The caregiver's hormone system co-regulates the baby's, and the content of this 'parental' interaction has a major effect on the structure of the brain which is being created during the first two years after birth. Turn now to the second sort of knowledge referred to in Chapter 1, and consider the growth of the child's 'mind'.

Minds grow and develop in the context of other minds. The baby initially has no sense of what a 'mind' is – their own or others'. This 'theory of mind' will develop by engagement with other minds. Parents who display what we may call 'mind-mindedness' are aware of the child's mind and respond accordingly. This means they respond to the child not as an object but as a subject with wishes, feelings, capacity for pleasure, pain, affection and hatred. They respond to the child in terms of its current capacity for understanding and speech and its future potential. They recognise its need and drive to understand, its inner response as well as its behavioural reactions to frustration, fear, pleasure and abandonment. Sometimes these responses involve the adult simply acting on their natural impulses, and sometimes they involve the adult holding their own frustration (caused by the child) in favour of expressing their deeper drive to do what is right and respond to their child's experience. Meins (2005) followed more than 200 mothers and babies over a period of a year and a half. She found that of all the potential predictors of development (family income, parents' education, maternal depression, family support and so on), the best predictor of talking, playing and other cognitive development was the mother's 'mind-mindedness' – her ability to 'read' the child's mind and respond accordingly. Parental 'mind-mindedness' was found similarly to relate to the child's development of a 'theory of mind', to which we turn next.

The growing child forms its idea of what a person is, and what a mind is, by its experience of this adult mind and by what through the operation of the adult mind it discovers its own self to be. If all goes well, the baby discovers that there is at least one significant 'mind' which cherishes it, thinks about it when it is not present, is concerned about its feelings and well-being, and is reliable and predictable. Its own 'mind' is distinct from but in a predictable relationship to that mind – able to love and be loved, able to understand and be understood. Experiences which we as adults would call fury or anxiety (as well as contentment) may be all-consuming and seemingly eternal, but develop in such a way that the child finds it survives and is kept safe.

Bearing this in mind, it is profoundly disturbing to explore the experience of a baby for whom things are significantly wrong. Suppose that after birth, Tia were to come to hate the baby. When she looks at it, she hates it for the problems it has caused her, the interference it represents in her life; the dirt, restriction and tiredness it causes. The destructive, painful feelings provoked when the baby won't behave conveniently – when it cries through the night or, as a toddler, will not do as it is told – are not moderated by feelings of love, care and responsibility. When the child relates to this parent and begins to form a concept of what a 'mind' is, what does it discover? It discovers hatred towards itself, a wish that it did not exist, a desire to harm and distress. In this environment, what does it discover its own mind to be comprised of? Probably some satisfactions when it is on its own, but hatred, resentment, fear and alarm when relating to a 'significant other'.

What if one of the significant carers is violent and inflicts physical abuse? The concept of 'mind' discovered will depend on the individual situation, but may be such that expressing opposition causes physical retaliation and physical harm; perhaps 'minds' are dangerously unpredictable – friendly and unexceptional one minute and seriously dangerous the next.

In the situation of *neglect* rather than abuse or rejection, the child who has the capacity to develop a sense of mind looks to the adult to respond to its unformulated feelings and impulses and finds – nothing. Where the child in need of food, comforting or stimulation should meet a responsive parental 'self' which allows the child to form a sense of 'mind', instead it meets an absence. The child needs a context of 'minds' to form its own mind, but with neglectful parents, its mind has to grow in a void (Howe, 2005: 115).

Situations of sexual abuse of young children by carers vary enormously – they may or may not be accompanied by otherwise attentive affection and parenting, so there are many different effects on the child's sense of self and 'mind'. The growing child perhaps discovers that the carer from whom they learn will use the child for their own gratification, and in due course, create confusing conundrums, uncertainties and paradoxes instead of providing a secure, reliable emotional base.

People sometimes view the job of the child protection agencies as 'rescuing' children from abuse, particularly family situations of abuse. How do the previous paragraphs help to explain why even when it is an appropriate course of action, this 'rescuing' and placing with carers may be only the beginning of a very long task?

Possible answer: The emotional experiences of abuse or neglect (and their consequences) do not disappear because the child is no longer living with abuse. Early experiences of abuse may shape the child's expectations and experience of the world, its emotional makeup. A child's distrust or hostility towards adults may make it difficult for even well-intentioned carers to care for it, so the child with special need of stability may be faced with constant changes in placement.

Neglect and abuse are mentioned again at various points throughout the book – particularly in Chapters 3 and 7.

BEING A TODDLER

It was an early spring afternoon, but the sun beat down forcefully on the unshaded grass, creating the atmosphere of high summer. Jamie, now 22 months, had found a window wiper, a rubber blade on a short handle, and was swishing it vigorously over the miniature daffodils bordering the lawn. 'Oy, you're silly, you!' called his paternal grandfather, forcefully but affectionately, 'That's for windows . . . win-dows', the last word enunciated slowly as if to mimic speech rhythms from which Jamie had learnt before. Jamie stopped, and looked up for several seconds as his body straightened. His face was turned towards granddad – blank, you might have thought, his eyes wide and unblinking, apparently unfocused, his mouth open. Something was undoubtedly processed, however. He straightened completely, turned, and walked unsteadily but purposefully, negotiating the grass, the verge and a narrow path. His target was evidently the window of the patio door, for, having reached it, he intently rubbed the blade of the bone-dry wiper up and down its glass. There was a general cheer around the garden as Jamie laughed, cheerfully and enthusiastically continuing his work on the patio door.

A little while later, Jamie had spotted the narrow gap between the garden shed and the retaining wall. 'Oy, not there!' called his grandfather,

'You'll get mucky. Your mum'll be cross!' Jamie stopped, looked across again, this time his eyes clearly focused on his grandfather, and then he turned back to the enticing dark crack which invited exploration. 'Mummy poss!' he said clearly, and then walked rapidly to the site for exploration and clambered into the pile of mucky pots, spiders' webs and abandoned bamboo canes.

Had Jamie understood the meaning of the words used? Clearly he had – everyone was tickled that he had understood what 'windows' meant and made a link to the function of the wiping blade. They laughed because he had almost fooled them, choosing the very objects – patio *doors* – which have an ambiguous description in adult language. And there seemed little doubt that in saying 'mummy poss', he was reflecting back to granddad exactly what had been meant to be conveyed. Did he want to please adults, to obey direction? Well, in the first instance, yes, even though it disrupted his previous purposes. But in the second, the implied direction from granddad and the prospect of mummy being cross were no deterrent.

Not all toddlers experience exploration and learning as Jamie does. When he was that age, Tia's grandfather Bob would sometimes be left entirely to his own devices, to discover which items in the world taste good and which are bad, or which materials cut you and which are flexible. Sometimes his enquiries could be followed to their conclusion, and at other times they would be abruptly interrupted by a wallop to his head as adults stopped him doing something which they realised was dangerous.

ERIKSON'S PSYCHOSOCIAL MODEL OF EARLY CHILDHOOD

Erik Erikson (1902–1994) sought to find words and concepts that described human development (the same task that occupies you). His work was set out some time before the academic research discussed earlier about brain development and 'mind-mindedness'. Examining the lives of men and women of differing ages across cultures, he concluded that the key way of describing human development was to focus on 'identity' – our changing sense of who we are, what we are capable of, what we need, and what we most wish to achieve in our life. He tried to analyse the patterns of internal (psychological) development and how they had been influenced by significant people in the individual's environment and by cultural patterns, pressures and opportunities.

Erikson's view (1950/1995) was that at the stage of life just described, Jamie is gaining conscious control of his body, becoming aware of his independent identity. All this is illustrated in Jamie's slightly studied and careful standing up (he's controlling his own body, like a recently qualified driver with a car), the beauty of his maintaining balance as he arises from a squatting position (try it with a doll with human proportions – it's very hard!), his reciprocating non-verbal 'conversation' by performing the realistically irrelevant act of swishing the window wiper on the glass, his apparently conscious decision a minute later to go against the adult injunction about playing behind the shed. All contrast with earlier and later responses, but they arise from the former and will influence the latter.

Control over walking, running and jumping – greater control over limbs and movement – is one obvious example of increasing personal autonomy. Another which is relevant to this stage of life is control over bowels and bladder, which removes dependence on adults for the management of these bodily functions, another area in which the previous control of others over one's body is left behind. Erikson identified the experience of intentionally 'holding on' or 'letting go' as important aspects of social interaction.

Chapter 1

You can see that Erikson's ideas about this phase of life knit together biological, psychological and social factors, areas identified for study in Chapter 1. Biologically, before the brain, nervous system, muscles and bone have reached the right level of function, there can be no ability to walk and run, to control bowels and bladder. Erikson's conclusions about the component of identity which is built on the early experience of autonomy are about psychology. And he emphasised that the actual outcomes for an individual child are dependent on social factors – the behaviour and attitudes of adults and children around the child. Jamie's experience, for example, is so different from a child in an East European orphanage who lived his first two years almost entirely in a cot with high iron sides (see Rutter et al., 2000). So too, seventy years ago, was the experience of Tia's grandfather Bob, who was sat on a potty every afternoon at 2.00 pm until he performed, after which he was put down to rest on a camp bed, like the other twenty-five children in his day nursery. These ways of behaving towards children are in turn heavily influenced by the ideas of prevailing 'culture'.

The processes discussed in this chapter each have implications for understanding what can cause difficulties in early childhood development. Thinking in terms of co-regulation, or mind-mindedness (or attachment theory, discussed shortly) gives you ideas about the hurdles some children face, as well as the processes of productive development. For this stage of 'toddlerhood', Erikson summed up the characteristic positive developmental outcome as *autonomy*; the alternative, the negative outcome for the child who is made to feel dirty because he cannot control his bodily functions, or who is controlled by adults who want to rule his life instead of letting him discover his own freedom, is *shame* and *doubt*. For each child, the outcome of this stage will be some mixture of these characteristic qualities, depending on how positive or negative are the social demands.

This growth of autonomy as a component of identity, and the admixture of shame and doubt depending on circumstances, will build on the outcome of earlier stages. In turn, it will provide a more or less secure foundation for other components of identity which are characteristically embedded in later stages. The next section of the chapter broadens out from the example of the toddler to give an overview of Erikson's model of all the life stages.

Erikson's life stages

Do you remember the brief reference to stages of prenatal development in Chapter 1? In the first three months the baby's body is 'taking shape'. Typical errors at this stage tend to result in the body having the wrong shape – for example, when the drug thalidomide was mistakenly prescribed to many mothers early in pregnancy in the 1950s, limbs did not form properly and thumbs were sometimes attached to elbows. On the other hand, in the final three months the baby is growing in size and typical errors at this stage result in a low birth weight. Erikson's view of personality draws on a similar framework: he considered that there are stages of personality development, each with particular tasks, and errors at the different stages produce characteristic personality difficulties.

The previous section referred to his second stage, in which the child is developing autonomy; as discussed, the typical problems in development at this stage are associated with shame and doubt. Erikson considered that there are eight stages discernible in life, as outlined in Figure 2.1.

For each stage, there is a characteristic positive outcome when things go well (autonomy in the second stage), and a characteristic impaired outcome when there are problems (shame or self-doubt in the second stage). The drive to achieve the characteristic positive outcome, with the danger of the damaged outcome, is described by Erikson as a developmental crisis. For a number of thinkers, this is an important concept – it emphasises there are psychological 'crises' which are entirely normal and unavoidable, and are part of development. The first stage is early infancy. If the child has parents who attend to its needs, the positive outcome is the achievement of a sense of

Infancy	Consistent care lets the child find the world safe, nurturing and reliable
Early childhood	The child discovers control over its life and body, requiring parents who assist the child to manage itself
Play age	The child explores the world in its own way
School age	Acquisition of systematic knowledge and a sense of valued achievement
Adolescence	The stage of forming an independent adult identity
Young adulthood	A search for intimate and lasting relationships
Adulthood	A time of productivity and creativity, in family and work
Old age	The period when the whole of life can be reviewed and integrated

Figure 2.1 Erikson's psychosocial stages

basic trust in the world. The opposite outcome, in a developmentally unsatisfactory environment, is the failure to develop a basic sense that the world is safe – *basic mistrust.*

The model emphasises that developmental outcomes are social as well as emotional in nature, and depend on the social and cultural context as well as inbuilt patterns of development. Erikson therefore described his model as a *psychosocial* model.

Chapter
EB6

Refer to the technical summary in 'Essential background', section 6 for more detail. Erikson's stages will be referred to in appropriate chapters throughout the book. Two further examples are his description of the fifth stage of 'adolescence' and the eighth stage of 'old age'. He sees the positive outcome of adolescence as a coherent adult identity, more independent than previously from the influence of parents and teachers, and the negative outcome as role confusion. In old age he sees the positive outcome as a sense of completeness and integration, an ability to look back over the whole of life, and the potential negative outcome as despair – a giving up on life as meaningless and without value.

Erikson's psychosocial stages are referred to in Chapters 3, 4, 6 and 8, as well as in 'Essential background', section 6.

'STATES OF MIND'

The next sections introduce **psychoanalytic** ideas about development, beginning by emphasising the insights that come from careful attention to 'states of mind' from the first days of infancy through to the end of life.

Some aspects of development, such as changing height, increasing muscular strength and even intellectual performance, can be specified in quite measurable terms. On the other hand, your changing experience of life – the emotions you feel and how they develop over time, the interplay of inner maturation and external influence – is harder to quantify. 'States of mind' is a term used to draw attention to emotional and relationship aspects of developing experience.

Present-day states of mind emerge and grow out of earlier states of mind

Each state of mind emerges seamlessly from those before it. A psychoanalytic understanding emphasises how, in some way which is not easy to specify, present-day states of mind still contain echoes of earlier states of mind. Waddell (2002) quotes the poet T. S. Eliot: 'Time present and time past are both perhaps in time future' ('East Coker' from *Four Quartets*). To a degree – just how far you will make your own mind up about – your experiences in the present are made from the same fabric as earlier states of mind, and what you experience now is part of what will shape your experience in the future.

Think of two brief examples of Jamie's behaviour given earlier in the chapter – at 11 months he crawled out of a strange living room and then scuttled back to the safety of his mother's knee; at 22 months in his grandfather's garden he first conforms to adult guidance as it leads him to understand the external world (and receives recognition and enjoyment from the adults), and then goes against adult guidance in order to continue explorations further (and is met with good-humoured management by the adults). Both of these are part of a consistent pattern of experiences, and in psychodynamic terms they lay the basis for later states of mind in which competent protective figures can be relied on, exploration and learning can be enjoyable, and responsible adult figures protect without being aggressive. In psychoanalytic terms, a father responding to his child's needs will be drawing on 'states of mind' that have origins in his own childhood; how he was dealt with when he disobeyed his father's requests, and so on.

Tia's grandfather Bob, on the other hand, was brought up in the 1930s in an impoverished and very strict environment where the child's place, his duty, was to obey adults. In areas where they could exert control, adult caregivers regulated much of the child's life, even including his bowel movements. On his own, he had perhaps more freedom than many children today, and less interaction with his parents. But when with adults, behaviour which was not sanctioned by them, particularly 'disobedience' or expressions of resentment, was met with punishment which hurt (and of course provoked the urge to complain further). As he explains in his own way (see Chapter 9), these attitudes were influencing him as he tried to deal with his 'rebellious' daughter Bella (Tia's mother). Difficult childhood experiences do not predict the future – Bob himself could have rebelled against these attitudes and determined never to inflict them on his own children. It would be no surprise to a psychoanalytically minded listener, however, to hear Bob describe how in dealing with his daughter he couldn't get away from the underlying feeling that it was dangerous to allow a child, particularly a girl, to express rebellious feelings and to be disobedient with impunity. It is often at times of stress that the least resolved aspects of earlier feelings are felt – as abandonment, rebellion, unconstrained violence or desolation. It is important that social workers understand the power of these primitive feelings.

Chapter 9

Social workers are human, and when they deal with the very emotive human problems which are the day-to-day material of their work – mothers overwhelmed by their children, physical or sexual abuse of vulnerable people, dangerous and uncontrollable adolescents, mental health problems and intense family conflict, as well as friction within their work environment – their 'states of mind' in the present may have awakened highly charged elements which date from 'states of mind' much earlier in their lives.

States of mind contain unconscious as well as conscious components

In a psychoanalytic view, your present state of mind contains unconscious as well as conscious components. Nicola may joke with another mother: 'Do you know, I swore I'd never say that to my children, it used to get me so annoyed when mum said it to me – but when Jamie came back in yesterday with mud on his new trousers (after I'd told him to change first), I could just feel the words welling up – it was all I could do to stop myself.' She's taken by surprise at the way the interplay between herself and her mother from more than twenty years ago, the opposite of her conscious attitude to her son, is still active in her.

Chapter 1

These unconscious elements may not follow adult logic. You may recall that in Chapter 1, a component of Tia's expectations of her baby may have been that it will be the one person who will unconditionally love her, who will be *hers* – a baby content in its mother's arms or playing happily with her is the very symbol of love. But in reality the baby can't meet these needs. The baby will be totally self-centred: will make demands in the middle of the night, will sometimes scream and not be pacified, will reject Tia when she tries to be close to it. Perhaps Tia's state of mind in this situation will contain those components which derive from all the other times when she should have been loved unconditionally and was met with rejection, complaint, self-centredness and hostility. If you think about this, you will realise that, paradoxically, Tia as a parent is looking for a baby to meet the needs in her which should have been met by her own parents. This, of course, is a flashpoint for temper tantrums vented on the baby which can be quite abusive.

As it happens, this also provides the workers with the clearest indication of what they need to provide in order to prevent child abuse – it is to meet Tia's own needs for care and affection. A residential worker from her last accommodation may well say this without any theorising: 'She's still a child – she needs looking after and loving ... my worry is when she's frustrated, she goes into a fury, just like a little child.' One of the early workers in modern child protection put it like this: 'Most of the mothers in our study talked quite openly about my giving them the mothering they had never had before' (Davoren, 1974: 145; see also Chapman and Woodmansey, 1985: 3). This 'looking after', this 'mothering' in Davoren's words, does not mean intruding. In fact, as will be mentioned later in the chapter, it is quite likely that one of Tia's 'resilience' factors is her independence. The affection and unconditional care she is entitled to should value, respect and enjoy this quality in her. The mind-mindedness she needs requires someone to hold her in mind even when she is not physically present – someone who does not abandon her, who thinks about her and lets her know they are thinking about her, someone who is there when she does need someone to confide in. This is discussed again in Chapters 6 and 7, which refer to firsthand accounts given by young mothers in difficulty.

Chapters 6 and 7

Waddell emphasises that to acknowledge the power in the present of earlier states of mind is not **determinist** – everyone has a drive for development, and although unresolved emotional responses to adverse circumstances 'may imprison him within a regressive or self-protective mode', they may alternatively be 'part of a holding operation, relaxed in the light of later more positive experiences'. She goes on: 'Development . . . runs unevenly' (2002: 4).

Returning to the lack of intellectual logic in the components of a 'state of mind', one might well say that the different components follow the 'logic of emotions', but even this would seem suspiciously organised to some psycho-analysts. They would emphasise that in the unconscious mind you can hate and harm a person one moment and then expect them to be totally loving towards you the next; you are entitled to lie to and deceive someone as much as you like but they are expected always to be honest to you; you can bite and cut people, both out of love and hate.

And we can note in passing that these ideas can be applied to each social worker's development, to their states of mind in their work. The fact that they are being professional and responsible in their work does not mean that they too do not have other active parts to their state of mind. Their sense of wanting to be helpful may be linked with a wish to gain approval from the person they are working with – not a motivation they are acting out, but nevertheless a real component of their state of mind which may exert a pressure to do or say certain things. And many young social workers in their first appointments at a headteacher's office to discuss a child may feel school experiences come flooding back!

> This use of 'states of mind' recurs throughout the book – for example at the end of Chapter 3, discussing unrealistic guilt and self-attack; in Chapter 4 about ado-lescence; in Chapter 6 about sex; and in Chapter 9 about death and bereavement.

LOVE, HATE AND GUILT – SOME PSYCHOANALYTIC IDEAS ABOUT DEVELOPMENT

Both Melanie Klein and Erik Erikson regarded themselves as building on the work of Sigmund Freud, who initiated the programme of psychoanalysis. The previous few paragraphs have been a general introduction pointing you towards the ways any social worker may incorporate ideas about 'states of mind'. This final section, and the material in 'Essential background', section 4, summarises some more specific ideas about development. To do justice to their ideas, you must read further and discuss with people who work using these ideas. Good starting points for reading are Ruch, Turney and Ward (2010), *Relationship-Based Social Work: Getting to the Heart of Practice*, and Wilson et al. (2011), *Social Work: An Introduction to Contemporary Practice*, which are both psychoanalytically informed core texts focused upon social work practice. Another text, Cooper and Lousada (2005), *Borderline Welfare: Feeling and Fear of Feeling in Modern Welfare*, explores the appli-cation of psychoanalytic ideas to issues facing staff, managers and policy makers.

Chapter EB4

Melanie Klein was a child therapist who devised many of the processes of **play therapy**, which is widely used today. She regarded play as the child's natural medium of communication. She paid particular attention to the very earliest non-verbal emotional experiences of the child, and discussed how these continued into later life. Klein regarded states of mind as developing around key issues of love, hate and guilt. The baby's 'state of mind', however, does not have the separate concepts to distinguish 'body' from 'mind' or internal from external. The experiences − of feeding, feeling full, sicking up milk, feeling angry, wanting someone to stop what they are doing − are not categorised as they are later. In looking at children and their play, she considered that they do not separate what we would call bodily experiences from what we would call emotions in the way that adults do (though this overlap in 'primitive' states of mind can of course be very active in the present-day states of mind of adults as well). She would emphasise that the child's earlier experience is pre-verbal, so any attempt (as we are doing now) to discuss it can at best point towards something which can't be put into words. In paying attention to 'feelings', she would say she ended up paying constant attention to what a child thought was going on inside their body and that of their mother.

Looking at a baby who is upset, you will see that its whole body is taken over by rage. It is as if its whole world has gone bad. Equally, a contented baby is the very picture of peace. Using words, we can say that the enraged baby has its whole world taken up by these bad feelings, and as these become linked with the adult caregiver, it simply wants that person to be 'deleted', removed, destroyed. The very earliest feelings are not even associated with a whole person but with parts of a person, particularly the mother's breast. When it is content in its mother's arms, the baby wants nothing else than to be totally and forever united. To want totally and forever to destroy the very object which is also desired for total union does of course provoke great anxiety, an early problem for the developing self. Klein considered that the initial solution is to consider the bad person to be a different individual from the good person. This defence against anxiety she called 'splitting'. The time comes when this defence is no longer adequate, and the child can no longer ignore that it wants to destroy the very object of its total affections. These states of mind are found later in life, as people like to have heroes who are all good and villains who are all bad. Many analytically inclined people would see echoes of infantile 'splitting' in the enjoyment of the clearly presented 'goodies' and 'baddies' in fairy tales and films. Mothers will sometimes joke, 'Oh, I'm the wicked witch today, Cruella de Vil − can't do anything right.' The child is convinced the mother is totally against it, is deliberately out to refuse it what it wants at every turn. It is much harder to tolerate and sort out how to proceed in a relationship in which the other person is sometimes good and sometimes bad − adults and adolescents in difficult relationships feel consciously and acutely the dilemma first felt by the infant.

From this point of view, the ability to tolerate loving and hating the same person, to be depressed about that situation, to feel guilt and to want to make reparation are important processes. On the other hand, to have to avoid these processes at all costs, to defend against having to deal with them (for example, by idealising loved people and vilifying problem people), is an emotional restriction to living a full life. From this psychological perspective too, in which adult logic has not yet made itself felt, the *impulses* to harm and destroy are not clearly distinguished from the *actions* of harming and destroying. We see this confusion still at work in adult states of mind, when people think they are bad for feeling ungrateful, or angry with their children.

In this tradition of developmental understanding, other important ideas include those about 'being held' and 'being held in mind'. The fragmentation referred to in the last paragraph – of feelings of love and hate, of people being in parts – needs somehow to be counteracted. Melanie Klein's view is that the infant makes no distinction (as we can do as adults) between the 'bodily' facts and 'psychological' facts. Much of what we as adults would describe as psychological features are experienced by the child simply as experiences of 'themselves' – body or mind or whatever (we are back again to the lack of words to use for early experience). Physical holding may play an important part in enabling the 'person' to be held (and later on, the emotionally responsive parent or social worker may 'hold' the person psychologically without physically holding them). The sensitive parent 'holds the child in mind' even when they're not physically together. For example, if at work or in college you ask mothers what their children are doing, many will tell you straight away, and will say what the plans for the child are for the next few hours. It is this holding in mind which enables the child progressively to develop a life away from parents.

Many people who have not had an adequate experience of parents holding them in mind need to have this experience later in life in order to feel integrated and safe and competent in the world. One of the features of good social work is that workers often demonstrate by their responses to, and actions on behalf of, service users that they are doing this. Unfortunately, institutional services often fail to provide this holding in mind, or may neglect the implications for staff. It is a process rarely recognised or expected in other occupations, and it will not show up in measurable targets or job descriptions. Wilfred Bion's view is that the sensitive parent (or staff caring for disturbed or overwhelmed people) acts as a 'container' for the emotions which are beyond the coping abilities of the person they care for. Staff or carers who are appropriately providing this function are likely to feel preoccupied by the welfare of those for whom they are responsible and are entitled to support that will enable them to leave their work worries behind.

The importance of staff support is referred to again in Chapter 4 (references to work with adolescents); Chapter 6 (about sex); Chapter 9 (about death and dying); and Chapter 10.

In general, the ideas discussed so far relate to the very early experiences which persist as states of mind. Many would be seen as explorations of the first stage of psychological development as Sigmund Freud (1905/1991) understood it. He considered that the states of mind in this first stage relate to gratification, pleasure and frustration which come through the mouth (his 'oral stage'). The echoes of these states of mind in adulthood are understood to be features of life such as comfort eating, sexual kissing, and a whole range of impulses including those expressed in the mother's words to her baby, 'I could eat you all up!' The next stage of childhood as he understood it was associated with pleasure or control exerted around defecation and bowel movements. The later states of mind associated with this stage are the pleasure in being messy, or the inability to keep things from becoming messy, or a need to control everything and a fear of 'letting go'. Apparently it is common in cultures throughout the world for the terms associated with holding on to things, being mean, to be like our slang 'tight-arsed' or the more polite term derived from Freud's ideas, 'anal retentive'.

Freud's view was that boys were faced with a struggle as to how to detach from their identification with the mother as love object and instead identify with the father. He linked this to the boy realising that he could not have the mother for himself because he had a rival, his father; finding ulti-mately that he could never overcome his bigger and more powerful rival, the boy resolves the situation not by getting rid of his father but by identifying with him, a defensive process described as 'identifying with the aggressor'. He saw this as a necessary stage in development, after which the boy could allow his developing sexual energies to be associated with his penis (but not as in an adult sexual relationship – simply as the focus of his sexual energy). After this, internal struggles could lie dormant ('latency period') until the emergence of full genital sexuality in which sexual energies are invested in other people.

To make more sense of these ideas of Freud, that psychosexual stages are at the centre of psychological development, it is worth understanding two concepts in rather more depth. Freud, and the later psychoanalytic tradition based on his ideas, regards the driver for development to be a psychologi-cal force which is present at the very beginning in the baby's urge to feed and develop, and later in the drive to procreate and reproduce. His view of 'sexuality' is much broader than the simple idea of genital sexuality. 'He sees it not just as an animal instinct but as specific to human culture and the form of conscious and unconscious life we lead within it . . . it is not one drive but a compound of many "component instincts"' (Minsky, 1996). This force he saw as developing over time, changing its source, its aim and its object, finally arriving at the form of adult sexuality. This cluster of forces, drives and instincts he called 'libido'. Second, it is important to recognise his conclusion that much of what goes on in psychological life is unconscious, possibly such that it can never actually be brought into consciousness, only ever inferred.

The basic ideas of psychoanalytic theory are summarised in 'Essential back-ground', section 4.

KEY POINTS

- Present states of mind contain elements deriving from the past.
- Kleinian psychoanalytic approaches regard the forces which shape emotional development to derive from the conflicts around destructive and loving feelings. They place emphasis on guilt and self-destructive impulses.
- Freud's psychoanalytic work focused on libido and sexuality as the forces which have to be managed by the growing person and society.
- Impulses and drives are as likely to be unconscious as conscious.

Both of these psychoanalytic thinkers emphasise the centrality of basic bodily experience in our 'psychic' life. Both, too, and particularly Melanie Klein, are important for emphasising that adult states of mind which embody, reflect, or echo early infantile experience contain non-verbal and non-verbalisable experiences. As a social worker, it is often important to recognise this – if you expect someone to put their feelings accurately into words, you may be expecting the impossible. To ask someone, 'What are you feeling?' or, 'What did you feel about that?' may be a sign that you are not in touch with their state of mind. It is quite possible for you to be in tune with their experiences (as a mother can with her baby) and to demonstrate this attunement, but the communication will not necessarily be through words. This is evident in examples throughout the book, such as those in Chapters 4 and 9.

Chapters 4 and 9

ABOUT YOURSELF

'CHILD'S PLAY' – AN ACTIVITY

Think of a time in your childhood. In your imagination, spend a few minutes locating yourself. As a child of this age, you will draw a person. You have three minutes to do this – this enables you to draw quickly and intuitively. Follow your first impulses rather than taking time to 'correct' anything or trying to produce an artistic finished product.

When you have finished the picture, it can help to write quickly on the back any words which come up for you in connection with it.

Suggested questions:

- Every picture tells a story – I wonder if there is a story to tell about this one?
- Would you say this person is a boy or a girl? A man or a woman?
- How old would you say s/he is?
- I guess the person has a name – what will you call him/her?

- I wonder what s/he likes to do especially? Is there anything in particular s/he's proud of?
- The child who has drawn this, or the person who is drawn, like everyone, has probably had tough times. What might worry him/her?
- Does this prompt any thoughts about Melanie Klein's concept of states of mind and their persistence/evolution through life?

ATTACHMENT – AN INTRODUCTION

In developing her ideas, Melanie Klein focused very much on the inner world of the child. Waddell (2002) describes this as recognising that the mind is 'a kind of internal theatre, a theatre for generating the meaning of external experiences'. Winnicott (1979: 177) believed she became capable of exploring this internal drama of the pre-verbal infant only by being 'temperamentally incapable' of allowing the importance of the real external environment. John Bowlby took psychoanalytic thinking in a very different direction from Klein's speculations about the unknowable unconscious mental life of the infants.

Bowlby's work started from the experiences of children in institutions, recognising that however well fed and clothed they were, what they were often missing was what was then called 'mother love' from whoever was to provide it – whether the birth mother, a nanny, a foster carer or a widowed father. His work over seventy years ago set off a tradition of research that tries to combine statistical and observational studies with standardised testing to explore the needs of children for attachment. This perspective started within psychoanalysis and is still combined with psychoanalytic approaches by many professionals, but is also an independent tradition in psychology, not necessarily linked with psychoanalysis. There is a considerable body of recent research about attachment theory in its various forms.

In current attachment theory, *attachment behaviour* is seen as a biological instinct. An *attachment relationship* exists when one person responds in such a way that these attachment behaviours achieve their purpose. In childhood, 'proximity to an attachment figure is sought when the child senses or perceives threat or discomfort' (Prior and Glaser, 2006: 17). This proximity is expected to relieve the threat or discomfort. When there is no threat or discomfort, the attachment figure provides a secure base from which the world can be explored. The attachment system remains active throughout life: in adulthood, people may be mutual and reciprocal attachment figures.

Many attachment theorists regard various related features as comprising an 'attachment system'. There is also an 'exploratory system' which drives exploration and enquiry physically, intellectually and socially (that is, in relationships). In the examples given earlier in the chapter, Jamie's exploratory systems are at work when he crawls out of the living room to see what's outside in the hallway and beyond, and also when he's attracted to explore the dark corner behind the shed; by contrast his attachment system came into play in the earlier example when, realising he's not sure what might be ahead, he scurries back to hold on to his mother's knee, his secure base. The attachment system is constantly at work in the background, using the secure base effect and scanning the environment in case attachment behaviours are needed. In this view, attachment behaviours are incompatible with the activities of the exploratory system. So, for example, if attachment needs are unmet (if a child is newly placed with foster parents, for example, and has not yet become confident in them as attachment figures), the child may not settle to school work which requires the active application of exploratory systems. The child's systems will be searching for the secure base and will be activated (realistically or not) to get out of the current situation.

The quality of attachment is said to be represented in the child by an **internal working model**, which is a set of beliefs and expectations about relationships (Shemmings and Shemmings, 2011). This contains behavioural (not necessarily verbal) answers to questions such as: Is the attachment figure usually available when needed? Is the child likeable and valued so that the attachment figure normally wants to protect and reassure? Is the relationship reliable? Attachment theorists believe that this 'working model' the child develops is influenced particularly by the degree of **attunement** which the attachment figure shows towards the child – the degree to which the adult is in tune with the child's state from moment to moment. You will see that this has obvious links to the ideas of 'co-regulation' and 'mind-mindedness' discussed earlier in the chapter.

The internal working model develops over time depending on actual experiences – this is one of the research topics in attachment theory – but is heavily influenced by early attachment relationships (or their absence), whose impact may be hard to change.

Before reading the essay below, you should review 'Essential background', section 2 and be sure that you understand it.

Chapter
EB2

TAKING IT FURTHER

UNDERSTANDING ATTACHMENT

Background

Attachment theory emerged from psychoanalysis out of a resolve to ground developmental theory on a more 'scientific' basis (Bowlby, 1979).

This section offers an overview of attachment: it summarises attachment as viewed as a form of animal behaviour; it outlines the biological processes which have been linked with attachment; it expands on the inner psychological experiences of attachment; it discusses attachment through the life course; and it discusses attachment as a social construct. It concludes with the answers given within attachment theory to four commonly asked questions: Is there a critical period during which a child must form attachments? Does attachment research indicate that those who don't form attachments are doomed to be antisocial? Does deprivation of childhood attachment cause mental illness – in other words, is attachment theory deterministic? Do attachment research and attachment theory hold that there is a single essential attachment (to the mother) and that the constant presence of the mother in childhood is essential?

Early research included observations of children who were in hospital and had been separated from their caregivers. One of the early insights of attachment researchers was that separation from the attachment figure, if not properly attended to, resulted in a characteristic sequence of responses:

- The protest phase
- The resignation phase
- The detachment phase

In the first phase, protest behaviour such as crying and screaming is designed to bring the attachment figure back. In the phase of resignation, the attachment relationship is considered still to be psychologically present, but the child has given up on the possibility of bringing the attachment figure to them so becomes listless and apathetic. In the third phase, 'detachment', the child is considered to have shut down its attachment systems and to have separated psychologically from the attachment figure. These phases were originally recognised in institutional care, and the remedial focus of the work (Bowlby and Robertson, 1953) was first to draw people's attention to the existence of these phases and to demonstrate that the sequence was not inevitable if the child's attachment needs were attended to. At the time of this early work on attachment, 'detachment' in institutions such as hospitals or residential schools was commonly identified as 'settling down', because the protests stopped; and the subsequent lack of consideration for other people, the affectionless response, was attributed to various personal failings of the child.

Attachment and animal behaviour

Different species have their own characteristic behaviours: robins (and others) defend their territories; salmon born in Scottish rivers migrate as young fish thousands of miles across the ocean, stay in their adopted land for three or four years and suddenly return, identifying the river where they came from and swimming upstream against ferocious currents, to lay their eggs in the river where they were conceived. Attachment theory arose at a time when interest in animal behaviour became a discipline that invited much attention and the question was asked: if we regard humans as displaying behaviour like other animals, do we have characteristic behaviours, and if so, what are they? In many species, for example, mothers consistently show particular behaviours after birth – is this true of humans? Among other related matters, Klaus and colleagues (1970) reported that after birth, if not constrained, typically mothers' handling of their babies followed a pattern, starting at the extremities (hands and feet) and moving inwards then to rest on the baby's torso. If left on their mother's tummy, the baby progresses by small push-ups to the mother's left breast and begins within about thirty minutes to mouth the nipple.

Researchers systematised the findings of a variety of studies to hypothesise that among other psychological systems the child has two linked systems – one of exploration and one of attachment. When the attachment system is aroused, it produces a variety of behaviours (see 'Essential background', section 2) to do with keeping the child safe and close to a protective adult. These behaviours are incompatible with the exploratory system whose function leads to behaviours that involve exploring the world independently and making sense of it. Put another way, it is only when the attachment needs are satisfied that the exploratory system can function properly.

Chapter
EB2

Attachment and biology

Initially, the baby is incapable of regulating its own feelings. However, as described earlier on pages 35–36 of this chapter (referring to work by Schore, 1999, 2001a, 2001b; Fonagy, 2016; Gerhardt, 2015), the levels of hormones which regulate emotions are found to vary in tandem between the brains of infants and their attachment figures. This minute-by-minute 'co-regulation' is seen by attachment theorists as the mechanism through which the developing child comes to self-regulation of emotions. At first, over- and under-stimulation have to be regulated by interaction with the caregiver, and gradually the regulatory process becomes internal and independent. Correspondingly, early relational trauma and lack of adequate experience of this co-regulation lead to enduring problems in affect regulation – the inability to settle the arousal experiences of aggression and fear.

The phase of development when this is at its peak is also the phase (the first two years of life) when physical brain development – growth and structure – is at its peak. The pattern of growth is that multitudes of cell connections (synapses) are constantly made, but only those which are constantly reused survive. Schore's view is that the experiences which are important in this process of structural development in the brain, 'far more than the stimulating mobiles and toys of the cot', are the relational experiences with attachment figures. After he has referred to the possibility of trauma from the physical and from the interpersonal environment, he states that in causing problems for brain development 'social stressors are far more detrimental than non-social aversive stimuli' (2001b: 205).

Schore lists in detail the relevant areas of brain development that are at their peak in the first two years after birth. Amongst many others, these include the organisation of the cortical limbic areas (Schore, 2001b: 217) and the right hemisphere of the brain (ibid.: 231–236). He describes what is known about the effects of relational stress on the biological development of these brain structures, and goes on to describe the effects of physiological impairment on personal functioning. Damage to the orbital prefrontal limbic system, for example, 'disrupts the behaviours of social bonding, and causes failure to acquire complex social knowledge', and efficient functioning of the right hemisphere 'plays a predominant role in the physiological and cognitive component of social processing'. He emphasises that attachment trauma is not an isolated incident, identifying the evidence that it is a continuing failure of the conditions for adequate brain development. Bringing the different studies together, he argues strongly that developmental neuroscience now offers explanatory pathways linking early failures in attachment functioning (and abuse) with impaired brain development associated with later problems in such areas as regulating emotion, cause–effect thinking, and recognising emotions in others. As life proceeds, the individual is likely to be less able to articulate their own emotions, may have a less coherent self and autobiographical history, and may appear to have a lack of conscience.

Resilience

However, although some children undoubtedly suffer long-term effects of abuse and neglect, others develop relatively unscathed. An important area of research has been the identification of factors which lead a child to thrive after abuse. These are generally categorised (see Howe, 2005) as:

- Individual characteristics including intelligence, humour, and creativity.
- Family and social support such as external positive support care.
- Community well-being and stability.

This 'resilience' research, and its translation into practice, is important because many childcare reports and studies have focused on 'risk' rather than resilience, and this can easily lead to unbalanced childcare practice. Newman (2002) reviews the research literature on resilience, and points out that three forms are generally identified: qualities which cause children not to be affected even though they are otherwise in a 'risk' group; coping strategies created by children who cope satisfactorily with chronic stress; and features which enable children to develop positively even though they have experienced trauma which leads to damaging outcomes for other children. Good attachment relationships in general create resilience against many later adversities (Cicchetti and Rogosch, 1997; specifically in relation to later mental health difficulties, see Svanberg, 1998). However, where these are missing, for example when children have been abused or have been brought up in care with multiple and impermanent caregivers, some children display resilience against the adverse effects. Howe (2005: 219) points out that the resilience factors for these children seem to cluster more around the individual characteristics such as independence rather than the external social factors which foster resilience in the non-maltreated children. This means, for example, that in developing work with someone such as Tia (the example used in this book) much effort should be put into supporting and valuing her evident qualities of independence of spirit and self-sufficiency, as well as supporting her use of potential attachment figures and allowing the creation of supportive social networks.

Attachment as psychological experience

There are many aspects to the psychological experience of attachment. In the early stages of life, it allows the child to discover that feelings of rage or fear which seem all-encompassing will in fact move on, and need not cause lasting damage. The child without this experience of natural regulation is left carrying the heightened arousal with no adequate resolution. It is through the constant repetition of this cycle (and a related cycle of positive stimulation) that attachment is built up.

There can be some confusion about whether a relationship is an attachment relationship. For example, is a schoolteacher or child-minder an attachment figure? Hazan and Zeifman (1994) pose four questions that express the core features of an attachment relationship:

- Whom do you like to spend time with? (Proximity seeking)
- Whom do you miss most during separation? (Separation protest)
- Whom do you feel you can always count on? (Secure base)
- Whom do you turn to for comfort when you are feeling down? (Safe haven)

Besides survival value, these characteristics obviously have important psychological meaning for the child. Insight into this is given by an observation procedure in which researchers created a scenario where children's exploratory systems and attachment systems are briefly aroused simultaneously. The child is observed in a sequence of six stages, beginning when the child is settled, playing with its primary caregiver, progressing through a stage when a stranger enters the room and the mother leaves, and finishing when the mother returns.

The researchers (originally Ainsworth et al., 1978) found that children's behaviour fell into more or less distinct categories. Based on these behaviour patterns, they postulate that children tend to have one of four 'internal working models' of attachment. These 'models' involve a representation of the child itself, of the attachment figure and the attachment relationship.

Figure 2.2 overleaf outlines the four main attachment styles.

The basic attachment patterns have been found in every culture in which attachment studies have been carried out (van IJzendoorn and Sagi, 1999). There is a remarkably consistent split between secure (60 per cent) and insecure (40 per cent) attachment patterns (Shemmings and Shemmings, 2011). The largest study to date had over 8,000 participants across the US and found that 59 per cent had a 'secure' pattern, 25 per cent had an 'avoidant' pattern, and 11 per cent were 'ambivalent' (Mickelson et al., 1997). This left approximately 5 per cent who were 'unclassified', of which many would be consistent with a disorganised attachment style.

It is important to recognise that the four attachment styles are descriptions of behaviour rather than clinical diagnoses. Attachment styles should be understood as the child's attempt to maximise their caregiving environment based upon their previous experience rather than as pathologising labels. The

Attachment style	Core features
Secure	The child explores freely when the caregiver is present using the caregiver as a secure base. May show distress at separation. Always greets the caregiver on reunion. If distressed during separation, seeks contact and comfort during reunion then settles down to continue play.
Avoidant	The child seems unresponsive to the caregiver's presence or departure. On reunion, is slow to greet, ignores or actively avoids caregiver.
Ambivalent/ resistant	Child resists active exploration and is preoccupied with caregiver. Upset at separation. On reunion both resists and seeks contact, showing anger, passivity or clinging. Does not easily return to play.
Disorganised	This pattern represents the greatest levels of insecurity. The child neither plays freely nor responds to the caregiver in any one coherent mode. At reunion, children show confused and contradictory behaviour, e.g. looking away when the parent is holding them, approaching parent with a flat, depressed emotion. Most children display a dazed facial expression or display odd, frozen postures. May cry and then hit, may 'freeze', trance-like, may move in slow motion or other stereotyped manner; may show fear of parent.

Figure 2.2 The four main attachment styles

child who demonstrates a secure attachment style regards the attachment figure as reliable and predictable in their wish to respond and reassure them.

By contrast, the child who demonstrates an insecure avoidant attachment style is likely to have experienced care that is consistently unresponsive: for example, a primary caregiver who is experiencing depression, which robs them of the energy to be able to respond to their child's distress. The child has learnt that the caregiver is unable to respond to their needs and is likely to respond badly to their negative emotions, so the best way to manage this is by suppressing or repressing difficult emotions.

A child who demonstrates an insecure ambivalent or resistant style is more likely to have received care that is responsive at times, but not consistently so: for example, a caregiver with substance misuse problems that mean that they can respond appropriately at some points but not when they are heavily affected by drugs or alcohol. Children with an ambivalent/resistant attachment style are likely to plunge into expressing their emotions without considering the effect on others. They have learnt that the best way to respond to caregiver unpredictability is to be more unpredictable themselves as this maximises the caregiving environment.

The first three attachment styles are organised in the sense that they enable the child to make the most of their caregiving environment. Patricia Crittenden reminds us that we should not focus on trying to eradicate insecure attachment: 'Anxious attachment is not the problem: danger is the problem, and that is what we, as professionals, should focus on. Change the danger, not the child' (Crittenden, 2016: 21).

For children who demonstrate the fourth attachment style, disorganised attachment, one of the most damaging aspects is that the behaviour is not coherent and does not maximise the caregiving environment. The child has learnt that their primary caregiver is frightening so that when they are distressed, moving towards their caregiver increases their anxiety. Mary Main describes this as 'fear without solution' (Hesse and Main, 1999). A child who demonstrates a disorganised attachment pattern is likely to have a caregiver who responds to the child's fear by making them more fearful, possibly because it reminds them of their own difficult earlier experiences. Disorganised attachment behaviour is only observed in infants and toddlers for a short time, before it is replaced by a more organised insecure attachment pattern, sometimes a secure pattern (Shemmings and Shemmings, 2011).

Disorganised attachment is seen to be particularly relevant to social work as there is a strong correlation between child abuse and disorganised attachment. Wilkins (2012) highlighted that some studies have found that 80 per cent of maltreated children demonstrate a disorganised attachment pattern. Shemmings and Shemmings (2011) as well as Wilkins and other practitioners suggest that disorganised attachment, along with other care-giver characteristics (unresolved loss, disconnected/extremely insensitive or dissociative caregiving and low reflective function), represents the most reliable indicator of child maltreatment currently available. In this context, of course, 'although a majority of maltreated children are often judged dis-organized/disoriented (D) in the strange situation . . . there is no reason to presume that the converse holds; that children who display D behaviours have necessarily been maltreated', write Granqvist et al. (2016). They identify a number of reasons unconnected with maltreatment which explain why chil-dren's behaviour is categorised this way in the observational procedure, and emphasise that this cannot be used to deduce parental behaviour in other situations. They warn that 'it is crucial to recognize that some misapplications of ideas relating to disorganized attachment have accrued in recent years (e.g. in the context of child removal decisions)', and that these have harmed vulnerable families and resulted in violation of human rights (Granqvist et al. 2017: 536, items 7 & 8).

One of the key theorists in attachment theory is Patricia Crittenden, who worked with Mary Ainsworth. Crittenden has developed the dynamic maturational model (DMM), which presents an alternative to the traditional four attachment styles outlined above. She argues that the term 'disorganised attachment' is unhelpful because it suggests that the behaviour is chaotic and irrational. Whilst not denying the reality of the behaviour described using this term, she prefers to see it as behaviour that is organised under extreme conditions.

Attachment through the life course

To theorists who use the concept, attachment is evident throughout life. Attachment systems are particularly activated at times of distress such as illness, or indeed in the social crises which are the routine material of social work – and if they carry out their work appropriately, social workers can sometimes be understood to be meeting attachment needs (or supporting others to meet those needs). The *Handbook of Attachment Theory and Practice* (Cassidy and Shaver, 2016) contains several reviews of attachment research in adult intimate relationships, same and opposite-sex. Howe (2005: 5–6, chs 5–9) writes particularly about research investigating the influence of parents' attachment style on their childcare style, and attachment theory has long been used in studies attempting to describe and account for the experiences of bereavement in adult life (Parkes et al., 1991). The responses of bereavement – searching for the lost person (sometimes taking the psychological form of constant sightings of the dead person), anxiety and anger – are analysed as related to the characteristic responses of the child when the attachment relationship is broken.

Attachment as a social construct

The ideas we now call attachment theory have links with social practices. They were used as part of the justification for improving the care of young children in hospitals, residential nurseries and orphanages. Recognising the importance of attachment needs resulted in changed attitudes towards the presence of parents, who may previously have been seen as disrupting the routines of the hospital. These ideas were the theoretical underpinning for closing residential nurseries, in which children were not able to form attachment bonds with a staff member. They provided a 'legitimated' rationale for providing supportive social work for families who had difficulties with their children.

In fact, attachment theory has become one of the dominant theoretical frameworks in UK social work with children, and this has meant it has been brought in to support practices both good and bad. For many children unable to live with their birth families, it was of benefit that they were found alternative families rather than placed in institutions. But Phil Frampton (2004) argues forcefully from his own experience and that of children he lived with that the closure of children's homes and the insistent search for alternative families created disruption, endless delays and moves, broke up his friendships and did not provide stability and security. Barth and colleagues (2005) argue that 'attachment' is constantly used to explain and tackle difficulties faced by children in adoptive families that should be dealt with in different ways. And O'Connor and Nilson (2005) argue that, too often, the human appeal of the word leads social workers to use 'attachment' ideas that are 'a loose metaphor' as if they were rigorous theory. Critics (such as Burman, 2016) regard attachment as one of a long line of instruments to monitor and control women's lives and child-rearing activities; as relating to social forces which have the aim of controlling and subjugating women's lives, not promoting the welfare of children.

This links to a more general feature of attachment theory as a social construction. Necessarily, the terms the theory uses have their meaning in relation to other terms in a particular culture at a particular time. Attachment is centrally concerned with relations between children and their mothers, fathers, grandparents and other carers. Burman (2016) finds it indisputable that children need 'warm continuous and stable relationships', but argues that the interpretations of this in attachment theory form part of a patriarchal system of organisation designed to define women by their childbearing, ensure their economic subjugation and keep them away from paid employment. In a similar vein, others have argued that the theory is based on idealising a particular 'atomised' version of family arrangement – mother and father living in a home independently of other people. This form of family is associated by critics of the theory with white English-speaking patterns. By setting this up as the 'standard' form, it is argued that the theory ensures that other childcare arrangements – such as those in which an African 'village' as a whole is said to rear its children – are defined as inadequate. In summary, the theory is said by these critics to incorporate terms and meanings that arise essentially in a sexist or racist culture.

Attachment theory is a hypothesis that links various observations. The previous three paragraphs have referred to its possible links with social practices beyond the factual study of human development. Within the formal and rigorous study of development, it is well established as a model, but there are disputes. One way of summarising these is that various different aspects of social influence are grouped together into one entity ('attachment'). In this view, social influences on brain development, responses to separation from loved people, the need for continuing relationships, the variety of problems in institutional upbringing, possible continuities of attitude between childhood experience and parenting, parents' feelings towards their children, and so on, are amalgamated into a single feature. Meins and colleagues (2003) find that 'attachment' as a scientific construct lacks discriminative ability: it has too many features rolled into one, and current research is better separating them out and examining them independently (this is illustrated by Meins's own research (2005) which specifies the behaviour that displays parental mind-mindedness and examines its effects). Some, for different reasons from those who regard the theory as privileging Eurocentric or patriarchal society, would nevertheless argue that constructing 'attachment' in this way leads to a neglect of other approaches to child-rearing and other significant influences. Harris (2009), for example, argues that there is an overemphasis on the relationship with parents and insufficient attention to the influence of peers. Thompson (2005) edited a collection of papers in which researchers presented both sides of this debate. His introduction (2005: 102) is a summary of the issues involved.

Attachment is a widely researched area. Although the critics may present their ideas as undermining its foundations, many of the issues on which they focus are regarded by others as areas for attachment theory to explore. Indeed, the research interests of the critics are often 'congenial to the concerns of attachment theory' (Thompson, 2005: 102). Cassidy and Shaver (1999) present authoritative summaries of research about areas such as gender differences in attachment, differences in attachment to fathers and mothers, the nature of ties to day carers, cross-national comparisons of attachment patterns, attachment patterns in group child-rearing, attachment to people who are not physically present (such as grandparents who live in the parents' country of origin) and so on.

?

Questions

Here are some commonly asked questions about attachment theory, and the answers as given by attachment theorists (in drawing up this summary, we have made particular use of Sroufe, 1988: 22–27):

Are attachments necessarily with the mother?

No. But they commonly are because mothers often undertake the majority of childcare. Early formulations of the theory (Bowlby, 1951) observed the chaotic and socially destructive lives of children deprived of attachment. The difficulties in relating to others which underlie both mental illness and socially problematic behaviour were seen as a consequence arising from the need for attachment not being satisfied. This need was presented as like any other essential for healthy development (such as vitamins in the right quantities). The children were seen as needing the experience of 'mother love', whoever was to provide it; whether the birth mother, a nanny, a foster carer or a widowed father. The attachment relationship was not seen as something provided only by biological mothers, but as something that mothers do normally provide. The absence of this experience (of devoted caring) was described as 'maternal deprivation'. Increased clarity came with the analysis that children in barren institutional settings were deprived both of a continuing devoted affectional relationship and of a host of other inputs – play materials, appropriate verbal stimulation, encouragement and so on. They also suffered a range of destructive inputs – punishment, harsh and depersonalising regimes, poor food. Further analysis emphasised the distinction between the loss of or serious interruption to an existing relationship (as when a child is in hospital or a residential school) and the experience of never having a particular affectional relationship (both were originally termed 'maternal deprivation').

Do babies form attachments to a number of people?

Yes. A number of attachment researchers (see Prior and Glazer, 2006: 18–20) believe that the evidence shows that babies initially form one main attachment; after this, their capacity to form more increases. One area of research is how children seem to use different attachments for different emotional and behavioural purposes.

Is there a critical phase when attachments must develop or the baby is harmed?

Attachment is not a 'critical period' theory. Children who have had poor early attachment experiences are quite capable of developing secure attachments later. There is, however, a phase when the child's systems are at their most ready for developing attachment, and research shows that there tends to be continuity over time in the attachment patterns laid down (Prior and Glaser, 2006). Later attachments are more difficult if early experiences are adverse. An example of the flexibility of attachment systems is shown in Steele and colleagues' findings (2003): that in a study of sixty-three 'late-adopted' children there was a strong tendency for the attachment style of the child to change to become like that of their adopted parents, and less like that of their birth parents.

Is attachment theory deterministic – if attachments are not formed does this cause mental health problems later?

Disrupted attachments and destructive behaviour within attachment relationships are significant risk factors for certain later problems. These include antisocial behaviour, difficulties in bringing up children and mental health problems. But there is no simple cause and effect relationship. Where attachment difficulties are regularly associated with these problems, so also are problems such as childhood poverty, lack of consistent intellectual attention, disruption to living arrangements, and adverse adult and peer cultures. Severely institutionalised children such as those in East European orphanages have suffered numerous other adversities – neglect, abuse, malnutrition and lack of stimulation – alongside the deprivation of an attachment relationship.

The children adopted in England from these institutions have been systematically studied by the English and Romanian Adoptees Study Team, headed by Michael Rutter (2001; Rutter et al., 2000). Among their findings is evidence that better outcomes are associated with shorter initial exposure to institutional regime, and earlier adoption.

Conclusion

'Attachment' has a natural appeal to workers in many areas of social work. It highlights an area of need which can otherwise be neglected in favour of more concrete and observable services and it helps social workers understand the development and responses of people who have had disruptive attachment experiences. It provides a particular perspective on the relationship provided by the social worker. However, whilst it is invariably helpful in providing a framework for positive interventions, its use has been criticised as having hidden ideological roots and as being scientifically debatable. Caution should therefore be exercised before using it in processes which could intrude negatively on someone's life, particularly if its use involves claims to 'expert' evaluation not otherwise available (such as using a supposed expert evaluation of the quality of attachment to justify the removal of children).

SUMMARY

This chapter initially focused attention on infancy and early childhood.

It referred to brain growth, which continues at least until the third year, and emphasised the research which shows that emotional interaction is a key component in shaping brain development. These ideas were presented using concepts from attachment theory – asking you to think about the need for a 'secure base' and about the child's working model of 'minds' and of relationships.

The example of a toddler drew attention to the increased sense of control over the body which is experienced after early infancy, and referred to Erikson's naming of this sense of autonomy as a characteristic of this stage of life.

This led to an account of the framework, using the growth of 'identity', which Erikson used to make sense of human development through the course of life. He identified eight key stages, in each of which there is a characteristic challenge or 'crisis'.

Next, the chapter considered another set of ideas which highlight how early experiences influence later development – Melanie Klein's psychoanalytic concept of 'states of mind'.

Chapter
EB2

The concluding section took the basic account of attachment in 'Essential background', section 2 further by setting it in its contexts. These contexts are: animal behaviour; biology; psychological experience; attachment through the life course; and its interaction with society.

FURTHER READING

There are many suitable textbooks giving more detail about development in early childhood. These texts also include more detail from a generalist (not a social work) point of view about psychoanalytic theory, Erikson's model and attachment theory. The following, also referred to at the end of Chapter 1, are written in an accessible and engaging style:

Boyd, D. and Bee, H. (2015) *Lifespan Development*. Seventh edition. Boston: Pearson/Allyn and Bacon. A readable and engaging textbook set out to take the general student systematically through the subjects.

Holt, N., Bremner, A. J., Sutherland, E., Vliek, M. and Passer, M. (2015) *Psychology: The Science of Mind and Behaviour*. Third edition. New York: McGraw-Hill Education.

The following stimulating and thought-provoking books, written for readers with a more specific interest and experience in the helping professions, are accounts of development using the models discussed in this chapter:

Howe, D. (2005) *Child Abuse and Neglect: Attachment, Development and Intervention*. Basingstoke: Palgrave Macmillan.

Gerhardt, S. (2015) *Why Love Matters: How Affection Shapes a Baby's Brain*. Second edition. London: Routledge.

Shemmings, D. and Shemmings, Y. (2011) *Understanding Disorganized Attachment: An Evidence-Based Model for Understanding and Supporting Families*. London: Jessica Kingsley Publishers.

Rayner, E., Joyce, A., Rose, J., Twyman, M. and Clulow, C. (2005) *Human Development: An Introduction to the Psychodynamics of Growth, Maturity and Ageing*. Fourth edition. London and New York: Routledge.

Music, G. (2017) *Nurturing Natures: Attachment and Children's Emotional, Sociocultural and Brain Development*. Second edition. Abingdon: Routledge.

Crittenden, P. M. (2016) *Raising Parents: Attachment, Parenting and Child Safety*. Second edition. Abingdon: Routledge.

Controversies within social work about the uses and abuses of neuroscience. Although the development of neuroscience has led to breakthroughs in understanding, the use of neuroscience more widely in social policy has caused controversies. This fascinating text describes key debates that this provokes:

Wastell, D. and White, S. (2017) *Blinded by Science: Social Implications of Neuroscience and Epigenetics*. Bristol: Policy Press.

Technical textbook information on the development of the brain:

Abbott, R. and Burkitt, E. (2015) *Child Development and the Brain*. Bristol: Policy Press.

On the internet:

www.netmums.com

Questions

Read the following, which is the summary of a real situation, and answer the questions that follow.

In a fit of temper, Mandy pushed her first child Freida (in a buggy) into the road, in the path of a speeding car. Fortunately, the subsequent episode at the hospital revealed only minor injuries, but this was the culminating incident in a series of problems and Freida was taken into care. Mandy had consistently refused to talk constructively to any of the social workers; she was exploited by men, erratic in her lifestyle and had an explosive temper. She first came to the voluntary organisation for which you work, providing assistance for families, a fortnight after Freida was removed from her care. Mandy was angry, suspicious and non-communicative. Freida, her first child, was later adopted, against Mandy's wishes.

Over the subsequent year, Mandy revealed a little more about her life, and it became clear that she had been abused and rejected from an early age. Three years later she became pregnant with her second child. There were many worries and dilemmas for the social workers and health service staff who were involved, but she kept the child and continued to use social work help. She was by then more able both to express her anger with staff and to seek help from them about the practical, relationship and child-rearing problems she faced.

1. What are the impulses of the mother (Mandy) to which attachment theory draws attention?
2. What are her needs?
3. What may be the role of the social worker in relation to her impulses and needs?
4. Can the social worker meet attachment needs without emotional involvement?

For you to research

Prepare a poster or brief report on one of the following:

■ Why play matters – the function of play in early infancy
■ Erikson's psychosocial model of development
■ Cross-cultural research into attachment

CHAPTER 3

The developing child

In this chapter you will find:

■ **Middle childhood: 'the play age'**

■ **Intellectual (cognitive) development from baby to adulthood: Piaget and Vygotsky**

■ **Learning and behaviour ('learning theories')**

■ **Education and social factors**

■ **Abuse and its effects**

■ **In more detail: guilt, conscience and morality**

INTRODUCTION

The playground was a seething mass of children. The volume was right up – a hubbub, a cauldron of yelling, of shouts, cries, and screams. Organised yet disorganised – a skipping game, a chasing game, a pull-his-coat-and-whirl-him-round game. The noise could be heard in the streets all around. Without a moment's thought, Bob flung his arms out wide to imitate an aeroplane and made a screeching noise followed by a machine gun – 'Eeeooow . . . rat-tat-tat.' His playmate flung his head up, his arms back and pretended to collapse, dead, on the ground. The year was 1939.

The noise in the playground was little different fifty years later when his granddaughter Tia was at school. But she had decided to stay indoors this playtime, with her friend. They sat side by side. They'd shared a snack bar, and Tia took a small doll from her pocket and settled it on her knee. 'She's a princess really,' she said, 'but she don't know it yet. She's gonna find out later.' They both looked at the little blonde figure. Tia put into words the question that had been bothering her all through the last lesson. 'How can you not have a granddad? My mum said, 'Shame she hasn't got a granddad', to that lady'. 'P'raps he's dead', said her friend. 'I've got one alive and one dead. Why don't you ask her?' 'No', said Tia. 'Don't think she meant that. Think she meant I hadn't got one at all. Don't think she'd tell me if I did ask.'

The adult world intruded with an abrupt instruction. 'Right, you two girls – Out! Outside and get some fresh air.' For a moment, Tia's impulse was to retaliate following the dislocation of her train of thought. But her friend had taken her by the hand. Holding tight to her doll, as if her grip would use up some of her rebellion, she made her way to the playground.

Chapter EB3

As the child moves out of the toddler stage, she consciously creates her own world out of the reality of the environment. In Erikson's terms (1950/1995), she is in a third stage, the 'play age' in which she has the experience of acting effectively on the outside world. Observing this with a slightly different perspective, attachment researchers note that her attachment relationships are the result of a two-way influence, in which her use of the attachment figure is consciously proactive, using and attempting to change the individual personal qualities of different attachment figures according to whether they are assets or problems for her. She modifies the attachment figure's behaviour, as they modify hers. As Bronfenbrenner points out (1979/2006 – see 'Essential background', section 3), the individual is part of a system in which each part influences others, thereby creating 'feedback loops'. That is, to a degree, the parent who interacts with the child is the parent the child's interactions have created.

From the many topics relevant to childhood, this chapter introduces the following: the development of thinking processes, known as cognitive development; behavioural learning; schooling/education; abuse and its effects. The chapter concludes with a more detailed look at the development of guilt, conscience and morality.

COGNITIVE DEVELOPMENT

How does thinking develop?

When Tia's mother, Bella, was a newborn baby, the barking of a dog meant nothing to her beyond a sense impression. When she was 2, her mother was amused that when she was taken to the zoo, she called yaks and camels 'moo cow'. Naoko's mother at that age called any four-legged animal 'inu', the Japanese word for dog. By 15, on opposite sides of the world, they were enthusiastically discussing the different merits of Elvis Presley and his rivals. As their children grew up, they discussed with their friends what behaviour was acceptable and what was not. They had very different ideas about the proper balance between individuality and conformity, and how to deal with difficult behaviour.

So, as people grow there is a change in the power of their thinking processes. One area of developmental study is to describe and research this change. What is the best way to describe the changes? Do they occur at the same age for everyone? If not at the same age, do they occur in the same order, perhaps at different speeds for different people? How much does the development depend on teaching or the educative behaviour of parents? You must think about the possible answers to these questions. As an active student of human growth and development, you should then find out if there are people who have systematically carried out observations and experiments which lend weight to one answer or another.

One of the most widely researched approaches puts the emotional and social influences on one side and studies cognitive development in itself. This field of research, associated particularly with the work of Jean Piaget (1896–1980), concludes that the development of thinking can be described in ways that occur in all children in the same order. To make more complete sense of this in the real world, it will be necessary afterwards to put back the influences of biology, the emotions and social context. Aspects of biology relevant to understanding cognitive development include normal or abnormal brain development, the impact of alcohol, or the effects of different types of brain damage; relevant areas of emotional and social influence include the effects of emotional abuse, neglect, disrupted attachments, different educational systems and cultures.

Piaget and later researchers

Piaget's research methods may have particular appeal for social workers, as he did not try to give all children standardised tests, nor did he aim to measure what they got right and wrong at different ages; instead he focused on understanding how they view the world – on understanding the thought processes of individual children. This section of the chapter will explain cognitive development by summarising how Piaget made sense of his enormous research material (he published more than fifty books and 500 papers as well as editing thirty-seven journal volumes), and then commenting on some of the ways in which other research has confirmed, modified or developed his findings.

For thinking to take place, he theorised that experiences have to be represented, organised and interpreted. These three processes link to the mind's increasing ability to structure and analyse its experience of the world (Piaget, 1950/1997; Piaget et al., 1995). The box overleaf summarises the stages in this development as identified by Piaget.

He found that children tend to make the same mistakes in thinking at similar ages. These typical mistakes gave him essential clues about the nature of children's thinking. Here are three examples which are characteristic of Piaget's work, relating to the different stages of development he identified. In the very earliest stages, one lack of competence is that the baby doesn't know about objects which persist – it doesn't know that if two toys go behind a screen, there is something wrong if there is only one toy when the screen is removed. A little later, a common 'mistake' is that viewpoints are always related to the child themselves, not to the viewpoint of the other

Chapter
EB5

The sensori-motor stage (0–2 years)

■   In the first stage, structure occurs simply in body experience and behaviour – typical, for example, of a baby and young child. The level of the child's intellectual 'processing' is simply the organised pattern of behaviour in response to particular objects and experiences. Examples and substages are given in 'Essential background', section 5.

The pre-operational stage (2–6 years)*

■   At the second stage, from about the ages of 2 to 6 years, actions, objects and experiences can be present in the conscious mind because the child develops the ability to symbolise external events mentally.

The concrete operational stage (6–12 years)

■   In the third stage of cognitive competence, the mind has processes which allow these representations in the mind to be manipulated mentally – 'If Helen cut the cake in two, she could eat half of it now and still have some for another time.'

The formal operational stage (12 years onwards)

■   Fourth level: at first, the manipulation just described is applied to concrete objects (as in the example), but in the mature stage of development, after about 11 or 12 years of age, general concepts can be abstracted from the individual examples and manipulated in their own right, as happens in mathematics or moral discussions. Problems can be solved by abstracting principles from examples, logically manipulating the principles, and then reapplying them back to the individual instance.

* The second level has this apparently unhelpful label because the final stages involve the ability to perform mental operations with concepts – so the second level is 'pre-operational'. At the third level, mental operations are performed, but only on concrete ideas, not abstract concepts.

person – a child may know that she has a sister, but deny that her sister has a sister. Until a certain age, if children see a quantity of coloured water poured from a shallow dish into a tall narrow jug, they say there is more liquid in the tall jug.

Many other researchers performed related observations and experiments, so current ideas are not identical to those of Piaget. For example, modern techniques for studying babies show that some idea of how objects can be expected to behave are present much earlier than Piaget thought – if a 'trick' is performed so that two objects are taken behind a screen and then another two, and when the screen is lifted there are only three objects visible, a baby pays much longer attention to the 'peculiar' situation than to the 'predictable' one (see, for example, Baillargeon, 1987 – at the time of writing there are papers by her and about her work on the website of her *Infant Cognition Lab*, Baillargeon, 2017). At some level, the baby has recognised there is something odd – there is evidently some awareness of objects and their properties, not just the experience of bodily sensations that Piaget thought was occurring.

Errors in the child's thinking can cause it to misinterpret the world in ways that cause anxiety. Especially if they go unrecognised by adults, the anxiety may persist into later life. For example, a child who disobeyed its parents on the day it later heard of the death of a grandparent may come to believe it caused the death by disobedience.

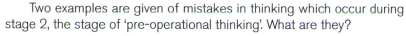
'Essential background', section 5 summarises the four main stages in logical thinking that Piaget identifies and picks out some of the characteristics of substages within each.

Two examples are given of mistakes in thinking which occur during stage 2, the stage of 'pre-operational thinking'. What are they?

Looking Closer

SOME SOCIAL WORK EXAMPLES ABOUT COGNITIVE DEVELOPMENT – APPLYING THE WORK OF PIAGET

Example 1: A parent who uses drugs may leave her young son with friends, promising him, 'You stay here with Jan for two nights. Then I'll be back and you'll be in your own bed again as soon as I get back. Two nights only, you'll be OK with Jan.' A social worker supervising the situation may need to recognise that neither the parent nor the temporary carer realise that the child has not yet developed an understanding of 'two nights'. A sense of duration linked with counting does not exist. The experience for the child is abandonment and unpredictability. Perhaps the child becomes fractious and unsettled because all it knows is that the familiar situation has ended, with no real idea of what the future holds.

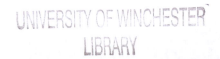

Example 2: A childcare social worker may need to be alert to a situation where a parent or other carer is demanding impossible things of a young child because they are expecting the child to 'learn' generalised rules or instructions before the child is capable of that level of abstraction.

Example 3: A social worker is responsible for helping a child understand why she was removed from her parents, who abused her. The worker needs to appreciate that the child's cognitive development may lead her to imagine at this stage that she has been removed because she caused a problem for her parents (because she is cognitively unable to see the world from a perspective other than her own, referred to above). The workers or carers have a responsibility to go over the reasons for the move in different ways in the succeeding months and years as the child's capacity for understanding develops – as she goes beyond this 'egocentric' logic, as she develops the ability to think 'what if?' ideas, and as she develops the ability to abstract general ideas from particular instances.

Note that in this example, for the moment, we are focusing on the child's cognitive inability to see the world from multiple perspectives. At all stages of intellectual development, however, there are also emotional and social reasons why people may blame themselves when things go wrong. These processes – and how they should be tackled – are further explored later in this chapter.

See 'The psychodynamics of conscience and guilt', pages 91–95.

Vygotsky

Piaget presents a universal model – the development of thinking operates similarly across cultures, and is driven by the internal development of the child (in fact, in Piaget's view, its biological development). Vygotsky (Vygotsky and Cole, 1978) understood that cognitive growth has to be understood in the context of what the child's culture values – complex forms of thinking have their origins in social interactions. More knowledgeable members of the culture, whether parents, siblings or teachers, structure the child's learning in a process Vygotsky called **scaffolding**. He refers to the area of development which is beyond the child's current ability to do alone, but within their capacity to do with assistance, as the 'zone of proximal development'. Good education provides scaffolding for development in this zone.

Strengths and weaknesses – Piaget and Vygotsky

Piaget's work has been influential in UK educational thinking for many decades, and numerous researchers in Europe and America have built on and successfully tested his ideas. His work has led to an enormous volume of research about child development which has amplified his work in some areas and corrected details in others. Vygotsky on the other hand died in 1938, his theorising comparatively unknown outside the closed culture of the Soviet Union, and it is only relatively recently that much more interest has been shown in his work. Both emphasise the active role of the child in its intellectual development; the role of the teacher or parent being to capitalise on this and provide the framework for it to be as fruitful as possible. Piaget, we might say, regarded each child from birth as a kind of scientist, trying to make sense of the world around it, trying (as no doubt you do) to construct a model of the world it experiences which makes sense. Vygotsky's theory emphasises in particular the role of culture and social interaction in making this possible and identifies the function of 'scaffolding' in the child's learn-ing. He saw learning as a continuum from birth to death, and did not focus on particular 'stages'. Vygotsky was aware of Piaget's work, but built on it in a specific direction. To a degree, both contrast with the simpler forms of behavioural learning theory, discussed later in this chapter, which emphasise the need for youngsters to be trained and given knowledge, without any great theoretical interest in the stages at which the capacity to learn and conceptualise occur.

Bronfenbrenner (1979/2006), whose work is explained at greater length in Chapter 5 and 'Essential background', section 3, complements them both by emphasising the role of a host of different systems – from the family system, through the school and government policies, to the society's culture – in shaping the development of thinking. His work constantly acknowledges how he built on the work of Vygotsky.

Chapters 5, EB3

Stage theories such as Piaget's should identify stages which apply across all domains of development (his theory does not say that children will be at one level of development when they study science, but another when they think about relationships). The universalist nature of his claims means that there should either be definite ages at which the stages occur, or there should be a consistent order in which they take place. In fact, researchers have found that young people (and adults) may function at the level of 'formal operations' in some areas of their life but not in others. Hunter-gatherers show sophisticated formal reasoning in their hunting, but failed the 'formal operations' problems devised by Piaget (Flavell et al., 2002). So achieving this stage in the way described by Piaget may in fact be 'gradual, haphazard and often limited to particular domains' (Smith et al., 2011). Critics (see Eysenck, 2000: 417) argue that he confused 'performance' with 'compe-tence' – performance is what is done on a particular (experimental) occasion, whilst 'competence' is the underlying ability, which may be demonstrated in familiar, readily understood situations. It is argued that the stage theory is arbitrary – he underestimated the differences within stages at the same time as he overestimated the differences between stages.

The puzzle of how to describe human development, which is so 'plas-tic' (changeable according to culture and environment) and also regular and stage-related, is a theme which can be found in the work of many developmental thinkers and researchers. As you examine different theories of development, you will find that some (such as Erikson and Piaget) are criticised for being too committed to identifying stages, ignoring the diversity which is found in psychosocial experience and behaviour – while others are criticised for failing to take account of the sequence in which changes occur, not being clear enough about which changes become possible at which stage, and which changes are ruled out until a certain level of maturity is reached. In its outlines, the next area to be considered – behavioural learning – contrasts with Piaget's work in being essentially unconcerned with universal developmental stages. Its core concern is with the way in which behaviour is shaped by environment.

LEARNING AND BEHAVIOUR

The most basic form of *learning* is habituation – in which the system learns not to respond to constantly repeated stimuli. The first time a cat hears a loud new doorbell, it may jump. The second time, it cocks an ear. After the bell has sounded on half a dozen occasions, the cat ignores it.

Beyond this simple form of learning, there are three main models of learning which describe scientifically how the environment shapes behaviour. Boyd and Bee (2015) are reluctant to describe them as developmental theories because they do not place their main attention on age-specific changes. In this, they contrast with theories of cognitive development such as those based on Piaget's work. However, classical conditioning, operant conditioning, and social learning undoubtedly provide one accurate way of describing why people display the behaviour they do, and what changes that behaviour (their strongest proponents may go further and say theirs is the only worthwhile account).

These three models, each of which is well established by experiment and observation, are termed **classical conditioning**, **operant conditioning**, and **social learning**. There is a large body of knowledge about this science of behaviour in general, and specifically its application to planned behavioural change. In this section we will introduce the theories and indicate their applications, including the most common present-day form – that of cognitive behavioural therapy. Basic technical details are summarised in 'Essential background', section 8.

Chapter
EB8

THREE TYPES OF BEHAVIOURAL LEARNING

Classical conditioning

Initially, and biologically, a cat responds to the smell and taste of the food being put in her bowl. A year later, her bodily systems respond to the noises of the food being prepared, the sound of the refrigerator opening and the spoon scraping the tin. This is 'classical conditioning' – the response which belongs naturally to food becomes triggered by a sound which always accompanies it.

And an example in social care: Bob used to respond with fear and anger when his father came home and shouted at him. By the age of 4, the sound of his father entering the house and slamming the front door was enough to make his body tense.

The principle of classical conditioning is that a naturally occurring response ('reflex') gets triggered by an 'artificial' signal (stimulus) which has become constantly associated with the naturally occurring one.

Operant conditioning

Nicola's son Jamie is clean and dry, day and night, by 2 and a half. In the previous six months, Nicola focused a lot on this; she gave Jamie lots of praise and attention every time he used the potty or gave signals that he wanted to go, or was dry through the night. Tia's daughter, on the other hand, still uses disposable nappies at 3 and a half. The disposables mean she is unaware when she wets herself, and there is no different response from those around her whether she is wet or dry.

Think about classical conditioning as being about what happens before the behaviour in question, and operant conditioning as being about what happens *afterwards* – behaviour which is reinforced tends to persist. This definition is not precise – classical conditioning is about the *association*, not the timing – but it conveys the idea of a 'signal' for the behaviour.

Social learning theory

Behaviour is also learnt through watching others – the young black woman's self-confidence derives from watching her mother and other admired role models overcome adversity and be proud of their status.

Going beyond classical and operant conditioning, Albert Bandura's social learning theory (1977) pointed out the mechanisms at work in learning when there is no external reinforcement. In this view, all behaviour is acquired, but it is learned by observing other people and modelling behaviour on theirs. Behaviour is regulated to a large extent by *anticipated* consequences. Cognitive abilities are emphasised more than in the other two models – cognition allows humans to have insight about likely consequences based on observation of others. When the behaviour of prestigious individuals achieves results desired by others, that behaviour is likely to be recreated.

Learning theory is sometimes applied directly using the ideas of operant and classical conditioning. Social workers, however, are probably more likely to encounter it in the form of **cognitive behavioural therapy** (CBT).

The technical descriptions of classical and operant conditioning deliberately make no reference to thoughts or emotions. They refer to external (environmental) stimuli which happen before behaviour, and the external reinforcements which follow behaviour. CBT, in contrast, incorporates cognitions (thoughts) and emotions into the stimulus–behaviour–reinforcement schemes. It makes use of the insights from cognitive therapy (developed particularly from the 1960s – see Beck and Weishaar, 2005), which explored the way in which changing negative thinking can alter behaviour or mood. For some problems, emotions are inserted into the scheme for changing behaviour – for example, teaching the individual to recognise that the behaviour which produces negative consequences is preceded by particular feelings, and creating a learning schedule for the person to act on when they experience these emotions. In other problems which appear to be primarily about feelings (such as panics or depression), the therapy installs behaviours which are such that the problematic emotions do not arise. In other situations, work is put in to reframe the cognition, and this avoids the negative feelings which may be unwanted or may lead to unwanted behaviour. Like other behavioural models, the basic processes are **didactic** – the expert teaches techniques for the management of a problem – but the manner in which it is implemented may involve attention to the relationship and mutual exploration of the meaning of the issues to the person concerned. A simplified scheme used to describe the framework leading to CBT is shown in Figure 3.1.

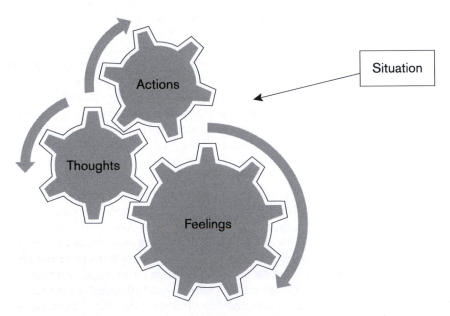

Figure 3.1 Scheme used in cognitive behavioural therapy

As an example, cognitive behavioural therapy might be offered to a student who becomes immobilised at the prospect of academic assessments. She suffers enormous stress because of this and in tests achieves below her ability as demonstrated in other settings. Cognitive behavioural therapy might proceed by giving her weekly 'homework' in which she practises making statements which reflect her true ability, not her perceived incompetence. This results in the confidence to continue realistic preparations for her assessment and allows her to experience the assessment itself as something she expects to complete well, rather than a mountain that she can never climb properly.

Cognitive therapies explored the way in which changing thinking can alter behaviour and emotion (who will learn maths better – someone who believes they are no good at maths, or someone who expects that if they are shown, they will learn?). In summary, cognitive behavioural therapy combines behavioural therapy with cognitive therapy.

Understanding learning theories of behaviour

Behavioural learning theories and applications are environmental in their core philosophy. Their strongest proponents, sometimes called 'radical behaviourists', would argue that all behaviour is learnt and problematic behaviours can be tackled by appropriate re-learning (see, for example, Skinner, 1971). To simplify, the baby is understood to enter the world with a mind which is a 'clean slate'. From then on, the experiences of life take over to shape the child – 'give me a dozen healthy infants, well-formed, and my own specified world to bring them up in and I'll guarantee to take any one at random and train him to become any type of specialist I might select – doctor, lawyer, artist, merchant-chief and, yes, even beggar-man and thief, regardless of his talents, penchants, tendencies' (Watson, 1930, who admitted he was writing a little ironically – his earlier studies were about instinctual behaviour in birds). There are extensive empirical studies of behavioural learning, and the outcomes can usually be translated into readily understandable everyday logic. However, there is also significant scope for error in translating everyday experiences into the technical language of learning theory. A commonly quoted example is that of the child in the supermarket who pesters her mother incessantly until she is given sweets, at which point she becomes quiet. The process at work here is that the child is shaping the mother's behaviour by negative reinforcements – the reinforcement for the mother's behaviour is that the nasty feeling is avoided if the sweets are bought and given. So 'negative reinforcement' shapes (produces) a behaviour, different from 'punishment' which extinguishes a behaviour. Researchers study which type of reinforcements are most effective and which schedules of reinforcement are most effective for which types of behaviours (Eysenck, 2000: 233).

Behaviour which is reinforced tends to persist and behaviour which is punished or not reinforced tends to weaken or be extinguished. The problem with punishments in social life is that they can have varied and not necessarily advantageous effects. The behaviour which is extinguished may not be 'behaviour X' (hurting little sister) but 'behaviour X when someone is watching'; punishments have effects other than extinguishing the 'target' behaviour. For example, they are likely to instil fear, secrecy, resentment or rebellion into a relationship which an adult wishes to be caring, trusting and reliable; the punishing parent has trained the child not to reveal in adolescence the very matters the parent may wish the child to talk about, and punishment may be a positive reinforcement of a valued 'anti-authority' identity.

Boyd and Bee (2014) concisely summarise the ways in which classical conditioning offers explanations for the development of emotions and emotional bonds, as the parents or other carers become constantly associated as triggers for pleasurable feelings.

Reflective thinking

'Behavioural learning' principles are sometimes used to shape behaviour in education, child-rearing, or social welfare. Can you give examples? Are there examples of your own behaviour that have been shaped by rewards and punishment?

In order to be effective, does behavioural shaping require the consent of the person whose behaviour is targeted? Does this raise any ethical questions?

SCHOOL AND EDUCATION

Education is a major influence on development. This is so even if schooling is absent or problematic, as is the case for many children with whom social workers are concerned.

Schooling and its system of measuring interacts with the child's age-related cognitive abilities discussed earlier. Children who, because of the administrative system's cut-off age, entered school a year ahead of children only a week or so younger were found to be using more advanced cognitive processing and memory approaches. But bear in mind also that many parents and teachers will be able to tell you of the lower self-image and related academic performance of these youngest children in a class, who may be developmentally a year behind the oldest children, and suffer as a result. Crawford and colleagues (2007) found that younger children in a year class consistently scored lower in academic measures than the older children. Considering various implications in detail, they suggest that children's scores should be age-adjusted, so that young children in a class who obtain the same raw score as older children would be awarded a higher exam mark.

Role of school in social and emotional development

Once children begin schooling, it becomes a major context of social and emotional life alongside neighbourhood and family. It is the place of affirmation or failure, of happiness or unhappiness, of friendship or isolation. It is a major culture in which the child is embedded – both peer culture and official school culture. This culture may be one in which they function smoothly and are at ease with larger society, or it may become one which targets them (because of skin colour for example) or prizes self-destructive behaviour such as the use of drugs, and is hostile to wider social structures. Teachers may be concerned that the low achievement of some groups of students is heavily influenced by a peer culture which negatively targets school success, where achieving large amounts of money fast through gang or drug activity is enforced as the 'normal' aim of a boy in opposition to an interest in learning and academic subjects.

Bronfenbrenner's ecological model, explained in Chapter 5 and 'Essential background', section 3, emphasises the interaction between these influences. In this view, what happens in each face-to-face setting (family, friendship, classroom) is important, but so is the relationship between those different settings – whether family and school are delivering similar messages with similar values or are antagonistic to one another, and so on. Furthermore, the model draws attention to the way in which what happens to the individual in their several face-to-face groups is affected by what happens in the wider networks in which they are embedded. A society full of prejudice and divisions is likely to produce a schooling system that reflects those problems.

Chapters
5, EB3

Social workers will be particularly concerned with the problematic areas of school life – bullying; educational achievement of abused children and children in care; drug-taking and drinking; and disruptive or violent behaviour in school. Bronfenbrenner's model is sometimes used as a way of setting out the factors involved in these problems and the points at which intervention is necessary. For example, the *Assessment Framework for Children in Need* (Department of Health, 2000) uses an ecological model in assessing the needs of the child (individual, family and environmental); Morrison and L'Heureux (2001) similarly examine suicide risk and necessary interventions among gay and lesbian teenagers; and the work by Moore and Glei (1995) uses Bronfenbrenner's approach to create a model which examines positive indicators and resilience as well as risk factors. The 'Sure Start' programme in the UK (Belsky et al., 2007) was directed at improving children's prospects by intervening simultaneously in the different interlinked areas which contribute to outcomes.

Education and social difference

There are many complex relationships between the social position of a child in society and their educational outcome. Whether these 'differences' are described as 'inequalities' depends to a large degree on whether an explanatory model is used to account for them, and if so, what explanation is chosen. Some of the differences in sociological view represent differences in the degree to which authors regard people as 'acted upon' by social forces and structures, or as 'individual actors'.

Jencks and Phillips (1998) describe the analysis of social statistics in education as 'a statistician's nightmare'. A number of variables, such as class, ethnicity, gender and family characteristics, are clearly relevant, but educational outcomes often depend not on the variables themselves, but on their interrelationships (both Bangladeshi and white girls achieve better than boys, but whereas Bangladeshi girls achieve better than white girls, the reverse is true for boys — see Table 3.1). The educational relationship with the variable has changed over time (boys used to do better than girls, but now the reverse is true), the interrelationships have varied over time, and unfortunately it is not easy to establish whether the educational outcome measures (such as 'A-level passes' in the UK) are stable or are changing over time. Any theory of what 'causes' the differences has to account for all these features and many more. As with all inter-group population statistics, perhaps the first caution is to be clear what difference in 'variation' is being referred to alongside a difference in 'average'. Two populations may have different average scores, and yet there may be more variation within each population than between them. You may recall that the 'Taking it further' section in Chapter 1 explained that the balance of factors that account for individual differences may be different from that for group differences.

The social factors that have been examined in relation to educational outcomes include social class, gender, family income/poverty, ethnicity and various features of family structure and functioning. Other significant variables examined include pedagogical (teaching) methods, school structure and organisation, educational system (for example, selective, non-selective, single-sex or mixed, public or private). These are in addition to 'individual' variation such as disability, specific learning difficulties (such as dyslexia), experience of abuse, and the relation to subsequent economic and social achievement. Outcomes have been studied in relation to children who are in public care and in different sorts of care (fostering, residential care or adoption, for example).

In the 1970s, the sociological concern by feminists was with the low achievement of girls in the educational system compared with boys (see, for example, Weiner, 1994), which they usually saw in terms of inequality, attributing the difference to sexism in education. By 2007, the statistical picture was reversed, with girls on average being likely to achieve more highly on measures such as GCSE grades A*–C or A-level passes or entrance to university. This time round, concern about boys' low achievement was criticised by some feminist writers: Abbott and colleagues (2005: 91), for example, who regarded it as a 'moral panic'. The difference between boys and girls is different for different ethnic groups. Grouping women from non-white 'ethnic minorities' together, they had a higher participation rate (58 per cent) in higher education (university) than – in order of participation – men from non-white ethnic minorities (55 per cent), white women (41 per cent) and

Table 3.1 Percentage of pupils achieving five GCSE grades A*–C

Ethnic group	Percentage
Black	59.2%
Asian	67.2%
White	62.8%
Chinese	82.8%

Source: Office for National Statistics (ONS, 2017i). These statistics are available online, and more detailed tables are presented by the Office for National Statistics (ONS, 2017i).

white men (34 per cent). However, Pakistani and Bangladeshi women are much less likely to participate than men (Botcherby and Hurrell, 2004). White men are the largest priority group to improve access and increase participation rates in higher education. The situation is different for achievement at GCSE level, where likelihood of success follows the pattern shown in Table 3.1.

These percentages refer to categories of very different sizes, using ethnic categories which are artificially constructed and are ambiguous, representing varying degrees of social reality; 'ethnic identities are not fixed' (Heath and McMahon, 2001), but are in constant flux.

In relation to future life course, the analysis by Heath and McMahon (2001) concluded that educated people from a minority ethnic background (particularly Indian and Chinese) received the same benefits as those who categorised themselves as 'white', but those who competed in the manual labour market were disadvantaged in outcome. That is, at the upper end, educational achievement works to assure entry into higher status jobs in the same way as it does for whites, but at the lower end, it is less effective in preventing social exclusion.

In addition, gender and ethnicity then interact in a complex way with social class. Educational achievement has always been systematically linked with social background – as researchers at the Joseph Rowntree Foundation summarise the relevant research, 'low income is a strong predictor of low educational performance. White children in poverty have on average lower educational achievement and are more likely to continue to under-achieve' (Hirst et al., 2007).

One cultural view of education has been that it is the way to improve society (latterly there is also a prominent view which conversely holds failings in education responsible for social ills). But increased meritocracy, widening access to higher education, and improvements in measured educational attainment of working-class children have consistently failed to affect relative achievement in respect of social class. Policy changes designed to reduce inequality in educational outcomes consistently leave class differentials untouched, and may even widen them. Halsey and colleagues (1980) found that improvements in the mid-twentieth century had done 'little to iron out class differentials' (see Bilton, 2002: 271–275). Both in the UK and elsewhere, changes in education consistently benefit middle-class compared with lower-class children, even when the aims of changes are explicitly to affect social structure by increasing mobility.

Ethnicity, gender and class are understood by sociologists to be ways in which our society structures itself. There are many other factors which influence the lived experience of a child at school, the development fostered or hindered, and the measurable educational outcomes achieved. Sometimes the reasons for this and the way the factor operates are obvious; at other times a statistical correlation is known, but there is no convincing cause-and-effect explanation which accounts for both the correlation and the different achievements of those in similar situations. Parental expectations and support are influential, as is the level of parental (particularly the mother's) education. Peer group norms towards learning are significant, as are attitudes of teachers, both towards individual children and about groups of children.

As discussed in Chapter 5, the educational development of children in care is particularly likely to conclude with low achievement, and only 6 per cent enter university.

The social research data on education expands constantly and rapidly. It is too extensive and complex for one person to summarise. Each area is the subject of constant debate and exploration, but it is clear that, looking at society as a whole, there are social patterns to the different experiences and outcomes for children, some of which have been described in the previous paragraphs. These patterns of difference are clearly not arbitrary individual effects, but external social processes that have been put forward to explain inequality have generally been found inadequate. Sexism in the curriculum and racism in the treatment of pupils are unjust and reduce performance, but changes in educational outcomes over time, and differences within groups, have been found not to be accounted for by variations in these factors. Some sociologists (see Bilton, 2002: 290) then look for other ways to formulate the processes which are at work; others attempt to quantify some of their influences, like the Joseph Rowntree Foundation (Hirsch, 2007) stating that 14 per cent of variation is a result of school factors. In general, it is clear that any blanket explanatory social account of difference will be, as Heath and McMahon (2001: 23) comment in relation to ethnic differences in the workforce, 'at best a half truth'.

Reflective thinking

In your view, what are some of the factors that affect success and happiness in school?

ABUSE IN CHILDHOOD AND ITS LATER EFFECTS

There are many behaviours towards children which needlessly hurt or harm them, and circumstances which avoidably damage their development. All of these could potentially be called 'child abuse', but it might be thought that there is a dividing line such that all those of a particularly severe nature are called 'child abuse' in an objectively defined way. This is not in fact so – there is no objective way to define what is commonly called 'child abuse'.

From what we know, few human societies have not had the expectation that parents will love, cherish and prize their children; most have regarded it as a praiseworthy responsibility for adults in general to protect children from harm. But this leaves enormous scope for differing attitudes towards children across cultures; even for the celebration (as desirable) of practices which are grossly harmful to children. The Spartan Greeks left baby boys on a mountain so that only the strong would survive (the others presumably crying themselves to coma and death), and then brought them up to value fighting above all else; mothers and grandmothers in some cultures think it desirable to genitally mutilate their daughters; in English public schools teachers have viewed regular corporal punishment as beneficial. The Victorians thought children should be protected and nurtured, but, as described in the work of novelists like Charles Kingsley (*The Water Babies*) and Charles Dickens (*Oliver Twist*), they tolerated child labour, child exploitation and child prostitution. What is defined as unacceptable 'child abuse' varies from society to society and from decade to decade. Judging by history over the last century, there is every expectation that practices which are tolerated with little comment today will be condemned as obviously neglectful or abusive in a decade's time.

> There are references to child abuse in Chapter 2 – 'states of mind' and 'attachment'; in Chapter 4 – an example involving teenagers, one of whom ran from genital mutilation, and one of whom is a teenager in care following abuse; in Chapter 5 – a young man with learning disabilities; in Chapter 6 – intimate relationships in adulthood are coloured by childhood sexual experiences; and in Chapter 8 in relation to mental health.

Current UK law and social policy refers to duties of 'child protection'. The Children Act 1989 places a general duty on all public bodies to safeguard children and to promote their welfare. So the first step in preventing child abuse is to provide support for children in need and their families. 'Safeguarding' children from harm includes a duty to investigate any instance where there is reason to believe a child is suffering significant harm. Where appropriate, children become subject to a child protection plan. Court orders such as a care order are issued if a court is satisfied that the child is suffering significant harm, and that this will continue unless the order is made.

The philosophy of current regulation and policy is that children will only be protected from abuse if all the community's resources are involved – if schools, health services, social workers, and a variety of parental support services are working together. Partly as a result of this, the work of child protection is heavily regulated and directed by procedure. Studies show that in comparison with other European systems, UK social workers are much more driven by the law, procedures, coordination and regulation. In a cross-national comparison (Hetherington et al., 1997), these issues consumed much time and emotional energy for English social workers. Workers from countries in mainland Europe, by contrast, spent more energy discussing what was happening to the different people in the families they worked with, and what might help to produce change – although the researchers concluded overall that there is a clear commonality about the way in which social workers from the countries surveyed approach the dilemmas of child protection. As we shall discuss shortly, remedying the problems of child abuse is a long-term task, one that requires a perspective of ten or twenty years. Unfortunately one major current problem in the UK is that the teams dealing with these situations are often staffed with the least experienced social workers, who may not stay in their posts long – childcare is the area of social care with the greatest problems both in recruitment and in retention. So although it is an area with a particular need for very experienced staff who have long-term knowledge of the families and children concerned, the severity of the work and the current context and practice of child protection make it hard to achieve this.

Current approaches identify four types of child abuse: physical abuse, sexual abuse, emotional abuse and neglect. These are overlapping categories – for example, by definition someone who is sexually abused is also being emotionally abused. We have already seen that society's definitions of what is abusive in these categories vary over time.

When the state takes care of children who are abused, it has to take the responsibility to halt the damage in the present; but also to provide something better in the future, and to help undo the damage which has been caused. This tends to be very difficult. An abused child has often been brought up to realise that those in the world who seem best suited to care (parents) turn out to be destructive. This 'internal working model' of relationships ('Essential background', section 2) makes it unsurprising that adults who offer care might not be trusted. This may test subsequent carers (and their families) to the limits, as foster parents or residential staff initially offer genuine concern, but find it met with mistrust and secrecy. In addition, the difficulties presented by the child, or the problems of organising personal life through a public system – with its regulations, varied policies and changing staff – or unexpected events in foster carers' own family lives, frequently result in these children lacking a consistent caregiver. The initial difficulties experienced by children who have been abused are compounded by their experience that when they expose themselves by trusting someone to care for them, the relationship does not last. Although there may be pressure in formal planning meetings to focus on risk to physical well-being, measurable educational outcomes or

Chapter
EB2

difficulties in placements, one central priority for social workers responsible for a child's well-being is to understand the impact of life events on the child's internal world. Responding in a restorative way will not necessarily be best served by referring to another professional for 'treatment' – this is one area of many where a competent social worker needs to have therapeutic skill and the ability to support others in work which has a therapeutic outcome.

There is no single pattern to the after-effects of abuse. The most severe experiences of physical abuse lead to death or permanent injury. For some children facing problems at home, school may be a welcome refuge; but for others, constant emotional pressure inside the family leads to a lack of resources to cope in a polite, well-mannered way in school – frustration resulting in outbursts and aggression. Sexual abuse may lead to an inappropriate precocious sexualisation or an aversion to sexual contact. It may lead to lack of trust and difficulties in later intimate relationships. All forms of abuse may well lead to an inner lack of confidence that is covered up in later life, but continues simmering under the surface. In many of the adult mental health situations in which social workers intervene, this vulnerability will be a factor. Faced with difficulties with their own children, parents who were abused may be beset by doubts about their ability to be good parents. Hearing the frequency with which sexual offenders describe having been abused themselves, they may worry that their own experience of abuse will lead them, despite themselves, to abuse their own children.

IS CHILDHOOD ABUSE A RISK FACTOR FOR BECOMING AN ABUSIVE PARENT?

This is a complex subject to cover, but the main message is that people who were abused as children should not worry that this alone will lead them to abuse their own children. Whatever the increased risk, there are other factors involved. Statistically, many people who physically abuse children were abused as children themselves. The situation in relation to sexual abuse is gendered: the majority of children who are sexually abused are female, but the majority of adults who sexually abuse are male, so there is no straightforward non-gendered causal link. However, some authorities see boys' childhood sexual abuse as a risk factor, and 'boys who do sexually abuse are likely to have grown up in a climate of violence and poor care' (Bentovim, 2002). These statistics, however, do not relate to the likelihood that a child who was abused will themselves abuse children, as shown in Figure 3.2: the size of the overlap area in relation to the left-hand area gives no information about its size as a proportion of the right-hand area. As is to be expected, the size of the area of overlap is not accurately known. Findings vary from about 9 per cent to 30 per cent (Rezmovic et al., 1996), with a large number of studies reporting in the range 9–16

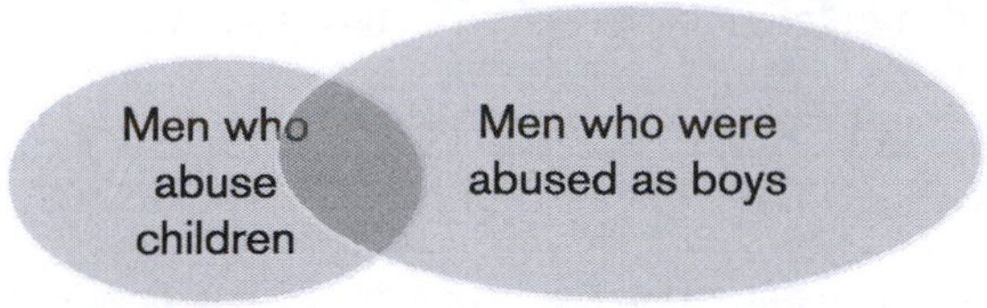

Figure 3.2 Risk: the overlap represents a different percentage of the right- and left-hand areas

per cent. There is vigorous debate among experts as to whether male sexual abuse in itself should be considered to increase the likelihood of later sexual offending.

For a view that supports the contention, see Glasser et al. (2001); opposing it, see Boyd and Bromfield (2006); reviewing the evidence as inconclusive, see Rezmovic et al. (1996). The issues are analysed by Gelles (1998: 18), who insists that the question to be addressed is not, 'Do abused children become abusive parents?' but 'Under what conditions is the transmission of abuse likely to occur?'

In the last two decades, childcare research has taken particular interest in the protective factors causing '**resilience**' – the ability to adapt success-fully and to overcome adversity. These protective factors include intelligence and the availability of a protective, concerned adult who is not part of the abusive situation. Howe (2005: 219) summarises further aspects of this research by suggesting that it may be that different factors build resilience for maltreated and non-maltreated young people. For children who have been abused, self-reliance, self-confidence and autonomy seem to be of high importance – 'independence' personality factors – rather than the rela-tionship factors prominent for children in general.

Good parenting provides the child with a confidence in their own worth; abusive parenting can instil the message that the individual has no basic worth and that behaviour which is self-destructive or destructive of others is only to be expected. The challenge for the after-care of children who have been harmed is to provide an experience sufficiently enduring and loving that it makes real inroads into the problems created by destructive parents. Because it is often unrealistic for this restorative task to be completed dur-ing childhood, and because 'parenting' in the best of situations continues into adulthood, the state's duty of care for children harmed by their par-ents must have a perspective that continues in a supportive, therapeutic and non-stigmatising way into adulthood.

- What elements in how and when you learnt can be understood in terms of Piaget's stages of cognitive development?
- What elements can be discussed in terms of operant conditioning? (Behaviour which is reinforced tends to persist – see box on page 73.)
- No doubt you remember your school achievements partly as the result of your own efforts (or lack of effort!). But what were the social influences that also determined your educational outcomes?

The final section of this chapter is a more formal review of ideas about guilt, conscience and morality. In the course of the preceding sections there have been several references to people inappropriately blaming themselves – in the examples used about Piaget's work and in relation to the lack of self-confidence that can be caused by abuse. We could have added that many people subjected to abuse blame themselves for the incident itself – 'I know he went too far, but I have to say I did deserve some of it' – so the following section is concerned both with the development of morality and with the nature of guilt.

TAKING IT FURTHER

GUILT, CONSCIENCE AND MORALITY

Introduction

A person may feel guilty or blame themselves in circumstances where they have done nothing wrong. Another person's behaviour, by contrast, may be self-centred, showing no sense of respect for the rights or property of others. A social worker may have to deal with both issues – of unrealistic guilt and of a lack of 'moral' standards – in the same person. To give a rather dramatic quotation, psychological researchers in a youth offending institution found that in response to stress, a 'characteristic inmate reaction pattern could be described as anxious, acquiescent, self-demeaning, and depressive-like' (Hokanson et al., 1976).

This section of the chapter outlines some models that have been put forward about the development of thoughts and emotions related to morality. The areas touched on are only a small component of the study of antisocial behaviour and criminality, and the essay should not be seen as an introduction to that subject. The first part is concerned principally with cognition, and the second with one approach to the emotions of guilt and self-attack.

Overview

This subject touches on a range of philosophical issues about morality. An absolutist view of morality holds that there are standards which are above personal wishes and cultural conventions. This view has the advantages of matching the everyday meaning of 'morality'. It allows one's moral values to be applied to another situation and culture (so that one can view a family's 'honour killing' of their daughter because she has been raped as barbarous and immoral) – maintaining that there are values which transcend local practices. These absolute moral values may be understood as coming from a religious authority or from the 'natural law'. A relativist view points out that in reality, these authorities prescribe different codes as moral – so how can they be right? Who has the authority to decide between contradictory moral codes? Such a view points to the conclusion that 'moral' standards are always constructed by society, and vary according to the local culture. The literature on ethics, the philosophy of morality, analyses these views and others. Each generation of philosophers adds its own contribution to these issues; some building on earlier insights, some proposing new formulations and some adopting one stance, some another.

It is not the purpose of this essay to explore these philosophical questions, but they often underpin and complicate the discussions which follow. They point to a further range of questions which could be asked. Sometimes a thoughtful practitioner may feel that the pragmatics of the situation make such discussions entirely hypothetical. At other times, the same person may acknowledge that it is important to consider these angles.

The first part of what follows presents the conclusions of Piaget, Kohlberg and Gilligan about the stages children go through in coming to an adult understanding of 'right and wrong'. Originally, learning theories of behaviour were not primarily about cognitions, but about the emergence and maintenance of behaviour through reward and punishment. However, Bandura's 'social learning' theory and the development of cognitive behavioural approaches are nowadays central to understanding how 'prosocial' or 'antisocial' attitudes are developed, and the essay considers the place of these approaches. The second part of the essay considers psychoanalytic views which explore the continuing emotional dynamics of the development of guilt and shame.

Piaget and Kohlberg – 'Where do rules come from?'

Developmental psychologists who studied cognition also examined the cognitive aspects of moral reasoning. Piaget joined in games of marbles with children. As if he was ignorant of the rules, he asked them questions such as: 'Where do rules come from?'; 'Who made them?'; 'Can we change them?' From the results of these and other observations of children of different ages, he formulated the theory that children went through three stages in their reasoning about morality and rules.

Up to the age of about 5, children are 'amoral' and show little awareness or concern for rules. Next, in a stage of 'moral realism' (up to about 10), children consider that rules are simply part of the world, unalterable, and given by a higher authority such as God or parents. Piaget quotes a child who was asked about making up a rule: 'If I made it up, it wouldn't be a rule.' Finally, children come to realise that rules are changeable; they are created by people, and in a game, can be changed by mutual agreement. Piaget termed this stage 'moral relativism' or 'moral autonomy'.

Piaget further examined the basis of children's moral judgements. He told them stories such as those in the box below and then asked them questions.

1. A little boy called John is in his room. He is called to dinner. He goes into the dining room. But behind the door there is a chair and on the chair is a tray with fifteen cups on it. John does not know that all this is behind the door. He goes in, and the door knocks against the tray. Bang go the cups! And they all get broken.
2. There was a little boy called Henry. One day when his mother was out he tried to get some jam out of the cupboard. He climbed up on to a chair and stretched out his arm. But the jam was too high up and he could not reach it. While he was trying to get it, he knocked over a cup. The cup fell down and broke.

Piaget first checked that the children had understood the stories and then asked them which child they considered the naughtiest and why. In the stage of moral realism as described above, children tended to say that the child who broke the most cups was the naughtiest. The sheer amount of damage is the measure, not whether the act was intentional. By contrast, older children tend to take motivation into account, deciding that whether someone is morally culpable or not depends on their intentions.

In a further series of observations and theorising, Piaget examined children's ideas about punishment. For example, describing a child who had damaged the toy of another child, he asked which would be the fairer punishment – to replace the toy with one of their own, to pay for it to be repaired, or to be forbidden to play. Younger children tend to think that the last punishment should be made, because it makes the person suffer – the greater the misdeed, the greater the suffering which should be inflicted. Older children tended to consider that 'the punishment should fit the crime'; they took motivation into account, and thought the purpose of the punishment would be to ensure the rule was observed next time. Piaget found that younger children tend to believe in 'immanent justice' – breaking the rule will always result in punishment, and justice is the natural order of things. Older children have learnt that rule violation will often go unpunished, and tend not to believe in immanent justice.

Kohlberg was a Jewish psychologist. In the decades following the Second World War he worked in America and led a free-thinking series of seminars. He presented children of different ages with a story in which there is a moral dilemma. Perhaps the most famous involves a fictional character Heinz who has a sick wife; the chemist stocks the necessary drug, but it is too expensive for Heinz. The question presented by Kohlberg as a moral dilemma is: 'Should Heinz steal the drug?' His research was not interested in the judgement made by the respondents, but in the reasoning they gave.

He identified the following stages of moral reasoning:

Level 1 – Preconventional Morality: This is similar to Piaget's stage of moral realism. Kohlberg thinks of this level as applying to most children under 9 years of age and to some adolescents, and to adolescent and adult offenders. Morality at this level is external. The child conforms to rules in order to avoid punishment or to obtain personal rewards.

Within this level are two stages: one where obedience is valued for its own sake, and the criteria for what is right and wrong are determined by what is punished; and the second where rules are followed if they are in the immediate interests of the individual – 'It's not good to steal from a shop. It's against the law. Someone could see you and call the police.'

Level 2 – Conventional Morality: Morality is considered to consist in obeying the laws of society and religion. The purpose of morality is to uphold the rules, to avoid censure from legitimate authorities, and to gain their praise and respect. Laws are regarded as necessary to ensure the good order of society, and are in the best interests of everyone.

Kohlberg differentiated two stages to this level of moral thinking. In the first stage, actions are regarded as moral if they live up to the expectations of the family and a sense of being good is valued in itself. In the second stage, this widens to include wider social groups and society as a whole.

Level 3 – Post-Conventional or Principled Morality: In this level, the individual recognises that conventional morality may not always be right, that social rules may not always be moral. There have to be general moral rules underlying specific injunctions. If an individual's principles are in conflict with society's rule, then the individual's moral principles should take precedence.

Here, too, Kohlberg identified two stages. In the first stage, a social contract orientation means that individuals generally act in a utilitarian way ('the greatest good for the greatest number') but do recognise that some values are not relative, such as each person's right to life. In the second stage, individuals adopt and follow ethical principles that they have chosen as part of a thought-through system of values and principles.

Kohlberg considered that the identification of how people develop their moral thinking had implications for education. He linked his ideas about moral development to the stages of cognitive understanding.

Difficulties with the schemes of Piaget and Kohlberg

It can be seen from the sample 'vignettes' that the ideas of Piaget, Kohlberg and the cognitive theorists are heavily linked to concepts of 'justice' as the measure of developing morality. But in everyday social work this is only a small part — usually a very small part — in the moral judgements with which social workers are involved.

Sometimes, it is true, they will be faced with dilemmas about the requirements of justice. The study by McAuliffe and Sudbery (2005), about moral dilemmas experienced by Australian social workers, reported tensions when the agency required them to support one course of action (for example, the separation of Aboriginal siblings in foster care) whilst their professional judgement was that this violated clients' rights. But more usually the moral qualities of social workers consist in having the persistence and strength of character to find creative solutions, regardless of the expectations of bureaucracy. These qualities are in play when social workers take into account the needs of everyone involved in a complicated situation, and in the degree to which they put themselves out to obtain what people need. A heightened emphasis on accountability within public organisations can raise anxieties within practitioners and managers and increase the temptation to engage in defensive practice as a means of protecting oneself at the expense of service users (Whittaker, 2011; Whittaker and Havard, 2016). Strength is often needed to avoid this and to be able to use supervision in difficult situations. It is demonstrated in the energy put into finding caring solutions; for example when an ageing husband wishes to remain at home but his wife feels unable to look after him any longer. This mature morality does not link in an obvious way with questions about which punishments are most just, or with the basis of fair rules. Indeed, it is not clear how verbal answers relate to a person's moral behaviour in complex life situations.

Carol Gilligan (1982/1993), whose work will be referred to again in Chapter 4, about adolescence, regarded these anomalies as being caused by using a 'male' conception of morality, based on rules and justice. This contrasted, she argued, with a woman's morality, which would be more focused on care and relationships. Her criticisms were prompted because Kohlberg and Piaget found that girls and women tended to take longer to reach the later stages of moral development. This was equivalent, Gilligan considered, to describing women as 'morally immature'. The schemes she developed paid more attention to care and the preservation of relationships as elements in morality. Continuing research generally has not supported her idea that males use a 'justice' orientation in their morality and females a 'care/relationships' orientation (for a summary, see Boyd and Bee, 2015). However, her emphasis on care and relationships as core components of morality seems self-evidently relevant (as acknowledged by Kohlberg et al., 1994).

Emotions, empathy and interpersonal responsiveness are given considerable importance in the final section of this discussion section. They are one strand of several that highlight the difficulties of taking those studies of cognition and verbal statements as valid measures of moral development.

Chapter 4

Another is to note that the significance of these statements for moral development cannot be assessed without considering matters of moral philosophy and moral relativism or absolutism. For example, Kohlberg's 'moral' dilemma about Heinz may have a different meaning in cultures where it is a moral principle to revere one's elders – in such cultures, 'moral development' may require a different answer in Kohlberg's example depending on whether the sick person is a spouse or a parent. There are many other problems in taking 'moral reasoning' as understood by Piaget and Kohlberg to be a valid indicator of 'moral development'. It may be, for example, that the primary purpose of statements about what ought to be punished is not to express dispassionately a person's moral principles. Instead, the statements may be a way of criticising the actions of others (the rule-breakers themselves or the judiciary). Accurately describing one's own moral principles is a different task.

Nevertheless, cross-cultural and cross-gender studies have in general supported the findings of Piaget and Kohlberg: that reasoning about punishments and rule-breaking develops in stages, and that these are broadly comparable across culture and gender. Further, there are some messages for social work and education from their research. Continuing studies have found that adolescents with the highest level of moral reasoning are also those who show the most prosocial behaviour, and that lower levels are associated with antisocial behaviour (Schonert-Reichl, 1999). This supports the ideas of Kohlberg that there are significant implications for education, including the educative processes that take place in interventions linked with social exclusion or youth justice. The lessening of egocentrism which Piaget associated with greater cognitive development and with greater empathy has also in Kohlberg's view to be enhanced by opportunities with peers and adults for 'meaningful dialogue about moral issues' (Boyd and Bee, 2015). Koenig and colleagues (2004) found that at the age of 5, abused children had less understanding of situations such as cheating, stealing and other rule-breaking which other children recognised as producing guilt and shame.

As so often in matters affecting social work, developmental understanding involves an appreciation of the interaction of cognition, emotion and social experience.

Behavioural and learning theories

Behavioural and learning models offer their own perspectives on 'moral' behaviour, whether in relation to users of the social work service or social workers themselves. Mechanisms of reinforcement can be used to account for both antisocial and prosocial behaviour. Whether considering youth offending, the adult justice system or good operational practice, the use of motivating rewards or punitive sanction are two ways of accounting for (or shaping) behaviour. Skinner (1971) considered that 'moral' behaviour arose because parents and other authorities punish children for morally unacceptable behaviour. He regarded 'moral' categorisation as an obstacle to achieving a free and dignified society, and described punishment as a primitive and ineffective mechanism. He was equally critical of many fashionable alternatives to punishment, which he regarded as 'unscientific'. From a moral point of view, one of the potential limitations of classical conditioning is that it selects for behaviour which pleases someone else. This is not a basis for ethical behaviour or moral motivation.

Learning models are expanded by taking account of cognitions. A cognitive behavioural approach with a youth offender, for example, might aim to change the thinking patterns in which the offender views an innocent victim as a victimiser of himself, or regards himself as having an entitlement to property which actually belongs to someone else. It might develop thinking which results in greater empathy and reduces the risk of hurtful behaviour. Results of two related evaluations of cognitive behavioural interventions with offenders showed contrasting results (Friendship et al., 2002; Cann et al., 2003). (For a summary of cognitive behavioural approaches, see 'Essential background', section 8; Scott and Dryden, 2003; McGuire, 1995).

Chapter EB8

Bandura's social learning model incorporates the dimension, always important for social work, that the individual learns by observing significant others. The growing child's behaviour reflects not just what adults are 'training' in him, but even more fundamentally the principles underlying the adults' behaviour. Whatever 'good' behaviour a parent attempts to instil by beating a child, that child also learns about authority figures' apparent 'right' to inflict violence. This observational learning from respected adults is clearly a major influence on the development of moral attitudes in children; it is potentially a major dynamic in effective social work practice with people who harm others (the parent who hurts their child learns more from how the social worker treats their own 'delinquency' than from the social worker's child-rearing instructions, which they have usually heard many times before), and observational learning from respected colleagues and supervisors is a major factor in the development of mature professional ethics.

The psychodynamics of conscience and guilt

Social workers are often concerned with 'conscience' and 'guilt' – whether dealing with behaviour which damages other people or with an individual's sense that he has done wrong. It is one aspect of Jordan's statement (Jordan, 1991) that 'moral issues haunt social work; social workers stalk moral problems'. It affects the workers themselves because at times they are likely to feel that they have failed someone even though they have done all they could. Social workers may berate themselves about small details; after an interview, feeling, for example, that they have said the wrong thing. And faced with greater tragedies – the suicide of someone with whom the worker has been closely involved, or the removal of a child after months of effort to keep the family together – self-examination may take the form of feelings of guilt or failure.

So as well as moral *reasoning*, the development of moral *emotions* needs to be understood by social workers. The account which follows presents concepts about the dynamics of conscience and guilt which have been found useful in practical social work – relevant both to the users of the service and to the experience of the workers themselves. Particular use is made of the psychodynamic insights of Colin Woodmansey, who built on the ideas of Sigmund Freud. As 'Essential background', section 4 explains, Freud's psychoanalytic ideas have been taken in many different directions – there is no single 'authoritative' account of psychoanalytic thinking.

Chapter
EB4

Broadly, Freud regarded 'conscience' as having two components. The *ideal self* (or, using psychoanalytic terminology explained in 'Essential background', section 4, the *ego ideal*) is the person's picture of who they would like to be. The *superego* is the component of the conscience which forbids bad actions.

In Woodmansey's view (1966, 1972, 1989) true moral values come from the positive motivation of 'doing to others as you would wish others do to you'. In ordinary 'good enough' development, it comes from wanting to be like the parent or other authority figure who is experienced as helpful, admirable and caring. This, in his terms, is part of the basic ego which develops naturally when a child is competently cared for. If parents trust their own best instincts (they sometimes need support to be sure of what these are), they have no need to be frightened of the child's basic impulses, including aggressiveness and selfishness. Common sense and attentive care of the child lead to appropriate development. For example, any child may snatch a toy from a brother or sister if they want to play with it (or if they want to make their sibling cry). If parents problem-solve appropriately, they do not need to punish the child, and in due course the child reaches a stage where it defers gratification of its own immediate wishes out of regard for other people – just as, in fact, the parent did for him.

However, through a process that Woodmansey describes as 'the internalisation of external conflict', another part of the self may develop which is hostile towards the child's own basic impulses. It is this part, called by Woodmansey the 'hostile' or 'punitive' superego, which is at the root of self-attack, self-punishment, guilt, and unrealistic self-criticism. Woodmansey suggests that the interaction to understand is that in which a parent, determined to stop a child in some strongly motivated behaviour, uses punishment and deterrence until the child obeys. Since a healthy child will at first resist such attack, 'punishment and retaliation will provoke each other in turn until the child can stand no more . . . yet, he will often be unable to escape'; his own impulses are each time to complain further, which attracts a further dose of punishment from the adult. Woodmansey suggests that the child fortuitously finds a way out of this cycle. The child turns its anger on itself, regarding itself as the cause of the problem, and since the fight can't be continued on two fronts at once, self-directed aggression has the by-product of removing the child from conflict with parents. The cost, however, is that the child's ego is split – one part owns the natural impulses, while the other, the punitive or controlling 'superego', becomes antagonistic and controlling towards aspects of itself.

The aspects of self (actually unproblematic, but experienced as dangerous) which tend to attract this self-punishment and self-criticism are those which have provoked rejection or punishment from the parent. These are commonly: aggressiveness – the child's tendency to be angry when thwarted, for example; the need for comfort (if this is met with rejection); and untidiness or sexual impulses. The punitive/controlling state of mind – an 'ego' in its own right, unsympathetic to the basic needs of the self – is likely to be recreated in other, similar situations later, causing self-criticism, repression and self-punishment in relation to natural impulses.

The core idea is that these two 'states of mind' have contradictory qualities and are mutually antagonistic. One state of mind is of self-attack, self-criticism; the other is the state of mind of being attacked. In a helping relationship, the two states of mind require different responses. One requires sympathy and support because they are constantly blamed for matters which are not within their control; but the other thinks the basic self is bad and deserves criticism or punishment. In the controlling state of mind, a woman vigorously and constantly cleans her house, reproaching herself that it is not clean (even though to an outsider it is perfectly presentable). In the other state of mind, she may feel depressed and defeated that however hard she tries, she always seems to fall short.

Although these states sound similar, as Woodmansey pointed out, in practice there is a difference in the way they feel. One is like the critical parent controlling and wanting to punish the child, keeping up standards by driving ever harder; and the other is like the hurt child being constantly criticised, feeling a failure. The latter wants warmth, care and reassurance, whereas the former despises such things. The 'punitive superego' wants – and offers – no sympathy for the weak, undisciplined self with whom it shares a life (and a body). The two states of mind do not exist simultaneously, and it is fruitless to respond to one when the other is speaking.

So when discussing difficult situations, there may be three elements to the social worker's conversation. One is the practical discussion of the outside situation, and the offer of assistance with appropriate plans or actions. The second is to respond to the punitive state of mind, and the third is to respond to the self-criticism and feelings of failure.

An example from social work in a children's hospital is given by Sudbery and Blenkinship (2005). A child had been severely burnt in a kitchen accident. Some exchanges in a conversation with the parents were about making financial applications (which the parents had never done before), and reassuring them that the circumstances of the accident were such that no one would blame them. In the same conversation, other exchanges involved acknowledging that 'it doesn't matter what anyone else thinks, you think you are to blame for what happened' (acknowledging, but not agreeing with, the views of the punitive superego). In yet other parts of the conversation, the social worker was essentially sympathising with the feelings of the parents, staying with them in their pain, and pointing out that it is unjust for them to be blamed, on top of that pain, when there was nothing they could realistically have done.

In summary, besides external relationships (which are often the obvious concern of social workers), people also have relationships with themselves, which can be amicable (accepting) or hostile (punitive). Mixed in with the practical problems presented to social workers, there are often difficulties in the relationship with the self. For effective social work, these are as important as the other problems. In day-to-day social work, the sensitive social worker may address the two sides of a person's self-attack without consciously thinking about psychological structures. Sometimes, particularly when practical help or sympathetic comments are missing the mark, it can be helpful to realise that in self-criticism there are two different states of mind being expressed – one punitive and one punished (in Woodmansey's terms, an ego and a split-off hostile superego).

Roberts (1994) suggests that staff in social work and other helping professions are particularly prone to self-questioning, and certainly their work will regularly provoke self-doubt. They are therefore entitled to supportive supervision which lessens their tendency to self-criticism, and this experience itself will directly increase their sensitivity and competence about the issues faced by the users of their service.

Cooper and Lousada (2005), using ideas from Melanie Klein, suggest there is another aspect to the experience of guilt in welfare work. They regard the ability to experience and withstand guilt as essential because otherwise policy makers and practitioners will go to unrealistic and potentially damaging lengths to avoid it. This is developed further in Cooper and Whittaker (2014), where this is explored within the history of child protection scandals in England.

History shows that welfare work and welfare policy sometimes fail people in severe ways. There are regularly reports of children who have been left at home only to be later harmed by the parents (or the removal of children from parents who in fact have not harmed them). To avoid 'guilt', Cooper and Lousada suggest, policy makers may engage in grandiose schemes after tragedies such as these. Faced with the enormity of the damage, policy makers may implement unrealistic and ultimately unhelpful reorganisations and procedural provisions 'to ensure this will never happen again'. This may well be impossible for anyone to guarantee, and the proliferation of reorganisation and ever-increasing regulations may hinder services rather than improve them.

Practitioners need to be able to cope with guilt because the experience of history is unfortunately that, even with good intentions, conscientious work and approved practice, they are likely to be avoidably harming the users of their service. In retrospect, during every decade 'good' social work and welfare practice has been harming people (even though it is only with hindsight that this becomes clear), so it is unlikely that it will suddenly stop. In the post-war years children from English inner cities were sent out 'to new lives' in the Commonwealth countries of Australia and Canada; unfortunately, the effects of the consequent exploitation, dislocation and lack of care still drive many of these lives sixty years later. In the 1950s, young children were still being placed in 'residential nurseries' entirely ill-suited to care for the emotional needs of young children; in the 1960s, social workers were still giving childless couples the joy of an adopted baby, and the child a chance of a good family life, but at the expense of young women who had given birth outside marriage, and who have continued to suffer through the decades since. None of this detracts from the essential assistance that has also been given over the years by social workers, but they have to be able to accommodate appropriate guilt for actions they take in good faith, which later turn out to have been against the best interests of the citizens they tried to assist.

Guilt, Melanie Klein's analysis suggests, is an unavoidable component of early childhood experience (coming originally from the realisation that the child has wished to harm and destroy the very person they love). Both then and later in life, it can be avoided only by using psychological defences that are ultimately unhelpful. If social workers themselves are at ease with this component of guilt, they will be well equipped to alleviate the unrealistic, punitive superego. In fact they will realise that if they perform this service properly for their clients (whatever harm they have done to others), they will, by however small or large a degree, make it more likely that the person will experience true reparative guilt. The victim and those concerned about her require the perpetrator to feel guilt based on the harm done, not on unrealistic self-criticism.

SUMMARY

Thinking ability develops from unreflective engagement with the material world through to the ability to manipulate abstract concepts. Piaget envisaged the individual as like a scientist gradually constructing a model of the world. He concluded from his research that thinking develops in universal stages from infancy to adulthood. At each stage, there are characteristic mistakes in thinking processes (cognitions). Vygotsky placed more emphasis on the culture in which knowledge can develop and the influence of significant adults such as teachers. He understood children to have a 'zone of proximal development', an area of learning they are ready for; good education should provide 'scaffolding' to enable this potential learning to take place. The tradition of research set out by Piaget has been fruitful, but many researchers have found that the description of stages needs modification, and that the precise nature of cognitive ability depends on tasks which are commonly performed and varies across different intellectual domains. Information-processing approaches place more emphasis on the development of functional components of thinking ability (such as short-term memory and working memory).

The chapter summarised three main theories of learning and behaviour. In classical conditioning, an artificial (conditioned) stimulus becomes associated with an unconditioned response – the dog begins to salivate at the sound of a bell. In operant conditioning, behaviour is shaped by the reinforcements which follow. In social learning, behaviour which is rewarded when others display it is learnt by observation. All are relevant to work in social care. Cognitive behavioural approaches also emphasise the cognitions which affect behaviour and emotions.

Education is a major location of social, emotional and intellectual experience for children. Statistics show clearly how educational outcomes are related to the way society is structured, through class, gender and 'race' for example. The pattern of these statistics seems to rule out any simple explanation of the causal mechanism through which educational outcomes are linked to social structures.

Abuse damages children, sometimes fatally, and tends to have lasting effects. Social workers need to be alert to these effects long after the abuse has ended. Current policy distinguishes physical abuse, emotional abuse, sexual abuse and neglect, but these are overlapping categories. It is important for social workers to understand 'resilience' as well as 'abuse'.

The formal essay discussed the development of cognition about morality and the emotions associated with guilt and conscience. Influential 'stage' models of moral cognitions have been put forward by Piaget and Kohlberg. Gilligan believes these are too focused on concepts of 'justice' and punishment, and highlights the importance of empathy and relationships. Cognitive behavioural work operates to change inappropriate thinking which is involved in antisocial behaviour. In relation to punitive guilt and self-reproach, social workers must understand that people have a relationship with themselves as well as with others, and this relationship with self can have a degree of self-directed hostility. They have to relate both to the punishing impulses of the individual and to the effects of being punished.

FURTHER READING

There are many readable accounts of cognitive development which build on the enormous quantity of research material. About cognitive development (the work of Piaget and later researchers):

Bee, H. and Boyd, D. (2014) *The Developing Child*. Thirteenth edition. Boston, New York and London: Pearson, pp. 140–181. There are two chapters devoted to cognitive development and a third that discusses moral development.
Piaget, J. (1973) *The Child's Conception of the World*, translated by Joan and Andrew Tomlinson. London: Paladin. The classic text of Piaget that outlines his ideas.

About all aspects of social work with children and families:

Butler, I. (2011) *Social Work with Children and Families: Getting into Practice*. Third edition. London: Jessica Kingsley.

About child abuse and child protection:

Howe, D. (2005) *Child Abuse and Neglect: Attachment, Development and Intervention*. Basingstoke: Palgrave Macmillan.
McCluskey, U. and Hooper, C. A. (2000) *Psychodynamic Perspectives on Abuse: The Cost of Fear*. London: Jessica Kingsley.
Wilson, K., Ruch, G., Lymbery, M. and Cooper, A. (2011) *Social Work: An Introduction to Contemporary Practice*. Second edition. Harlow: Pearson, pp. 488–498.

RESOURCES FOR PARENTS AND CHILDREN

About starting school (reassuring and funny story for children):

Child, L. (2015) *Charlie and Lola: I Am Too Absolutely Small for School*. London: Orchard.

About abuse:

Ainscough, C. (2000) *Breaking Free: Help for Survivors of Child Sexual Abuse*. Second edition. London: Sheldon.

The NHS NICE Clinical Knowledge Summary website has information on a wide range of topics about child health and children's medical conditions:

https://cks.nice.org.uk/

Questions

Based on the text:

1. The introduction to this chapter refers to features of early childhood identified by: (a) Erikson's psychosocial model; and (b) attachment theory. What are they? (The features are subtly different from experience in infancy.) Give a brief example to illustrate your answer.
2. Explain how the following topics, discussed on a television programme, relate to different models of behavioural learning:

    ■ 'In the old days', perhaps children's behaviour was better because policemen could administer a quick physical slap to young people who misbehaved.
    ■ Footballers should be good role models for young men; and ultra-thin fashion models influence girls in the wrong way.

3. 'People have a relationship with themselves as well as with outside people. This internal relationship, too, can be friendly and accepting or hostile and punitive.'
    Use this as the title of an essay. In the essay:

    ■ Describe some of the ways a relationship with self can be critical or punitive.
    ■ Give examples relating to the experience of social work students, practising social workers or their clients.
    ■ Discuss some of the possible origins of this harsh attitude towards the self.
    ■ Using a social work example (which may be from the literature or an anonymous account from your own experience), describe how services may either worsen the problem or help to remedy it; in your answer focus particularly on the contribution of the individual social worker.

For you to research

If you specialise in work with children, you will make more specialist and detailed studies later in your programme. Out of the many possible topics, here are some suggestions for student research and seminar presentation:

Chapter 9

■ Childhood disability – parents and siblings of a child with a disability
■ Mental health in childhood
■ Bullying (face-to-face and online)
■ The experience of learning disability in childhood
■ Dyslexia
■ The effects on children of parental separation and divorce
■ Children's experience of death (this is touched on in Chapter 9)
■ Children's play

CHAPTER 4

Transitions and adolescence

In this chapter you will find:

■ **Adolescence – biological changes; theories of adolescence; sexuality; Erikson and identity**

■ **Care leavers**

■ **Disabled people and adolescence**

■ **Hopson's model of transitions**

■ **Essay: Maslow, Rogers, and the development of the self**

EMOTIONAL BIOGRAPHY

Emma

Tia's friend, Claire (15 years), is in a relationship with a boy whom she met while she was at the children's home where she and Tia had lived. Claire was impressed with him and noticed how he wore nice clothes and bought her presents. He introduced her to his friends and felt the group accepted her so she spent more and more time with them as they 'felt like family'. After a while, they asked her to take 'something' to a rural town outside London and said that they would give her money, more money than she was used to. Claire suspected that it was drugs but she was afraid to ask.

Nicki

Nicki is 14 years old. Born into a male body, Nicki felt from an early age that she should have been a girl. She told her mother when she was 6, but her mother thought it was just a 'phase'. At the age of 10 years, Nicki's mother found her dressed as a girl and was shocked. The family doctor referred them to see a psychologist, who was very supportive. Nicki wanted to be female all the time so dressed as a female when starting secondary school. However, other children knew and Nicki was severely bullied at school and took several overdoses.

Vivian

Vivian had been 15. That was ten years ago now, a world away from her uncertain life in England as she awaits the decision on her asylum application. Back then, the struggle for power in Somalia had intensified over three weeks as the president clung to power. One by one, the small towns where Vivian's friends lived had changed allegiance, turning to support the rebels who promised to install a new, democratic government. Vivian's father had no real interest in politics, and Vivian understood even less. But her father had been faced with a choice between the burning of his house by the rebels or changing his allegiance away from the governor; and he saw the writing on the wall.

Vivian came home from school at two in the afternoon, hungry as usual; for in these troubled times food was short. She saw the men in uniforms at several of the houses, including her own. As she walked past the soldier he looked her up and down but said nothing. She was just in time to see her parents dragged away, still living. She never saw them again.

ADOLESCENCE

This chapter will outline various aspects of adolescent life. In presenting these ideas, we have as usual thought particularly about the people you will be working with as a social worker. Children who come into care will be teenagers before very long, and we refer briefly to some of the patterns of experience of adolescents in care. Young people may be both adolescents and parents, and the adults you work with will have had many and varied experiences as adolescents. Someone you see as a 90-year-old woman has spent her teenage years in circumstances that are both highly individual and shaped by historical and cultural patterns. Similarly, if you work directly with adolescents you are likely to feel that there are features of their life that are typical of their generation, and others which are specific to them and their individual difficulties.

Adolescence is defined by its stage as a transition between childhood and adulthood, but social workers are constantly dealing with transitions at all stages of life. This chapter outlines some theoretical approaches to understanding transitions. It concludes with a more academic discussion about the degree to which theories offering a universal view of human nature can capture the varied experience of people in different cultures and in different social positions.

Biological changes in adolescence

The idea of 'adolescence' and the concept of 'the teenager' have been invented (or 'constructed') by particular societies. Their meanings, and certainly their associations, are dependent on ways of living at particular times in history. This is discussed in the next section. Before that, here is a brief outline of bodily changes that tend to occur in the second ten years of life.

Growth spurt – the skeletal system. For many young people, there is a period over which they grow between 10 and 30 cm, sometimes 8 to 15 cm each year (Tanner, 1992, cited in Kagan and Tindall, 2003). For girls this typically begins in the eleventh year and is complete by age 16. Boys typically begin later and full adult height is achieved by about 19. Boyd and Bee (2014) describe the pattern of growth and comment that the sequencing of this growth may cause adolescents to look awkward, but actually their coordination is improving, sometimes because of the greater maturity of joints such as the wrist.

Brain development. There is increasing interest in and research about the development of the brain in this period. There are two growth spurts in brain development during the teenage years (Boyd and Bee, 2014). The first growth spurt occurs between the ages of 13 and 15 and occurs in the prefrontal cortex which controls executive processing and enables the conscious control of thought processes. This is followed by a further spurt in growth from the age of 17 into the early twenties, which affects the frontal lobes, areas which have particular importance in logic and planning (Boyd and Bee, 2014). The networks in the brain used by mature adults for decision-making may well be different from those used in adolescence (Blakemore et al., 2007). Once again, as described in the brief account of infant brain growth in Chapter 2, the process is one of massive growth of brain material which is then constantly pruned, with the surviving material and connections being made more permanent and enduring (Sowell et al., 1999; Paus et al., 1999). As with all accounts of brain functioning, these ideas have to come with the warning that we are still only just beginning to understand the brain and its links to behaviour, cognition and feelings; simplified accounts (for example, about different areas of the brain being used for different purposes) do not represent the immensely complex reality.

Chapter 2

Body fat and muscle development. Muscles also develop rapidly in adolescence, the increase being more pronounced in males than females. Boyd and Bee (2014: 116) quote research to show that between the ages of 13 and 17 the percentage of the body made up of fat rises from 21 per cent to 24 per cent among girls but drops from 16 per cent to 14 per cent in boys.

Sexual development. Human sexuality, as discussed shortly, is a complex mix of behaviour, emotions, personal relationships, societal attitudes and, of course, biology. Changes in the body's reproductive system are significant in adolescence. The pituitary gland produces hormones which trigger both the growth spurt and, in the first place, the growth of pubic hair. In girls, this and the early stages of breast development are followed about two years later by the first period. Irregular menstrual cycles are normal at first, and still into the third year of menstruation no eggs (ova) may be produced in about half of the monthly cycles (Boyd and Bee, 2015). Bee states that there is still uncertainty about the age at which boys' sperm becomes capable of fertilising an egg, but that it is usually between the ages of 12 and 14. In boys, the stages of genital development begin with the enlargement of the testes, scrotum and penis. The scrotum skin loosens, reddens and darkens. The development of a beard and the lowering of the voice occur during the later stages.

The ovaries, uterus and vagina, or the penis and testes, are described as **primary sex characteristics**; features such as the breasts, body shape, voice pitch and (in boys) beard are **secondary sex characteristics**.

The age at which puberty occurs is variable. It varies between boys and girls, between individuals, across subcultures within a society and between different societies. Some of the factors affecting this variation can be clearly isolated, whereas others are part of a complex and subtle interaction of biology, personality and society, and are the subject of much debate. The female body needs to have about 17 per cent body fat before puberty will begin, and about 22 per cent body fat for periods to continue. Young female athletes such as dancers, gymnasts and swimmers do not have these proportions of fat, and so menarche typically occurs for them around the age of 17. This is normal for their reference group, and indeed earlier puberty might be bitterly disappointing for them – athletes after their first period are taller, have significantly more body fat, and practise less (Boyd and Bee, 2014; Klentrou and Plyley, 2003). In most industrial countries, a random sample of 12- to 13-year-old girls will find some who are already completing mature puberty and others who are just beginning. Ninety-five per cent of girls have their first period between the ages of 11 and 15 (Boyd and Bee, 2014, quoting Malina, 1990). However, in 1850, the average age of menarche in industrial countries appears to have been about 17. Better nutrition is most often quoted as the reason for earlier onset of periods in global patterns, but Whitten (1992) argues that this is insufficient to account for the change, and believes that the worldwide spread of industrial chemicals which mimic hormones must also be involved (a classic statement of the evidence is found in Colborn and Clement, 1992). Stress in early childhood is one of a range of other factors which can bring on female puberty earlier (Chisolm et al., 2005).

Culture and adolescence

It is not just biology that is affected by different social conditions. 'Adolescence' itself is a social construct – it is created within a particular culture. How life is divided into phases is substantially different in different cultures. Some writers follow Aries (1996) in arguing that 'childhood' is an invention of the last 400 years. Certainly the idea of the transition from childhood to adulthood varies substantially. In many rural pre-industrial societies, children work at the same tasks as their parents, and are as responsible for family income, so the transition to 'adulthood' is stripped of many of the meanings that it has in present-day Western societies. In a number of societies, however, there are

rituals that mark the transition from childhood to adulthood. In modern industrial societies, formal ceremonies like the bar mitzvah or the requirement for
females to wear the veil are generally restricted to specific religious or social
groups. Sometimes, 'prom' dances or going away to university are interpreted
as fulfilling similar functions marking the beginning of a new phase of life.

In affluent Western societies, youngsters are dependent on their parents
for many years, and this extends the period of adolescence. In 1910 in the
UK, the majority of young people had started work by the age of 14, but their
wages were usually low and contributed to the family income (often given
to the mother). Girls remained in the family until they married, when they
became part of their husband's household. The extended period of transition
is a comparatively new phenomenon. The arrival of 'teenagers' with significant money of their own, creating a target for advertisers and producers of
goods (particularly music-related), was a new feature of the 1950s, following the Second World War. The situation today, with adolescents forming a
major and lucrative market for clothes, entertainment and lifestyle goods, is
distinctive to our culture and period of history. This drawn-out 'adolescence'
contains various markers of the arrival of 'adulthood'. The age of criminal
responsibility in Scotland is 8, and in England and Wales it is 10 (the lowest
ages in Europe). The age of majority is the age at which a person has the
majority of the – not the total – legal rights to manage their own body and
property, rather than it being vested in their parents, and in the UK it is 18.
Sex is illegal when it involves a young person under the age of 16 in the
UK. In a study to which reference is made later in the chapter, Singh and
colleagues conclude that surveys find 20 per cent of girls and 30 per cent
of boys report first intercourse before this age. However, an offence is committed if sexually provocative images of either are made or owned before
they are 18. Conviction of these offences bars the person from working in
many occupations. A driving licence can be obtained from age 17, the armed
forces can be entered from 16.5 (the lowest age in Europe), and the right to
vote arrives at 18. Young people generally leave home later than in previous
decades, and because of delayed entry into employment, increasing numbers
return home before finally leaving for good. Some of those with domestic
problems risk becoming homeless.

Modern British society is varied, made up of many micro-cultures with
expectations differing between groups. For some, adolescence is a heavily
sexualised period. In one subculture the dominant values may prize academic,
athletic or musical achievement, whilst in another these may be significantly
less important than social activities with peers, largely outside the supervision of parents and other adults. In one subculture, prestige or fear may lead
to physical violence, whilst in another the routines set by religion or other
established adult systems may provide a framework for the transition to independence. 'Young people who feel that they have been let down by authority
earlier need to have these feelings addressed before they can re-engage
with the system' (Frankham et al., 2007).

The physical changes described above can have different meanings for
different individuals and groups. Whilst puberty describes physical changes,

the emotional changes involved can be more complex. Whilst many young people have a gender identity that matches the sex they were born with (known as cisgender), some experience a dissonance, known as gender dysphoria. For 'Nicki' (described at the beginning of the chapter) the onset of male puberty is likely to be experienced as very distressing as it emphasises the dissonance she feels between the gender that she identifies with and the biological sex that she was born with. Young people may identify as being male, female, transgender or somewhere along the male/female spectrum (non-binary). Gender-variant is a general term to describe young people whose gender identity differs from what is normative for their biological sex in a particular time and culture.

Evidence from the education and poverty programme of the Joseph Rowntree Foundation (for example, Wikeley et al., 2007; Hirsch, 2007) suggests that learning that takes place in activities outside school is crucial to positive social development; on the other hand, Burton and Marshall (2005) found in a survey of 169 students in Glasgow that there was an opposite correlation for sport – for the boys in their sample, involvement in sport was associated with a greater likelihood of being involved in delinquent behaviour. Wikeley found that young people from families in poverty participate in fewer organised out-of-school activities than their more affluent peers.

In respect of adolescence, culture, then, both shapes and is shaped by the experience and behaviour of young people. Common cultural ideas about adolescence include that it is a time of fluctuating moods and conflict with or defiance of authority; a time when attempts to assert an individual identity may well create stormy situations – leading one writer to assert rather provocatively that 'youth on the other hand, is contemporaneously *expected* to be an age of deviance, disruption and wickedness` (Brown, 2005: 3). The next section begins by looking at the research evidence about these views.

Generational conflict?

Although the peak age for offending seems to be about 17 – and in 2005, 25 per cent of people between the ages of 10 and 25 reported committing an offence in the previous twelve months (Wilson et al., 2006) – research on the whole does not support the idea that adolescence is a time of particular stress or intergenerational conflict, except for a specific minority of people. On the other hand, reviews of findings about adolescent–parent conflict have interpreted it both as functional for the continuing development of the family and of society, and as crossing cultural boundaries; it is neither specific to 'individualistic' societies (like America or Britain) nor absent from 'collectivist' cultures (like China, where conformity is prized). There appear to be complex interactions between parental and child temperaments which vary with gender – for example, Kawaguchi and colleagues (1998) found that low adaptability in fathers and daughters was related to greater adolescent–parent conflict, but this was not the case for fathers and sons both low on adaptability. Some of their research about mothers echoes that of

Silverberg and Steinberg (1987), who found that it was mothers' temperament and emotional well-being that related to the intensity of adolescent conflict rather than fathers'. However, this is in the context of their finding that only a minority of American families (perhaps 10 per cent) experience a deterioration in parent–child relationships in early adolescence, and this is often related to difficulties earlier in childhood. As you may surmise, this is an area in which there has been extensive research and numerous different interpretations of the data.

The overarching message from much of the research is that: teens generally retain strong attachments to their parents; it is parents who worry more about conflict than their children; good early attachments to parents correlate strongly with adolescent happiness and well-being, as well as with educational achievement and (for girls) reduced risk of early pregnancy. These correlations hold across cultures, and when asked to identify 'someone you can talk to about problems/someone who makes you feel good', teenagers overwhelmingly put parents top of their list, above their peers (for information about various research studies, see Boyd and Bee, 2015).

The psychodynamics of adolescence

Many people regard it as true by definition that after adolescence the individual has the identity of an adult – normally regarded as responsible for their own body, property and actions, and entitled by right to various expressions of personal autonomy – and that before adolescence the individual has been building a different kind of identity as a child. This transition is often regarded as one of the core psychosocial features of adolescence, and it is discussed in more detail in the next main section of the chapter.

This section, however, points you towards the way other features of the internal world can be understood during adolescence. Adolescence reawakens 'states of mind' from the earliest days up to the present. In adolescence, the states of mind of an autonomous adult individual may alternate quite quickly with those of a child who needs comfort and protection, the state of mind which requires adults to take care of it. The person whose destructive and violent impulses in childhood were not met with containment and responsive care experiences frustration and contradiction as a threat to the self which will not be resolved. The natural response is fear, aggression and attack. The person for whom early experiences were genuinely life-threatening, and who as a child had to cope with the outcomes as best they could, may experience passing setbacks in adolescence as if they are a threat to the existence of the self. The young person whose emotions were never regulated in a caring, attentive and resilient relationship may express the fury of a child's tantrums but with the power and aggressive force of a mature body. A number of researchers and practitioners emphasise that in adolescence, dilemmas and challenges resolved in one way during infancy and childhood can come up afresh for new resolution as the person enters adulthood.

Chapters
2, EB4

As described in Chapter 2 and 'Essential background', section 4, attachment needs are understood to persist throughout life. The attachment relationship has the function of providing comfort in times of distress, protection from danger and a secure base from which to explore. As the years progress, the attachment bond increasingly does not need physical proximity to be effective – for the securely attached person (unlike for the 3-year-old), the parents may be taken for granted as a protective and caring force even when the young person is temporarily living away from them. On the other hand, the consequences of negative early attachment experiences may show themselves dramatically. Attachment theorists consider that one of the functions of attachment is to allow a coherent 'narrative' of the self to develop, and allow cognitive functioning to develop correctly (Holmes, 2000: 49–51). And conversely, a disrupted and destructive attachment-type relationship can hinder the development of a coherent sense of self and interfere with accurate thinking. The young person who does not know where he has lived at different times in his childhood, or who he lived with, who has been told lies about himself, told that he does not have the feelings he actually experiences ('Come on, stop being silly, you're not frightened at all – stop being stupid!'), or that those who care for him do not have the feelings they actually have ('I love you so much, you're the apple of my eye', said by a parent who is actually self-obsessed and unable to attend to the feelings of anyone else) may end up having significant difficulties in logical information processing, particularly under stress. The experience of duplicity, confusion and a lack of certainty about events as an endemic experience in early years can later be expressed as 'lying' and a lack of accuracy about facts in the present. Youngsters in trouble may come to believe their own falsehoods about what has happened on a particular occasion because 'facts' about personal life have always been arbitrary.

Unfortunately, it may be those who are most in need of a secure base (because of a lack of love, security or care in their childhood) who have most firmly decided that they no longer need or expect one, and therefore are least likely to find it.

Adults who are responsible for adolescents in trouble need themselves to receive ongoing support so that they can remain attached to the (often difficult) young person – caring and non-retaliatory even when faced with severe provocation. Persisting in this attachment is important for the happiness and security of the young person in the next phase of their life. Here are the words of 'Emma', who spoke to one of the authors (JS) when she was 21, some years after she had left the children's home she refers to (she had friends similar to the fictional 'Tia'):

> When I first went to X [home], I thought, 'Another home' – you know what I mean; it's going to be one of them again, where I would just stay so long then I would get moved. So when I was at X, everyone was my enemy . . . Me and Ann-Marie [staff member] never used to get on; I used to hate Ann-Marie. I have threatened Ann-Marie with a knife – I've bitten her and everything because I didn't like her.

So for me, for X [home] to put up with the way I was, I am quite surprised. For a child that can't think straight, and not being able to trust one person in their life because they have been moved about . . .

And it's weird how Ann-Marie and me now get on dead well . . . I was fostered with her after a while, for a year. It was hard when I had to move on, but she was like the mum I always wanted, even though I know she's not.

I speak to her on the phone, I guess every couple of weeks.

Sex and adolescence

Beckett and Taylor quote Cobb: 'Adolescents cannot simply add new sexual feelings to an old self', and go on, 'these feelings require a new self to be found' (Beckett and Taylor, 2010; Cobb, 1995). In general, sex presents quite a challenge for research. Discussing 'first sexual activity', for example, immediately highlights the fact that sexual expression is part of a continuum. Children are undoubtedly sensual; they will seek sensual pleasure and they will explore bodily and interpersonal sensation. Freud's idea of sex ('Essential background', section 4) understands adult libido to be continuous with life-promoting drives from earliest infancy, but with different pressure, aim, object and source. It is in later childhood and in adolescence that the overt power of sexual hunger and sexual experience becomes very evident – when desire can lead to a loss of equilibrium, but knowledge and the ability to manage emotions may be very variable. Chapter 6 discusses sex and gender more generally.

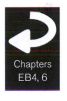

Chapters
EB4, 6

Singh and colleagues (2000) reviewed nationally representative surveys in fourteen countries (a total of over 25,000 young people), and found that in most countries, roughly one-third or more of teenage women and between half and three-quarters of men have had intercourse; in four countries (Ghana, Mali, Jamaica and Great Britain), about three in five are heterosexually experienced. In Great Britain and America, the relevant surveys referred only to heterosexual activity, so there is likely to be a smaller additional group who have been sexually active with someone of the same sex. In most countries, sexual intercourse during the teenage years occurs predominantly outside marriage among men but largely within marriage among women. According to the authors, who describe the UK data as among the most reliable in their study, about 20 per cent of women and about 30 per cent of men have sexual intercourse before 16, the legal age of consent. These figures are broadly in line with Wellings and colleagues' 2001 study of 11,161 men and women. This figure relates to any individual occurrence, not necessarily to a continuing pattern of behaviour – the study found that 'never-married young people are considerably less likely to be currently sexually active than to be sexually experienced'.

This summarises statistics which come out of the answers to question-naires in a very delicate area of life. To create a picture of what actually happens in any meaningful way requires a lot of other information about whether the sex is genuinely consensual, whether the contact is sporadic and with different partners or constant within a consistent relationship, and so on. In a longitudinal study of health-related matters in New Zealand, 54 per cent (211 out of 388) of women reported that they should have waited longer before having sex, and this rose to 70 per cent (90 out of 129) for women reporting first intercourse before the age of 16. It appears to be the case that for most women who have sex as adolescents, their first heterosexual contact is remembered as a negative experience. Based on her interviews with 400 teenage girls, Thompson's study (1990) described the most prevalent stories including negative themes such as boredom, physical and romantic disappointment, alienation from the body or coercion. No doubt this is partly a matter of their own bodily exploration and partly to do with the behaviour of their partners. The process of learning and maturation takes place in different ways for different people. Equally, young men who engage in early sexual activity may be unaware of the range of the emotional and sensual needs, of themselves and of their partners, which are potentially met through sexuality. Once again, the subject highlights the complex interplay of biology, bodily experience, emotion, interpersonal relationships and social attitudes which are involved in sex.

Most people, male and female, will find that some core aspects of their sexual experience of themselves are ignored, disapproved of or condemned by the majority culture in which they live; but this is particularly acute for those whose objects of desire are of the same sex – they may be deprived even of the acceptance (albeit often unspoken) of sexual reality which may be found in peer relationships. Gay and lesbian young people, and to a lesser extent anyone else who experiences same-sex attraction, have to affirm a large part of their sexual persona for themselves, without the support of social structures which validate their orientation, and in the face of 'cultural denial, distorted stereotypes, rejection, neglect, harassment and sometimes outright victimisation and abuse' (Morrow and Messinger, 2006: 179). 'I thought I was the devil's disciple', said a young Muslim man (BBC, 2017), 'I knew from about the age of 10 where my sexual attraction lay, but I was told that this was the work of the devil and I would go to hell'. Gerard Mallon (1998: 98) reports that in his interviews with young American people who were in the care system and aware that they were gay, a common description was that they experienced themselves as a 'throw-away child', part of the garbage, and those who did not experience this directly had kept the sexual part of their identity secret for fear of being treated in this way. In a study of gay and lesbian young people, the average age of awareness of their sexual orientation was 10, the average age of labelling themselves as gay or lesbian was 14, the average age of first disclosure to a friend was 16 and the average age of disclosure to family was 17. So these young people are forming a socially stigmatised identity at exactly the time when peer pressure to fit in is particularly strong.

> Lillian, now 25, was talking about her teenage years: 'In my first years at secondary school I was very shy. Then I was outed without my consent. My girlfriend gave me a kiss right in the middle of the playground.

I found it very hard to cope and . . . just put a cocoon around me. I became really, really butch. I wasn't going to let anyone . . .'. Her father was in the room during this conversation, and said: 'But then it was just so difficult. Everything was "because I'm gay".' Lillian argued back, 'Well, you said I'd just grow out of it, I'd get married, you wanted grandchildren.' Father: 'Well, yes, but, . . . and every parent wants grandchildren.'

McCarthy (1999: 13) in her interviews with women with learning disabilities similarly found that 'only a small minority' felt positive about their sex lives. In her concluding recommendations for policy and practice, she highlights the imperative need to protect these women from abuse and unwanted sex, and also the requirement that sex education should take the form of what her co-writer, David Thompson, calls 'erotic education' – none of her respondents, for example, knew either the name for or the existence of (let alone the potential of) their clitoris. These unsatisfactory experiences were with men, and she highlights the specific need for education and support for men with learning disabilities to reveal to them the satisfactions of giving pleasure and how that may be done.

ERIKSON AND OTHERS – ADOLESCENCE AND IDENTITY

What are the components of identity as it develops during adolescence? Carol Gilligan (1982/1993) emphasises that for women, these tend to include the maturation of their views about relatedness to other people. From the outset, she believes, women's object of identification has been their mother. If all goes well, they experience this woman caring for them, asking them sometimes to care for others, involving them in the tasks of caring. Important dimensions to the development of adult identity are relational responsibility, commitment and interpersonal sensitivity. Gilligan (a feminist researcher whose work is also referenced in Chapters 3 and 5) believes that women's voices are silenced, particularly in adolescence, by a male-dominated society in which adult autonomy is understood as separateness. She sees this understanding as a part of earlier developmental research which analysed typical pathways for men, who were said to strive for autonomy in ways that are less rooted in relationships.

Chapters 3, 5

Bingham and Stryker (1995) similarly emphasise that in the earlier stages of life the identity work of a girl is to develop a sense of self as a steady person who is capable of achievement, and in adolescence it involves tackling work which leaves her feeling worthy, entitled to assert needs and wants, and developing the confidence to cope with life in intellectual and social spheres. The positive outcome is to attain a sense of responsibility in being able to take care of herself and others.

Identity involves gender and sex, being a man or a woman in a particular society. Gilligan, Bingham and Stryker would all identify the developments just described as occurring in a context in which there may be a tendency to socialise girls to be more compliant and dependent.

Chapters
2, EB6

These ideas about adolescent development are placed by the authors in the context of the work of Erik Erikson, and to varying degrees in opposition to his ideas. He saw this fifth life stage (see Chapter 2 and 'Essential background', section 6) as one in which a distinctly new identity has to be forged, one more separate from the adults whose values and characteristics had formed the child's earlier identity. In his view, adolescence is the intermediate phase in which the child's identity and social roles are relinquished and an adult identity created. This is in preparation for maturity – living independently, being financially autonomous, playing adult roles in sex, work and family. The identification with the peer group so evident in adolescence provides a base, while the dependence on parents' definitions and evaluations of self is gradually left behind.

Erikson regarded this process as creating an identity crisis. It is no longer possible to rely on other people's perceptions of one's own identity, but security in self-definition, in a sense of one's unique characteristics and value, is not yet established. You may recall that he regarded crises as inherent in the process of development, and that each crisis can have a positive or a negative outcome. The positive outcome of this crisis he saw as a mature sense of self – and the negative outcome as role confusion.

In discussing 'identity' in this way, developmental theory refers both to what is created by the individual as a unique personal sense of security and confidence in who one is, independent of other people's perceptions, and to the influence of outside expectations, which are often based on ideas about group characteristics. Different writers on matters affecting social work emphasise different sides of this balance. Someone who has 'a strong sense of their own identity' is someone whose idea of themselves, their qualities, and how they should behave socially, is not thrown off course by other people's expectations; but people also talk of their identity 'as a Muslim' or 'as a black person', a man, or a woman – categories making heavy use of mutual social expectations.

CHILDREN IN CARE

For children in care[1] the path to adulthood is often more difficult than for their peers. Their developmental needs will not necessarily be met just because the state has taken responsibility. At the time of writing, 49 per cent of young people in Britain go to university. For care leavers, however, the figure is just 6 per cent. Very high levels of depression are found to be common. Statistically, in all kinds of ways, the risks of negative outcomes in adolescence are much greater for children in care. Of people in prison under the age of 20, 50 per cent were brought up in care. Payne and Butler (1998) argue that the health needs of children in care are not adequately met. Hobbs and colleagues (1999) put forward the view that the very fact of being in care should be regarded as a risk factor for abuse, on the basis that the rate of abuse is 3.9 per 1,000 in birth families, 39.5 per 1,000 in foster care, and 23 per 1,000 in residential care. Note that although these figures probably give an accurate figure of the risk of abuse experienced by young people, they require significantly more interpretation in order to be understood as giving information about carers' behaviour (see Sudbery et al., 2005: 73–90). Similarly, the other risk factors described in this paragraph are not necessarily caused by being cared for by the local authority – educationally, for example, children in care are perhaps 'low achievers' rather than 'under-achievers'. Nevertheless, these statistics show that special attention must be paid to the issues faced by children in care.

Earlier sections of this chapter referred to the process in adolescence of moving physically away from an attachment figure whilst keeping the attachment bond intact, allowing it to mature into a different form. What is the nature of the attachment which is being modified for the child in care, and what is the meaning of physical separation – living away – for such a young person?

Adolescents in general are reticent about sexual and emotional matters when talking with adults. Often, therefore, the carers of a young person in care who is subjected to violence, or drawn into child sexual exploitation (CSE), or who is suicidal, are faced with a challenging task. They must be able to allow the young person their burgeoning (if at times unrealistic) autonomy, and yet find a way of being available to discuss matters which may be of grave significance in the young person's life.

Teenagers examine their peers for any difference, and difference can single a vulnerable child out for taunts or insults. Equally, the individual does not want to be 'different' in any way which attracts low status. How then do children in care construct their social identity? Matters such as discussing where they live or inviting other people back to their house are everyday matters of social concealment or lying. The fabric of teenage life that builds identity, such as personal privacy or 'sleepovers', is not a matter of personal negotiation but a matter of state regulation and bureaucracy.

> Sue lay in bed, unable to sleep, fuming. She hated moving to a new place and here she was with new foster parents. It meant all that stuff at school all over again. They ask you where you live. What are you supposed to say? And you can just see the ones who are going to dig and dig and dig until they get it out of you. 'Bastards. Do they see it straight away? Is it like I've got "Child in Care" tattooed across my forehead?' she thought. This always made her think of something else. Her mother used to feel she had been through World War Three when she eventually got to her bar job in the evenings. Sue did everything she could think of to stop her going out. Her mum came to hate her for it. But after her mum had gone, Sue would go straight to her room, couldn't concentrate. And then every bloody time she'd hear those steps coming up the stairs, one by fucking one – she could hear every footfall of her stepfather.
>
> She had very little doubt that everyone who looked at her could see she was sexually abused, knew what had gone on. Just looking at her they could see everything.
>
> She didn't sleep at all that night, was up before anyone else but didn't show her face outside the room. Made an effort to get to school.

And then there's all that stuff – 'Susan Bates, why aren't you concentrating?' She knew what she wanted to say – 'Oh, just fuck off.'

The risk of poor outcomes for children in care varies considerably, even between neighbouring European countries, but it is easier to see problems than to be certain of the remedies. One approach has been to set governmental targets – for improving educational performance, for example, or reducing the number of moves experienced by children in care – with the threat of penalties if authorities fail. This, however, can have the paradoxical effect of care authorities being preoccupied with meeting government targets rather than with the individuals in their care. Children can become (in the words of a report into the management of child abuse – Butler Sloss, 1988) 'objects of concern' rather than individuals. Gaskell (2010) in her study of young people in care found that what they most wanted was for someone to care about them and to demonstrate this care – for example, by listening to them, by doing the things which reasonable parents do for their children. 'If the social worker had called, it would have shown they cared', as one young person said to her.

Chapters
2, 3

The particular qualities of resilience that are found in children who have faced exceptional adversity tend towards independence and self-reliance (Howe, 2005; see Chapters 2 and 3 above). The task for those responsible for 'looked after' children is to support qualities such as these at the same time as recognising that there are urgent unmet attachment needs. This delicate balancing act requires particular maturity. McMurray and colleagues (2008) found in their study that social workers tended to have a simplified view of the resilience of children in care that could lead them to underestimate the psychological challenges faced by those children.

ADOLESCENCE AND DISABILITY

Every individual is a complex mix of characteristics. A person whose body is not typical will have experiences in adolescence which have to be understood from a specific point of view. Most adolescents, for example, receive information about sex from their peers. Teenagers with disabilities will be bombarded by the same sexually oriented material – music, fashion, advertisements – as their peers; they are likely to be as interested as anyone else in the changes that occur in their bodies and emotions, but some, because of the very limited time ever spent away from adult surveillance, will miss out on these conversations. For teenagers with spina bifida, Blum and colleagues (1991) found, 'the majority of information comes from parents and teachers'. These adults may be unwilling to fill this particular gap, and the result may be that the teenagers experience loss, doubts and an unnecessary sense of difference.

Adolescents in general are expected to take increasing responsibility for their life decisions, leisure activities, healthcare, accommodation and work. They are expected to gain increasing control and authority over their bodies and their lives.

Nowadays, these expectations are no different for young people with learning or physical disabilities, to the extent that is possible given their impairment. In adolescence, however, teenagers with disabilities are likely to become aware of the obstacles they will experience in achieving their adult roles. They learn the challenging mechanisms involved in tackling these barriers. The law, education and employment will take the official view that all individuals are entitled to equality and access. There may be a dramatic difference, however, between the way things are organised for children and the way they are organised for adults. These discontinuities and disparities may make transition particularly difficult for people with disabilities, especially as changes in organisation and philosophy are determined according to chronological age, not the developmental stage and experience of the individual.

Many parents find that it is a constant battle to get their children who have disabilities the benefits and services they are entitled to (Sloper and Beresford, 2006). In general, however, services are intended to be person-centred and child-focused. Adult services may be organised on a basis that gives much less priority, even in principle, to continuity and the emotional components of care. An individual may need to make persistent efforts in order to be offered 'reasonable adjustments' for their capacity, such as low intellectual ability, in an educational or employment setting. Young people with disabilities are likely to be creating their identities and working out how to tackle barriers when they have restricted personal spending and have incomes (Hirst and Baldwin, 1994) below those of other young people.

There are different challenges according to the different ways a person's body or brain may differ from the average. Most people learn about sport and other social activities by watching others at play. An adolescent with severe visual impairment, however, may need to rely on someone else realising that they need explicit information and support. Adolescents with Down's syndrome may become aware of differences, and of sexual issues, but would benefit from support to understand and make sense of incidental social cues. Adults thinking about the sexual education of severely visually impaired girls and boys have to realise and be comfortable with the reality that they are much more dependent on learning through feeling and touch than through visual explanations. Teenagers who lack sensation below the waist are entitled to conversations about sexual needs, which apply to them just as they do to others – for example, the role of sexual intimacy in providing personal contact, reassurance, relief from anxiety and alleviation of stress, and the different forms this intimacy may take. For many young people with extensive physiological difference from others, the constant public gaze in therapeutic and medical examination may not have prepared them to construct appropriate personal bodily boundaries. A child with cerebral palsy may experience pubertal changes earlier than her peers, and this for a girl may increase her sense of being apart and different (Quinn, 1998: 123).

Measures of self-esteem comparing adolescents with disabilities with the general population present contradictory pictures. Hirst and Baldwin (1994) found that adolescents with disabilities were more likely than their non-disabled peers to report feelings reflecting a poor sense of worth. King and colleagues (1993), on the other hand, report roughly equivalent self-esteem measures for both disabled and non-disabled adolescents, indicating that when there are differences, they involve psychosocial characteristics of families, parental values and expectations.

Looking Closer

In Erikson's view, at adolescence the individual identity, previously shaped by the definitions of others, becomes an adult identity based on understanding one's own unique characteristics. Gilligan's work is based on the perception that this tends to set up a 'masculine' idea of rugged individualism as normal development. For many women, in her view, mature identity is based on 'relatedness to others'.

- Do these ideas fit with your experience?
- Are Erikson's ideas of identity formation in adolescence more applicable to that stage than earlier or later transitions?
- How far is individual identity separate from others' definitions and social expectations?

TRANSITIONS

Adolescence can be described as a 'transition' from childhood to adulthood. This chapter has referred to many different transitions that may take place – the transition from experiencing life in a child's body to experiencing life in a sexually mature adult body; for the disabled child, the transition from dealing with services organised for children to those organised for adults; the transition to the expectation of greater personal control over finance, or the use of time.

All social work is about transitions in people's lives. Successful family support work is concerned with helping parents and children to find a happier, more satisfying, less frightening life – less stressful and less unhappy. With a child coming into care (and all too frequently with children who are in care), you will be concerned with the move from one accommodation to another; with people with mental health difficulties you may similarly be involved in a change of support arrangements or moves in accommodation. With older people, you may be concerned with their personal transition from being able to manage their own lives to a state where they need to depend on others to some extent, or in their transition from independent living to residential care; you will also be responsible for the well-being of people who have been bereaved. You will often be concerned with untimely transitions (the death of a child before a parent, for example, or an adolescent being forced to live on their own before they feel ready for it). Frequently, too, you will find that the work you do in the present cannot ignore transitions – possibly untimely and poorly managed transitions – in the past.

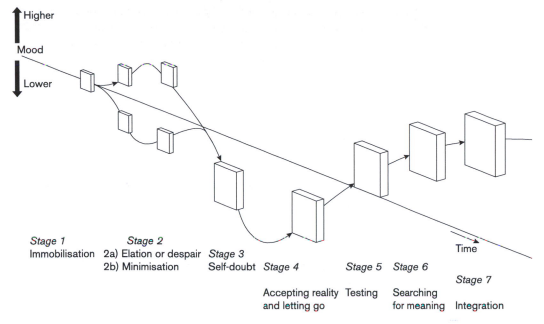

Figure 4.1 Hopson's model of transitions

Adams and colleagues define a transition as a 'discontinuity in a person's life space'. It is seen as a discontinuity either because general social expectations define it as a change, or because the person experiences it as such. Note that it can be triggered by the absence of an event as well as the occurrence of an event – for example, by not being able to have a baby, or failing to achieve promotion. Adams and colleagues present a simplified version of the stages involved in life transitions (Adams et al., 1976; Sugarman, 2009). They regard this cycle as applicable both to desirable and to undesirable transitions. Transitions may vary in intensity (moving up a year class in school is different from moving to live with an adoptive parent) and can take the form of experiences of varying length. Adams and colleagues suggest that the stages they identify are sufficiently frequent for most people to recognise them, although of course individual experiences vary significantly. These stages are set out in Figure 4.1.

Hopson's studies suggest that transitions are more stressful if they are unpredictable, involuntary, unfamiliar, of high magnitude, or frequent. He believes that every transition, however undesirable, offers the opportunity for personal growth and development.

1. *Immobilisation:* A sense of being overwhelmed: 'It can't be happening to me'; 'This isn't true'.
2. *Reaction:*

   (i) *Elation or despair:* a sharp swing of mood in the direction determined by the nature of the transition.

(ii) *Minimisation:* playing down the significance of the change, even to the point of denial. This may take the form of thoughts like, 'Well, it's all very well getting this great job, but now I've got to do it!' or, 'Well, it's not so bad really – life goes on.' Denial can have a positive function, enabling a person to cope with a situation that would be too overwhelming to face head on.

3. *Self-doubt:* a dip in feelings as the person becomes particularly conscious of the implications and challenges ahead. May involve feelings of depression, anger or apathy.

4. *Letting go:* The earlier phases involve much looking back. In this phase, the past is put behind the individual, who can now face up to the future. This is regarded as crucial in managing transitions. Levinson, whose work on adult transitions will be discussed in Chapter 6, describes it as a step into the unknown, as the person 'is cut adrift from the past, but cannot yet see the land of the future'.

5. *Testing:* Engaging with the new reality, the person tries out new strategies and approaches. New lifestyles and identities are sampled and discarded.

6. *The search for meaning:* a period of reflective thinking as the significance and personal meaning of the transition are explored.

7. *Integration/internalisation:* the final phase, involving the internalisation of the new meanings that have been discovered; the incorporation of these into behaviour, roles and outlook.

As with all the topics in this book, there is extensive literature exploring the subject further. For example, research has analysed the different factors involved in coping, identifying: the situation; the individual's characteristics; the nature of support available; the coping strategies adopted (Sugarman, 2009). Other studies explore which transitions tend to be most stressful (Holmes and Rahe, 1967), how transitions can be negotiated more or less successfully, and the vulnerability created by poorly negotiated transitions.

Looking Closer

Hopson analysed how the journey through the phases is affected by characteristics of the transition – whether it is positive, negative, sudden, unpredictable, frequent, of high intensity. Read more in Sugarman (2009).

Reflective thinking

List three transitions – including at least one that took place in your own life (for example, starting a university course) and one that would involve a social worker.

How far do you think the model proposed by Hopson fits the examples you have chosen?

The final section of this chapter is about the difficulty of describing 'universal' characteristics of human development. Thinking about the earlier sections of this chapter, what are some of the problems in describing 'universal' truths about human development? Write some general statements about adolescence, and then explain why they are not always true.

To give focus, the discussion refers particularly to 'humanistic' models of development. They are easy to understand, but have not been explained so far in this textbook. You will find a summary of them in 'Essential background', section 7, and the text below explains some of the concepts further. They are particularly good examples of attempts to specify development in universal terms, to find knowledge (as the title implies) which applies to all humanity.

Chapter EB7

TAKING IT FURTHER

ARE WE ALL THE SAME? HUMANISTIC MODELS AND THEIR CRITICS

The humanistic models created by Abraham Maslow and Carl Rogers have natural appeal in emphasising the common humanity of all people, the universal need for unconditional positive regard, and the desire in all people to achieve something worthwhile with their lives. For many, these ideas form a natural basis for social work. But they were originally developed in mid-twentieth-century America and were expressed in phrases littered with statements about 'man' and phrased with the gendered pronoun 'he'. Do such universalised formulations inherently (but sometimes covertly) privilege the cultural position of a particular commentator? Some have argued that they are based on a highly individualistic patriarchal culture, and result in superficially 'similar treatment for everyone' (thereby doing violence to the different experience of men and women, and the specific needs of different cultural and religious groups). This is an issue for all universalising theories of human need and development – here, the question is examined in relation to the humanistic models.

The humanistic model of development

'Humanistic' theories of development set out to emphasise the motivations, needs and achievements which are characteristically human. This discussion asks whether they succeed in creating a framework which applies to all people.

The starting point for the humanistic psychologists was that behavioural theories and psychoanalytic theories failed to capture the characteristics which make us distinctively human. Behavioural theory treated people as if they were no different from other animals, their behaviour simply the result of reward and punishment. Psychoanalytic theories emphasised hidden unconscious motivations, selfishness, destructiveness, conflict and negative attributes. What was distinctive about human development, this group of psychologists argued, was the struggle for meaning, the wish to lead a worthwhile life, the impulse to do good for other people even at a personal cost. As they might have put it, man's highest achievements are in the arts, philosophy, democracy, a civic community in which those with resources ensure that the vulnerable are protected and cared for. The various psychologists who set out this 'humanistic' approach tended to be active in helping occupations as counsellors or psychotherapists. Sometimes they worked on an individual basis (Rogers, Perls) and sometimes they worked with groups (Rogers, Perlman), espousing the power of the harmonious collective to promote growth in a way the individual 'expert' could not.

Chapter
EB6

This discussion will focus particularly on the developmental ideas of Carl Rogers (2004) and to a lesser degree on those of Abraham Maslow (Maslow and Frager, 1954/2003). Their ideas are summarised in 'Essential background', section 6 and in a number of accessible textbooks, usually in psychology (Eysenck, 2000: 27–30; McLeod, 2003: 140–160).

In this tradition core ideas about development are:

- The drive for growth comes from within the individual (so, for example, the counsellor or other helper is more like a nurturing gardener than a physician dispensing medicine).
- Each individual is inherently 'self-actualising'.
- For Maslow, fundamental survival needs (such as physiological needs and the need for physical safety) are the foundation on which self-actualising builds. Once survival needs are met, they are no longer motivating, for they are experienced only when they are deficits. The growth and self-actualising motivation, however, continues.
- For Rogers, all organisms, including 'man', fundamentally know what is good for them, and value whatever helps them achieve their full potential. Humans have a need for both positive regard (from others) and positive self-regard.
- During development, however, positive regard from others may come only 'conditionally'. The conditions attached may be out of accord with authentic organismic valuation – that is, ideas about who the child 'ought' to be, its 'ideal self', are out of tune with the real self. The bigger the gap between the socially induced 'ideal self', and the authentic individual, the 'real self', the greater the suffering. To survive, the individual has to use distortion and denial.

According to the research associated with this model, the key features of helping relationships are not the techniques used by the helper, but the qualities of the helper – that they give unconditional positive regard, show empathy and offer non-possessive warmth (amended to 'congruence' in later models).

In summary, then, the humanistic model of development is that everyone needs both positive regard and positive self-regard. If they are cared for and grow up in an atmosphere of acceptance, their own natural tendencies will cause the most valuable of human qualities to develop. If they grow up with conditions attached to positive regard (to be a good girl, a female must be clean, neat and submissive; to be a man, a boy must be aggressive, loud and never frightened), then they will develop a 'false self' as well as a natural self. This causes pain and social difficulty – there will be a split between what their natures want them to be and how they think they ought to be. An essential foundation for developing valued 'human' qualities is having basic needs met – physiological needs, safety needs, needs for care and affection.

Humanistic theory and social work

Many social workers find that these principles form an excellent basis for their work, transcending the difficult individual details they deal with, and stating principles that they find valid for all.

In ensuring that a family has a roof over its head, in ensuring a child lives in a safe, nurturing environment or that an older adult has appropriate accommodation, the social worker is providing for the most basic 'deficit' needs (Maslow's terms). This allows other development to take place. But the social worker is not simply a housing or finance officer. In listening to the bereaved person or to the adult who was abused as a child, attending to the mother facing the death of her daughter or to the older adult moving into residential care, the social worker is addressing their development. They cannot know what 'development' means for the individual, let alone create it, but they can ensure that their relationship is developmental – that it maximises rather than hinders the opportunity. Unconditional acceptance and empathy are small but much-valued contributions that assist people to find their own paths forward.

The general critiques of the humanistic model

A number of textbooks on human development (Boyd and Bee, 2015; Beckett and Taylor, 2010) do not refer to humanistic theory. Before considering the specific issue of universalisability, it is appropriate to note the general critiques. Although both Rogers and Maslow describe the characteristics of 'self-actualising' people, it is difficult to see how self-actualisation can be quantified, and this implies that the measure of failure to achieve it is equally elusive. The possibility of measuring whether a child is offered 'unconditional positive regard' over the course of its upbringing, and then measuring the outcome, is even more remote. In fact, although there is a body of outcome research about humanistic counselling of adults, the humanistic theorist would tend to regard such quantitative measurement as not respecting the essential nature of the approach. The humanistic school of psychology had its roots far more in existentialist philosophy, which emphasised the intrinsic value of authentic person-to-person contact, transcending concrete behavioural evaluation.

The model is chosen here, however, to illustrate a different set of criticisms, the criticisms which are applied to any 'universal model'.

Is this a universal model?

The most obvious way to check whether a theory applies across different populations and cultures is to conduct observations and experiments in which different populations can be studied. This has been done in relation to many models – attachment theory, cognitive development and bereavement, for example. In this way it can be established whether it holds for both men and women, Western and non-Western cultures, gay and straight people, and so on; and if so, what differences there may be. Like the generic criticism outlined in the previous paragraph, however, this will be beside the point in relation to humanistic theory – it could hardly be that men need unconditional positive regard, but that it does not matter to women!

It is a different kind of criticism that is being made. The critics argue that the apparent universality of the theory conceals its partisan nature. Because it fails to mention the specifically gendered obstacles to development faced by women, humanistic psychology may be seen as one of the apparently gender-neutral theories which in fact collude with the oppression of women – 'in all societies which divide the sexes in differing cultural or economic spheres, women are less valued than men' (Humm, 1992, quoted in Kagan and Tindall, 2003). It is argued that to be gender-neutral is to be gender-blind, and that any theory which does not mention gender is colluding with gender oppression.

Carol Hanisch wrote an article in 1968 (republished in 2006 with a commentary by her) with the title 'The Personal Is Political'. In other words, personal matters embody the structures of society. For her, as for a number of feminist writers who have used the phrase since, the 'political' includes the systematic oppression of women by men. This is seen as inherent to our society and is described as 'patriarchy' by these authors. Hanisch wrote, 'Women are messed over, not messed up! We need to change the objective conditions, not adjust to them. Therapy is adjusting to your bad personal alternative . . . personal problems are political problems.' As Morrow and Messinger (quoted in Kagan and Tindall, 2003) put it, 'The individual experiences of disease experienced by women have their roots in the powerlessness of women as a class.' For these feminists, a central feature of female development is the creation of a conscious awareness of this 'patriarchal' status quo. In this view, male gender power is seen as central to personal development. However highly girls achieve, Abbott argues that the educational system always disadvantages them (Abbott et al., 2005: 89). Societal power dynamics are understood to be inescapably bound up with personal relationships – for example, 'the question of whether heterosexuality is a tenable practice for feminists remains a source of contention' (Abbott et al., 2005: 228). From this point of view, a philosophy which centres on personal relationships and experience but makes no reference to the dynamics of **privilege** inherent in them is seen as inadequate.

Related critiques are made by those who regard society as inherently racist. If language and social structures (particularly in post-imperial and post-slavery societies and culture) privilege those seen as 'white', then components of personal development for others involve the challenge of this. The 'personal' conditions for this to take place, as specified by humanistic theory, should also specify that this political dimension is built into the personal.

Taken to its logical conclusion, similar criticism could be advanced in turn by those who regard present-day social relations as inherently 'disablist' or class-based or Islamophobic.

A number of such commentators quote Foucault as a thinker who emphasised that all concepts in a culture are interlinked, depending on others for their meaning. If apparently gender-neutral statements in fact refer to male hegemony in the culture, then close analysis will always show that gender-neutral statements of theory (such as those of the 'humanists') in fact privilege male experience and rights at the expense of females.

In detail, critics argue that the model presents the 'self' (understood to be 'self-actualising') as a kind of heroic male. For women, it is argued, the self is always experienced in relationship, not as an isolated figure who prizes above all else her ability to form ideas independently of others (Wine, 1989/2007). The process of development is inseparable from relationship. Black commentators have argued similarly that the African way of being does not privilege the 'self-actualising' individual (which is seen as a white Anglo-American concept) but places priority and value on the group, the common good, so the humanistic model prioritises the isolated individual in a way that is alien to African tradition. Finally it is pointed out that the attributes identified by Rogers (1961/2004) and Maslow (1954/2003) sound suspiciously like the self-description of privileged, white, middle-class, mid-twentieth-century America – with no sense of the power dynamic and oppression that maintain this privilege. The qualities are:

- Democratic, with a spiritual dimension which is not necessarily religious.
- Commitment to the well-being of others.
- Interest in culture and the arts.
- Ability to defer gratification for the sake of a longer-term good.
- Respect of others and tolerance for their views, combined with the ability to maintain a personal sense of integrity, even under pressure from others.

Remember that the accounts were developed in the years following Nazism in Europe, in which whole nations had shown how minds can be taken over by the power of a charismatic but murderous leader.

The argument is not with the words of the formulation, but that it focuses on personal interaction in a way that ignores, and indeed makes invisible, the social positions of the individuals involved. Those who adopt this stance see it not as the absence of something that can be added in, but as a blindspot of the definition. For these authors, the personal is intrinsically also the social, particularly in relation to the position of women and of people socially defined as 'black': a developmental model concerned with the personal which ignores positioning in society is unfit for its purpose.

The humanistic model values the ideal of a relationship-based self which seeks interpersonal integrity and satisfaction. A final critique comes from those who are sceptical of the existence of a core, integral developing self – as Bilton (2002: 331) summarises, 'Many postmodern social theorists have engaged in a sustained assault on the humanistic idea of a willed, creative, choosing actor ... As Foucault stressed, the very notion of the originating free-willed actor or subject is a historically specific construction.'

There are many counter-arguments. Feminists adopt a wide range of different viewpoints, and many regard the humanistic model – with its emphasis on equality, common humanity, empathy and acceptance, the centrality of 'human' contact regardless of measurable outcome or efficiency justification – as an excellent starting point. The idea of 'patriarchy' as a pervasive universal force to be blamed and fought against can be seen as simplistic. Human societies are created by both men and women, and different groups have different areas of privilege in different stages and segments of life, from the power and influence that women typically exercise over young children to the power of street gangs, policy makers, judges and lawmakers (Pollert, 1996).

Some have regarded the criticisms as misguided because they suggest that women are 'essentially' all the same, and essentially possess different needs and characteristics from men, rather than acknowledging the diversity of, and the impact of culture on, the way in which femininity is expressed and experienced. A similar criticism had been made by those concerned with cultural diversity – namely that the critique outlined above assumes the existence of an African 'essence', which is factually wrong and inappropriately based on stereotypes (Appiah, 1997). The criticisms, it is said, group 'women' or 'black people' together even more unhelpfully than the original reference to common humanity. If this criticism of humanistic theory stands, then the same arguments should be raised for children with disabilities, gays and lesbians, people excluded because of income and family background, people with learning difficulties, and every combination of these – there is no end to the divisions in society that every child has to encounter and rethink for themselves. Faced with this, it is argued, there is indeed value in underpinning such diversity with statements of common human need.

Whilst the 'postmodern' arguments emphasise the way our sense of self is constructed within particular social arrangements, social workers find that the people they assist need to be treated as authentic individuals with consistent identities and important personal histories. They experience themselves, in their work as well as in other aspects of their lives, setting out to achieve something of value, and to use their time and personal qualities in a worthwhile way – just as the humanistic models describe.

All social workers must grapple with some of the ideas presented in this essay. They will sometimes wonder what is the value of their work, and wonder what of its satisfactions are illusions created for self-regarding motives. Questions related to the issues discussed will arise in practice – as, for example, when there is a choice between recommending an adoption placement for an African child with white parents who appear fully capable of offering 'the core conditions', or waiting for an indefinite length of time to find a more 'culturally appropriate' placement.

SUMMARY

In adolescence, there is a spurt in the growth of bones and muscles. The proportion of fat to muscle changes – differently in males and females – and there are notable changes in the structure and size of the brain. These changes are triggered by the hormone system, and changes in the sex hormones are particularly distinctive of this period, as both male and female become adults capable of reproduction.

The age of adolescence varies in different cultures, as does its meaning and characteristics. How adolescence is typically viewed in developed industrial countries at the moment – including characteristics of 'teenagers' and older adolescents, duration of adolescence, the age at which it occurs – is not universal, but is distinctive of these particular cultures at this point in history.

Attachment needs persist through adolescence, and states of mind otherwise typical of a child and of an adult may alternate.

Adolescence is a time when the individual explores and begins to form an adult sexual identity.

Erikson's model identifies adolescence as the time when the child's identity, shaped by adults, is being left behind in favour of one formulated by the individual themselves (with peer influence). The chapter referred to the work of Gilligan, and Bingham and Stryker, who emphasised some of the ways in which females are fashioning new ways of relating to others, and exploring the ways they value themselves; these ideas are, to varying degrees, in contrast with Erikson's ideas that the adolescent's core development is in autonomy and independence.

The chapter referred to the particular challenges faced by young people in care and by adolescents with disabilities.

Adolescence is a transition, and social work often involves assisting people in transitions (such as bereavement). The chapter outlined the seven stages identified in Hopson's model of transitions. The student is directed to sources of further detail about this – how passages through transition are affected by the characteristics of the individual, the situation and the support available.

Finally, the chapter outlined some of the objections to one theory that attempts to provide a 'universal' statement of human development. The humanistic model emphasises people's drive to make something of their lives, the way they strive for higher qualities beyond basic survival needs, and the individual's need for unconditional acceptance in order to establish a resilient and rounded personality. An objection expressed by some feminists and some anti-racist commentators is that this ignores the social position of the individual, the distinctive features of women's (or, for example, African) experience, and takes no account of the way 'the personal is political'.

NOTE

1   The legal term for children referred to in this section is 'children looked after by the local authority', or 'looked after children'. The grammatical oddness of the briefer version can cause confusion in written text, and we have often used the less precise but commonly understood term 'children in care'.

FURTHER READING

About physical, cognitive and social development in adolescence:

Boyd, D. R. and Bee, H. L. (2015) *Lifespan Development*. Seventh edition. Boston: Pearson/Allyn and Bacon.

Social work or other professional practice with adolescents:

Briggs, S. (2008) *Working with Adolescents and Young Adults: A Contemporary Psychodynamic Approach*. Second edition. Basingstoke: Palgrave.

An excellent, down-to-earth and practical overview of the responsibilities of services in relation to adolescents with disability:

Quinn, P. (1998) *Understanding Disability: A Lifespan Approach*. Thousand Oaks, CA: Sage.

More detail and subtlety about Hopson's model of transitions – a good introduction to the literature on transitions:

Sugarman, L. (2009) *Lifespan Development: Theories, Concepts and Interventions*. Second edition. Hove: Psychology Press.

More detail about the application of transition theory:

Schlossberg, N. K., Waters, E. B. and Goodman, J. (1995) *Counselling Adults in Transition: Linking Practice with Theory*. New York: Springer.

For young people who are or have been in care:

Voice (formerly Voice for the Child in Care or VCC) joined the Coram group of charities and became Coram Voice: www.coramvoice.org.uk.

For young people who are gender diverse:

www.mermaidsuk.org.uk offer appropriate resources to young people, their families and carers, and professionals working with young people who are transgender or gender-variant.

1. What are some of the issues facing parents of an adolescent with Down's syndrome?
2. How would you summarise the changes ahead of the child who is about to make the journey through adolescence to adulthood?
3. In Rogers' humanistic model ('Essential background', section 7) people have a basic tendency to make something good with their lives. For this to be achieved, it is important they experience 'unconditional positive regard'. Those who are helping others need to offer empathy and unconditional acceptance. Illustrate how this model might apply in a social work situation. What might be described as the weaknesses of this model?

Prepare a poster or brief report on one of the following:

- Brain development during adolescence
- Adolescence and suicide
- Different routes to adult identity – Marcia's theory of adolescence
- Being black in a racist society – Phinney's model of ethnic identity development

CHAPTER 5

Living independently

In this chapter you will find:

- **Leaving home – young adults living independently**
- **Young people leaving care**
- **Living independently – and loneliness**
- **Prison**
- **Refugees, exiles and torture victims**
- **Globalisation and its effects – migration and cosmopolitanism, unaccompanied children**
- **After a child's death**
- **The impact of homelessness**
- **'You say things in my head, so I'm not lonely' – social work responses**
- **Bronfenbrenner's ecological model**

EMOTIONAL BIOGRAPHY

Nicola, aged 19 (eight years before the birth of Jamie)

Nicola settled into her seat as the train pulled away from the station. The two weeks since she had moved to Middleworth had flown by. Her parents had come with her a fortnight ago to help set up her new flat, and both her car and theirs had been crammed full. Her mum had rung twice since then. Truth to tell, although now independent, she had received substantial help from them during the move. Her first week in the new job had been hectic and at times intimidating, but she felt pleased with how she had coped. It would be good to see her mum and dad again, but she wouldn't see much of them this weekend, as the main reason for returning was her sister Katie's engagement party. The whole gang would get together again – that would write off Saturday evening and most of Sunday!

Bella, aged 19

Bella was quite clear in her mind. Her father had thrown her out. Initially she lived with her boyfriend David, and for a few months lived the life of a teenager that had been denied her whilst she was at home. After she became pregnant with Tia, she often felt unwell, and felt increasingly lonely and isolated. She knew in her heart that, for all his macho posturing, David was incapable of caring for her and a baby. Things got worse after the birth. David often stayed out; there were constant rows and many weekends when she did not know where the food would come from. Well, she'd moved out before, and she'd do it again. Offering to share the rent, she moved in with a friend. The one-bedroom flat, fifteen miles from her home town, was dark, damp and much too small for the two young women and their children. She was relieved when a year later she took tenancy of a housing association flat, even if it was on a large estate in an unpopular area. She had a deep love for her daughter, but longed for some respite from the constant demands. Tia was an attractive child with a ferociously independent spirit, and mother and daughter clashed constantly. Bella would fly into a rage at her daughter's defiance, but her threats did not work. Occasionally she thought of her mother. Her mother's last twelve months, when Bella was 15, when the cancer developed so rapidly, seemed to have been the beginning of the nightmare. She felt very alone.

Vivian, aged 25

The ball of Vivian's hand, her oiled palms and fingertips, moved slowly down her friend Ino's back. She concentrated on what she was doing, felt each bone from shoulder blade to base of the 18-year-old's spine, under the muscles and the dark brown skin. As well as giving comfort, she herself felt briefly reassured by the bodily contact. The project was based in the Red Cross Centre in London, and twenty minutes later she was speaking to the BBC reporter in the front office. 'I was told they hit my father with a sledgehammer. Sometimes it makes me sad when I give the massage.' The reporter said nothing; what could she say? Ino had come in: 'Everyone here has been running. Always running. At home, it was a month before they wanted me to be married. Two aunties were holding my legs and another was holding my hands. The older woman was between my legs and had started cutting, but I was fighting. Then when they saw all the blood they stopped. I have seen friends die from it. And so that night I ran. I came through many countries in Africa and Europe, and now I am here, and we wait for your government to decide.

They send us there, and they send us here. We do not know where they send me next week. Maybe they send me back. I live in a constant state of terrible anxiety, which is very hard to describe. It is the best thing that the Red Cross has organised this scheme that Vivian gives the massage. No one can solve the problem, especially until the government decide my application. But only someone who is in the same position, like Vivian, who is also a refugee waiting to hear whether she is to be sent back, only someone who knows can give you a little comfort. For that small time you are not on your own.' Vivian spoke quietly – 'When you're an asylum seeker, when you are abused, you're like a piece of dirt floating on the wave. You're running but you have no power. When I look after Ino or the others, for that moment I know I can do something – and for that moment, they know they are important.'

(For information about related Red Cross services, see British Red Cross, 2018.)

INTRODUCTION

This chapter is about 'living independently'. It takes its theme from the phase of life which often follows adolescence, but draws attention to the many other situations in which adults find themselves setting out on a new life away from their earlier social contacts and surroundings. For many people assisted by social workers, the subject has dark overtones. Problematic transitions disrupt social bonds and cut people off from the social networks which provided meaning, comfort and security in their lives. We look at loneliness, one aspect of which can also be a feature of many other social work situations.

It is the first of four chapters concerned with features of adult life. There are many different paths through adulthood. A choice, a chance event or illness combines with social circumstances to create a different future. History, politics, family traditions, gender, education and class all set the developmental scene within which an individual makes decisions. As with 'loneliness', some of the themes picked out in these chapters do not just apply to adults.

Chapters
1, 2, 3, 8, 9

THE NARRATIVES

The narratives at the beginning of this chapter are fictionalised. They are self-contained, for readers who are consulting this chapter in isolation, but they draw you into the life course of individuals. Tia, whom you first met in Chapter 1, is given some background: the circumstances in which she grew up as her mother Bella set up home on her own, and how this was closely tied up with Bella's relationship with her mother and her father Bob. Everyone's life is different, but nothing in these accounts would seem unusual to a social worker.

Chapter 4

Vivian was introduced to you as a teenager in Chapter 4. Since then, ten years have passed – years in which she has shown resourcefulness, strength and vivacity. Regrettably, neither her story nor that of Ino is unusual in terms of female development. Up to 500,000 women in the EU alone are subjected to or threatened by genital mutilation. The World Health Organisation (2017) estimates that 200 million women alive today have been subjected to genital mutilation in over thirty countries, and approximately 3 million girls undergo the operation each year. The United Nations Refugee Council estimates the number of people affected by conflict-induced forced displacement to be 66 million, the highest level of displacements on record (UNHCR, 2018). At the time of writing, 55 per cent of refugees worldwide come from three countries, Syria, Afghanistan and South Sudan (UNHCR, 2018).

The UK asylum system has received considerable criticism. For example, the Independent Asylum Commission report *Deserving Dignity* (Hobson et al., 2008) described the UK as falling 'seriously below the standards of a civilised society' and condemned its treatment of asylum seekers as 'shameful for the UK'. This has been followed by a campaign, 'Citizens for Sanctuary', to make the report's recommendations a reality (www.citizensforsanctuary.org.uk).

Waris Dirie (Dirie et al., 2005; Dirie and Miller, 2006) gives a first-hand account of the life of an African woman who has been subjected to mutilation as a girl.

LEAVING HOME: YOUNG ADULTS LIVING INDEPENDENTLY

The age at which young people move from their parental home, and the reasons and manner in which they do so, is widely variable. Besides personal variation, expectations change over time, and different cultures manage the process – if it is expected to happen at all – quite differently. Sneed and colleagues (2006) write, 'Although adolescence as a life stage is nearly universal, emerging adulthood is not. Emerging adulthood as a period of development predominantly characterises industrial societies in which marriage and employment can be postponed and education and exploration extended. In addition to these between-country differences, there are also within-country differences.' The process can be a time of excitement and satisfaction, as people manage their own affairs and experience freedom from following parental routines and expectations. But it can also involve loneliness and worry. Some surveys (such as Revenson, 1982) have found that young people are more likely to report loneliness than old people, and university counsellors remark on the way that parents who have stayed together 'for the sake of the children' may separate soon after the younger generation have left for university. Far from making it easy for children, this may in fact leave sons or daughters worrying about a parent. The situation may provoke anxiety about the well-being of a separated mother or father, or if concerns about a parent are well-founded (because the separation has been painful and disturbing) a child may abandon their developing independence in order to return home to the distressed parent.

Chapter 4

GENDER DIFFERENCES IN YOUNG ADULTS AND THEIR CONTACT WITH FAMILY – A RESEARCH STUDY

Sneed and colleagues (2006) found gender differences in the patterns of family contact after moving from home, and examined how this affected the younger generation's exercise of autonomy. Carol Gilligan was a member of the research team, and building on her ideas (outlined in Chapter 4), they identify '**instrumentality**' and 'separateness' as psychological measures that are conventionally seen as forms of autonomy. Instrumentality is broadly 'being your own person' and running your own life. It is measured in terms of being decisive, independent and making decisions without the influence of others, and was found to develop more quickly in males. Females, on the other hand, appeared more likely to value attachment, connectedness, empathy and intimacy as part of their mature personality, 'lagging behind' in instrumentality. You may recall Gilligan's thesis that women tended to be assessed by psychologists as immature, or 'maturing' later, because the measures used were geared to a 'male' concept of autonomy rather than a 'female' one (Chapter 4).

Previous studies had found that women tend to maintain closer relationships with their parents during the transition to adulthood than men (who tend to view separation from their parents during late adolescence as promoting increased independence). These studies also found that women tend to be more strongly affected by their relationships with their parents than men are. The findings of Sneed and colleagues were in keeping with this – they found that family contact tended to decrease more quickly for young men than for young women. In general, they found higher levels of instrumentality amongst men in matters of finance. As family contact decreased, 'instrumentality' increased over the ages from 17 to 27 for both men and women. Statistically, in general there was a negative relationship between family contact and 'instrumentality' – the more family contact a young person had, the less they showed independence in finance and relationship matters. There was a change in this relationship over time. For both males and females, as they grew older, the link between family contact and lack of 'instrumentality' weakened, so in the older groups, increased family contact became less likely to reduce instrumentality. In fact for men, at 27, the relationship between the variables changed round, so that increased family contact had a small positive effect on instrumentality. In discussing this, the researchers suggest that this concept of 'instrumentality' needs to be examined more closely. The existing psychological understanding of instrumentality is a kind of 'rugged individualism' prized by male culture, but they suggest there is another sort which is based on responsibility in attending to relationships, which is more likely to be typical of women, and is fostered in those mature men who have more contact with their family.

The study was based on single interviews with 200 participants, so the data are vulnerable to the effects of memory distortion, although the researchers took steps to minimise this.

A report by the Joseph Rowntree Foundation (Morrow and Richards, 1996) found in 1996 that while young people expected autonomy and independence earlier than in the past, economic factors and social policy had made them dependent on family support for longer, right into their twenties. They entered the world of employment later than previous generations, and policies to do with income and student support made them dependent on parents for longer. The report expressed particular concern that 'for children who are effectively "without kin" the "dependency assumption" is especially problematic: research has shown that young people leaving local authority care who have no contact with their families face a range of difficulties financially, socially and psychologically' (Morrow and Richards, 1996: 3). Another study compared the experiences of two large samples of young adults born over twenty years apart (Bynner et al., 2002). It compared data collected on all the 10,000 people who had been born in a single week in 1958 with that of nearly 16,000 people born in a single week in 1970.[1] It described how a larger gap had opened up between those who achieve a high level of educational qualification and those who do not, and noted that the 'poverty penalty' underlying this (people from poorer backgrounds were less likely to gain qualifications) seemed to have increased.

Two of the risk factors highlighted in the previous paragraph – the lack of kin and lack of higher-level educational achievements – bear heavily on children brought up in care. The next section summarises some features of the experience of independent living for young people whose upbringing has been the responsibility of the state.

Young people coming out of care

In their study of forty-seven young adults, Hecht and Baum (1984) found that disrupted attachments during childhood correlated with feelings of loneliness in early adulthood. If we think of loneliness in terms of Weiss's definition (1980) – 'loneliness is separation without an attachment figure' – these findings are hardly surprising. They highlight, however, the vulnerability of young people leaving care. These people, by definition, have experienced disrupted attachments, and, all too often, they experience the challenges of independent living without any continuation of such attachment figures as have been made available to them in alternative family arrangements during their childhood.

Most young people setting out in their independent lives have the emotional (and often practical) resource of their parents to keep in the background. Even when they rebel against the ideas of their parents, consistent relationships have existed as a foundation on which they can build their own. Those who because of earlier experiences are least equipped for living effective independent lives and coping with the emotional and practical complexities of life are unfortunately often sent out to manage on their own.

About a third of children in care move to independent living at just 16 or 17 (National Audit Office, 2015). By contrast, 50 per cent of young adults still live with their parents at the age of 22 (National Audit Office, 2015). One of the most important tasks for 'corporate parents' is to provide continuing resources for the vulnerable people for whom they have assumed responsibility as children. The Children (Leaving Care) Act 2000 sets out the statutory duties for local authorities to support care leavers, and the Children and Families Act 2014 introduced 'staying put' arrangements which allow children in care to stay with their foster families until the age of 21 years.

Chapter 4

Chapter 4 referred to some statistical outcomes for young adults who have been brought up in care. In relation to education, for example, 6 per cent of care leavers, compared with 49 per cent of the general population, go to university. Looked after children in England are now six times more likely than children in the general population to be convicted of a crime or to receive a caution (DfE, 2015a). Care leavers represent only 1 per cent of young people, yet they represent 11 per cent of homeless young people, 24 per cent of the adult prison population and 70 per cent of sex workers (CSJ, 2015). Although many people brought up in care are grateful to the foster carers and others who looked after them, these statistics point to the gap between what any parent would wish for their own children leaving home and what care leavers face as they set out on their own in what will often be a lonely and intimidating adult world.

Looking Closer

CORPORATE PARENT

This is a term used when the responsibilities of parenting are carried by an organisation, not a person – often used when the local authority has parental responsibilities. Even though this arrangement is usually made with the best of intentions (to protect a child who has been harmed by its own parents, for example), an organisation has salaried staff who take holidays, change jobs and work thirty-five-hour weeks; they have to obey written procedures and job descriptions. When an organisation is responsible, it is very hard to provide the kind of spontaneous, loving and flexible care an individual parent supplies.

The experiences of young care leavers from different ethnic groups

Using conventional categories, the proportions of children in care from different ethnic backgrounds differ from the proportions in the general population. Black children are more likely than average to be in care, and Asian children are less likely. Barn and her colleagues (2005) studied the post-care experience of 261 young people from different ethnic groups. They found that many young people experienced disruption and disadvantage during and after care; however, young white people fared the worst in terms of placement instability, early departure from care, poor educational outcomes, homelessness, and risk-taking behaviour including criminal activity and drug use. Africans and Asians experienced most stability in care and in education. 'For young asylum seekers,' the sponsors of Barn's research (2005) summarised, 'uncertainty about their legal status and their prospects left them unsettled and highly vulnerable to stereotyping and racism on a daily basis. Yet social work professionals commented favourably on the tenacity of asylum seekers in trying to put trauma and adversity behind them and work towards a positive future for themselves.'

Recent world events led to a significant increase in the number of unaccompanied asylum-seeking children (UASC) looked after by all local authorities in England: the number more than doubled, from 2,050 at 31 March 2014, to 4,210 at 31 March 2016 (ADCS, 2016).

Globalisation and cosmopolitanism

The economies of the world are closely interlinked. Features of the housing market or the level of debt in one country can have an effect on the living standard in many others. Political conditions in one country affect lives in many others. This and related effects are described as 'globalisation' (in terms of the theme of this chapter, it emphasises that people are seldom in fact living 'independently'). A number of sociologists use the term **cosmopolitanism** to refer to the extent to which individuals may live in one country or community, but have identity links, roots or cultural beliefs originally characteristic of another. They may or may not have a sense of loneliness or isolation in their current home. Globalisation is not only an external force, it is a 'force within' society, and this internal aspect can be called 'cosmopolitanism' (Beck, 2000). Naoko, the young Japanese woman referred to in Chapter 1, may call her apartment in England with Paul and their baby Ayu 'home' but she also refers to Kyoto in Japan as home. She has decided to settle here, but when she meets with others at a Japanese event, she knows there will be many who regard Britain as simply a place to work or study for the moment – next year it could be Germany or the USA or back to Japan. The money transfer of migrant workers has been described as the biggest force for wealth redistribution in the world at the present time. The concept emphasises that many people have a sense of identity and culture which is international and goes beyond where they currently live.

LIVING INDEPENDENTLY – AND LONELINESS

In the report of the UK Director of Children's Rights (Morgan and Lindsay, 2006) about young people's views of leaving care, loneliness is listed as the first of care leavers' 'top ten worries'. This is emphasised in a more recent Centre for Social Justice report, where a care leaver stated: 'The thing about being in care is it doesn't matter even if you have the greatest [foster] family in the world, if you don't know where you're from, who you are, you always have that sense of loneliness and being on your own . . . you need to be able to feel that you belong and that people are there for you' (CSJ, 2015). The remainder of the chapter looks at situations in which social workers encounter people who are 'on their own', either because they are physically separated from anyone close to them or because a problem leaves them with a sense of being alone in the world. This is an aspect of many and diverse situations – children leaving care, asylum seekers and refugees, parents whose children have died, men leaving prison, mothers in prison – but the text here focuses on loneliness as a common theme, and asks you to think about the response people will value from a social worker.

Loneliness is not the same as alone-ness. A person can feel lonely in the company of many others, or not feel lonely even though they keep their own company. Specific research findings related to this are set out, for example by Qualter and Munn (2002). Think about the different contributions of social and emotional loneliness in the situations discussed below. What should the social worker's contribution be to addressing those feelings? They should certainly be a component of the professional assessment you make as a social worker (independently of your employment procedures), but would they show up in the formal procedural assessment and prioritising you may be asked to complete?

Prison

Social workers often need to empathise with people for whom others feel little sympathy. There are many aspects of life for people who have been imprisoned in which they set out on a journey alone. This aloneness may be from the absence of someone who is felt essential for their emotional life, as we can see in the statistics that 66 per cent of women in prison have dependent children under 18, and each year more than 17,700 children are separated from their mother by imprisonment. On average women are held fifty-eight miles from their home, and 60 per cent of women are in prisons outside their home region. For 85 per cent of these mothers, it is the first time they have been separated overnight from their children, and they often have no control over who looks after their children in their absence (once a mother has been sentenced, only 5 per cent of children remain in their own home afterwards). Of men in prison, 49 per cent have children, and 45 per cent of men in prison lose contact with their families (Hansard, 2007; NACRO, 2000, quoted by the Prison Reform Trust, 2007). The aloneness is also particularly likely to be felt on release from detention.

Imagine you are a 21-year-old woman with a 2-year-old daughter (if you have followed the narrative, think of Bella, the mother of Tia). You have been sent to prison and don't know who will care for your 2-year-old daughter – you have never been separated from her even for one night. You don't really sleep for the first two nights. Write an imaginative account to represent thoughts and feelings that go through your head, particularly those about your daughter, as the lights are switched off on the third night.

Reflective thinking

Refugees, exiles and torture victims

In many fields of social work you may encounter people who have been forced to start a new life in an unfamiliar society with different language, culture and expectations. Hollander (2000) characterises exile as the situation in adult life which most closely echoes the child's loss of attachment figures. She views culture as providing a reliability and predictability of environment similar in some ways to the qualities provided in infancy by parents. 'Suddenly cut off from one's homeland, with its familiar and predictable language, cultural signifiers and social relations, the exile feels like a defenceless child.' She describes many details of the experience of being a forced exile. 'One might be able to understand the dictionary and yet not be able to understand much at all.' Although the results are sometimes described as 'post-traumatic stress disorder' she remarks that the new situation is itself an ongoing and traumatising situation. She describes how people may oscillate between idealising their culture of origin and despising their new (and often rejecting) society on the one hand – and recalling the terrors from which they have fled and identifying with the new situation on the other.

Some refugees may have experienced torture, or have witnessed the torture of those close to them, and all will have fled from deeply traumatising situations. The British charity Freedom from Torture (formerly known as the Medical Foundation for the Care of Victims of Torture) has five centres in major cities in the UK. It receives over 1,300 referrals each year, including almost 300 children and young people. These experiences are so traumatic, victims are unable to process them – in the psychoanalytic words of Truckle (2000: 174), 'things done to the ego which totally overwhelmed it'.

But it is not only in specific work with refugees that social workers meet people whose development has involved either forced migration or torture. Mental health workers will be involved with the psychiatric after-effects. Childcare workers are responsible for the care of accompanied and unaccompanied asylum-seeking children, who might have arrived alone from countries torn apart by the savagery of civil war and life as a brutalised child soldier, and are informed that after living here for perhaps four or five years, they will be returned to their country of origin when they reach the age of 16. Workers with older people will encounter English survivors of Japanese prisoner-of-war camps and also the children of parents whose lives ended in torture, such as the 10,000 children (now in their eighties) who came to Britain in 1938 as 'kindertransport', most leaving parents who were subsequently worked to death or gassed in concentration camps.

In a different context, a social worker might encounter some of the 150,000 children who were moved from Britain, aged around 8, without their parents, to Canada, Rhodesia, New Zealand and Australia between 1922 and 1967 (Parliament of Australia, 2001). Agencies such as the Child Migrant Trust are now concerned with the emotional and relationship consequences of the child welfare policies of that period, both for the children and their parents, which in the words of an Australian official enquiry, 'deeply scarred them and had an immeasurable impact on the rest of their lives ... We heard stories of children feeling worthless, vulnerable, stigmatised, unloved and being denied opportunities, and adult lives filled with poor personal rela-tionships, broken marriages, suicide attempts, uncertainty and insecurity ... a number of witnesses to the Inquiry have described severe and prolonged trauma' (Forde, 1999).

Refugees are frequently fleeing a situation in which emotional and physical abuse perpetrated by gangs of powerful people has forced them to escape into an uncertain future. However, many survivors of physical and sexual abuse (as adults or children) in this country will have been traumatised in similar ways. For many, with the return of these experiences as memories, they feel alone with impossible problems, and surrounded by people who do not understand.

Looking Closer

Work with older people who arrived in Britain as 'kindertransport' illus-trates how social workers need to understand development across the life cycle, not just the life stage defined in terms of their 'client group' (understanding the experience of childhood trauma may be relevant to sensitive work with older people).

After a child's death

The examples referred to so far in this chapter occur when people lose or become detached from their close social circle and are faced with forming new social links. Loneliness and isolation, however, can arise from the loss of a single significant person whose existence has been taken for granted, part of the social and emotional world. We have seen how the mental rhythm of mothers in particular (whether by biological fact or social arrangement) is closely mingled with that of their baby. When a mother sits on the sofa watching television, with her child in her arms, her brain is closely aligned with his, as it is when his cries alert her and cause distress or frustration. For most mothers and fathers, the well-being of their children, the tasks and responsibilities associated with them, form a major part of their mental life. Later on, for some parents, after their children have left home, comes the challenge of creating a satisfactory social existence. Specifically, however, the death of a child leaves a gap in their world, a gap that may not always be noticed in the future, but one that is always there. Bereaved parents are living without someone who seems an integral part of their emotional survival – 'it is why we feel so isolated from society, from family and friends' (White, undated). Other aspects of the death of a child are discussed in Chapters 7 and 9.

Chapters 7, 9

Homelessness

Some young people are forced to leave home. Centrepoint (2018) identified a range of issues faced by young people who become homeless, as listed in the box below. A main trigger for homelessness among young people is the breakdown of relationships with parents. A significant minority have experienced violence at home, and one in seven of the young people whom Centrepoint assist are refugees. Centrepoint stresses that few young people 'choose' to be homeless. They propose that the correct strategy for preventing youth homelessness is to identify the young people in these risk categories, and provide support to these young people and their families to tackle problems at an early stage. Homelessness is associated with poor physical health, and can precipitate a range of drug-related and mental health problems, as well as being caused by them. It is difficult to establish the rate of youth homelessness in the UK, but it was estimated in 2013/14 that 64,000 young people were in contact with homelessness services in England, more than four times the number accepted as statutorily homeless (Clarke et al., 2015).

KEY ISSUES FOR YOUTH HOMELESSNESS

The homeless charity Centrepoint identifies a range of issues related to young people who are experiencing homelessness:

- Relationship breakdown, often between young people and their parents or step-parents, is a major cause of youth homelessness. Around six in ten young people who come to Centrepoint say they had to leave home because of arguments, relationship breakdown or being told to leave.

■ Complex mental health and physical problems can also be a significant contributing factor. More than a third of young people who come to Centrepoint have a mental health issue, such as depression and anxiety, while another third need to tackle issues with substance misuse.

■ Deprivation and poverty. Young people are more vulnerable to having to leave home in areas of high deprivation and poor prospects for education and employment.

■ Gangs and crime. Young people who are homeless are more likely to be vulnerable to gang-related problems. One in six young people at Centrepoint had been involved in or affected by gang crime.

■ School exclusion. Being outside of education can be a barrier to accessing support for problems at home or health problems and to gaining employment.

■ Leaving care. One in four young people at Centrepoint have been in care and earlier traumatic experiences can make young people vulnerable to mental health problems and unemployment.

■ Refugees fleeing war and conflict. Young refugees make up 14 per cent of young people at Centrepoint, including young people who came to the UK as unaccompanied asylum seekers fleeing violence and persecution in their own country (Centrepoint, 2018).

Homeless adults without children are not a priority group for statutory services, and there is no reliable source of statistics on single homeless people. The risk factors for homelessness that have been identified by research (Fitzpatrick et al., 2000) are housing trends, labour market forces, poverty and the break-up of family relationships. There is little longitudinal research which points reliably to patterns and outcomes, but homelessness is associated with poor physical and mental health. Fitzpatrick and colleagues quote arguments that poorer physical health should be attributed to inadequate health provision rather than to homelessness in itself. The involvement of alcohol in a proportion of homelessness is widely recognised. For younger people, Quilgars and colleagues (2008) found that homelessness is associated with the break-up of existing social networks, but also with the formation of supportive relationships in new settings. Fitzpatrick and colleagues highlight that there is little reliable research about the friendship pattern of adult homeless people. Asylum seekers and people released from prison are particularly at risk of being homeless.

Social work responses

Social work is about the 'person-in-their-situation' (Perlman, 1957: 4). Typically, its purpose is to help when the life course of the 'person' becomes problematic because of their 'situation'. Feelings of isolation or loneliness because of the loss of a social network are common in episodes in people's lives when social workers become involved. If this 'aloneness' or 'loneliness' is one aspect of the problem, what response by a social worker can make a difference?

Practical responses

On some occasions, a social worker may help by introducing the person to a community resource, day centre or club which turns out to reduce the isolation, or by facilitating the provision of aid for mobility. Implementing the person's wish for more suitable accommodation may similarly result in tackling a problem of social isolation. In certain fields, introducing a person to self-help or specialist interest groups may turn out to be valuable, or, recognising a gap, the social worker may be instrumental in setting up a support group. There are, in short, various practical ways in which social work actions affect a person's life experience in this regard. Equally, it will turn out that there are many occasions when such interventions are inappropriate, irrelevant, undesirable, or impractical.

The social worker is unlikely to be the person whose physical presence reduces isolation (that is usually the role of companions, friends and acquaintances), but there are a number of settings in which arranging volunteer contacts and befrienders turns out to be useful. For example, in relation to postnatal depression (and other difficulties facing parents), Crispin and colleagues (2005), and the Home Start website, describe the kind of support which can be offered by volunteers. Dean and Goodlad (1998) examine the role and impact of befriending schemes in a variety of communities and for a variety of purposes. Some are based on a specific routine while others involve varied activities. Their study examined the ways in which these schemes enabled people to participate in community activities. The organisers, volunteers and users of the service all emphasised the importance of the relationship between the user of the service and the volunteer.

Relationship responses

Although there are many situations where the last thing people want a social worker to be is a 'friend', there are others in which the value of the social worker's 'befriending' should not be underestimated. The young care leavers quoted by Morgan and Lindsay (2006: 20) wanted practical support in setting up independent living, but they also wanted the social worker to 'like, be there for us'. At some time or other, most committed social workers have heard people who clearly appreciate the service offered say something like, 'I think of X more like a friend than a social worker'. There is much to understand in this, but if the service is offered correctly, the relationship is certainly not like other social friendships. It is not a symmetrical relationship, since the social worker has obligations which are not reciprocated by the person they see. Social friendships have elements of mutual support which are not in the professional relationship, and so on. Nevertheless, it is the word people choose, and it is not difficult to understand why.

It is a basic service to offer 'the hand of friendship' when someone has fled from persecution to what they hope will be a place of refuge after months of days and nights of worry, flight and fear. This is a first psychosocial gesture which underlies others. The social worker has to understand a wide range of possible 'pasts' and must do whatever will make a positive psychosocial 'future' more likely for the person.

When people feel alone with a problem that seems too much to cope with, some of the anxiety may be alleviated by contact with someone who is regularly emotionally available to them. Writing about the response to loneliness, Hobson (1974: 73) analyses what the professional offers as 'friendship of a curious kind'. He quotes the words of Bertrand Russell: 'In human relations one should penetrate to the core of loneliness in each person and speak to that.' This often rings true in social work situations. Hobson points out that this can only be done if the response is one of 'real true feelings' rather than the response of someone 'only playing a part'.

The detail of what happens within the relationship will be as varied as people are. The response will be conveyed by unforced body language – eye contact, a reassuring touch, the change in a tone of voice. In social work, perhaps unlike some disciplines with more circumscribed responsibilities, the communication may come through preparedness 'to go the extra mile', to do something which might not be directly prescribed by the role. The director of Children's Rights found in his investigation (Morgan and Lindsay, 2006: 20) that care leavers were particularly appreciative of this. For one person, a conversation may allow the worst terrors and fantasies of the sleepless night to be seen for what they are – unrealistic and unlikely outcomes. For another, the contact may leave them appropriately reassured that it is they who are 'OK' and it is the people who cause their problem who are unreasonable, destructive and harmful. The right words in a single conversation can remove the sense of isolation – a young Muslim described in a radio programme the reassuring effects of a conversation with someone at the end of a telephone (BBC, 2017): 'For a while I was just very upset because I thought, well if I am gay and gays go to hell, then ... then I am going to go to hell ... I was really worried that I thought maybe I was – umm – maybe I am one of the devil's own disciples because I had such a conviction that there was something wrong being gay, and I must be evil and then I am going to go to hell.' He describes the reassurance he gained from a helpful conversation with a professional person: 'And they [the person with whom he spoke] said, "God made love so how can it be a sin to love someone else?" and I thought, yes, it's not just sex, it's love as well, and then I went back to the Koran.'

'I'm going to Torquay, but it doesn't matter, because you say things in my head, so I'm not lonely'

Truckle (2000: 178–182) describes her work with a 22-year-old man who had learning disabilities. She reports the above, which he said to her over a holiday period. 'Donald' had been sexually assaulted in a residential setting, and had subsequently severely sexually assaulted his 3-year-old niece. A further incident of concern had involved a young woman of his own age. Here are some extracts from Truckle's description of her relationship with him:

> Donald was a normal adolescent, full of raging hormones and sexual feelings, heavily into pop music. Yet I discovered he did not have the most rudimentary sexual knowledge. No one had ever used the words 'erection', 'masturbation' or 'contraception' with him . . . I tried to explain to Donald that the female student's parents might be afraid that she would get pregnant. 'How?' he asked, looking bright eyed and alert. I explained to him in much the same way that I would to a five year old, but Donald's reaction was totally different from a child's. It was adult. 'Wow,' he said, with his eyes glistening with what I thought might be tears. 'I could make something as perfect as a baby.'
>
> I was also aware that Donald might be gay, so I decided to tackle both the female and male student in one fell swoop. I said to Donald that he had the same problem that any young man had: he wanted to be held and touched and made love to. He nodded. I asked him if he knew the word 'tactful'. Donald shook his head. I explained it and that he had to manage to get someone to have sex with him in a tactful way that didn't scare them, and allow them to say 'no'. We had by this time talked extensively about Henry, and how frightened and confused he must have been when he leaped on Donald's back and got shouted at [Henry was the boy who had three times sexually assaulted Donald in the residential college] . . . I reminded Donald of how confused and frightened he had been and said that this is what is meant by abuse, and if you really force yourself on someone, that is rape . . . Donald looked at me very sadly and said 'Like what I did with Geraldine?' [his niece]. We could then think about the abuse he had perpetrated on Geraldine . . . and at the same time he could identify with Geraldine in her pain, terror and horror at the way he had betrayed her trust.

Alleviating his 'loneliness' involved a genuine and fully human relationship. In the chapter we have quoted, Truckle discusses the appropriateness of expressing any feelings a worker has, but she leaves the reader in no doubt that if a genuine relationship is offered, it may evoke strong feelings in the worker – 'I said goodbye to him for the last time . . . I must admit I went away and had a private cry at the thought of him trying to reach maturity in a world that offered him so little help, recognition or respect.' If effective social work is offered, there will always be times when it will evoke such feelings – sometimes of care and protectiveness, sometimes of sadness, sometimes of anger, sometimes of self-doubt, and sometimes of horror. As the final section of Chapter 10 discusses, this is not a sign of weakness or unsuitability, and it is one reason why the worker is entitled to ongoing sensitive support.

There may be times when there is no practical arrangement which can alleviate the sense of being alone, and no emotional remedy that another person can offer for the harm or trauma that is being addressed. Nevertheless, inadequate as you may feel it at the time, the person you are working with may tell you that they value your relationship 'because you understand what's going on'. It is the quality of understanding which has left them feeling less alone. This is not always easy to get right, which is one reason workers should have received help for their own problems, in the process exploring what facilitates their own development and what they value in a helping relationship (this is touched on again at the end of Chapter 10). Paradoxically, the very sense of not understanding may be an important communication of empathy − after all, the person you are helping may not understand their own feelings and behaviour, let alone those of others, so why should you?

However, any worker wants to feel competent, and appear helpful; it may take a lot of confidence to provide authority, security and empathy at the same time as admitting that you don't understand. Patrick Casement (originally a social worker but now a widely respected authority in psychoanalysis) goes further; as he explores with great sensitivity in his book, *On Learning from Our Mistakes* (2002), it is by making mistakes with those we are helping that we develop greater empathy.

The biggest challenge is presented by a sense of aloneness in the wake of torture or abuse that cannot be alleviated at all. Hollander (2000) points out that when pain is inflicted from sadistic motives, its purpose is to dehumanise, and in many cases it succeeds. The victim is unable to share the experience and is cut off from subsequent human comfort. Social workers encounter this in relation to some forms of child abuse and domestic abuse, or when working with refugees or former Japanese prisoners of war. Writers such as Blackwell (1997) and Truckle (2000) write persuasively that, in this case, there is an ethical aspect to simply 'bearing witness' to the social atrocity that has been committed. This is one element of the social work with child migrants referred to earlier.

THE PERSONAL OCCURS IN A SOCIAL CONTEXT − INTRODUCING BRONFENBRENNER'S ECOLOGICAL MODEL

This chapter has been about experiences of being (or feeling) alone. These experiences arise from a social context − leaving home, leaving care, being in prison, or being tortured and fleeing for one's life. A social worker in particular has always to understand how individual experiences of development are inseparable from social processes − it is not enough to consider only the individual, even if the well-being of the individual may be the target of her responsibilities.

There are many different kinds of social processes – the interaction between a boy and his sister is one example, but at the other extreme, so is civil war and political violence. The word 'ecology' describes how living things fit in with their environment, and Uri Bronfenbrenner presented an 'ecological' model of human development. This model provides a scheme for understanding how different social processes influence development. Its main outlines are easy to understand, and fit quite naturally with the way social workers view their responsibilities.

A straightforward summary of the ecological model is provided in 'Essential background', section 3, and you may find it helpful to read this before the essay which concludes this chapter. The activity 'About yourself' also illustrates the use of Bronfenbrenner's model. The essay sets the earlier part of the chapter (very much about individual experience) into a social context by discussing the use of Bronfenbrenner's model in social work.

Chapter EB3

ABOUT YOURSELF

APPLYING THE ECOLOGICAL MODEL

The ecological model shows the various levels of the social environment, each of which affects our development. In written form, the model can seem intimidating to students, not least because of the unfamiliar technical terms from systems theory. In practice it is easy to understand and presents an approach very compatible with social work. The following activity should make its application clear.

1. Think of a period in your life (in view of the theme of this chapter, you may possibly choose a period when you set out to live independently, or when you were isolated or lonely). Draw some of the relationships which turned out to be influential on your development, or whose disruption had caused the loneliness. For example, see Figure 5.1. Each set of face-to-face influences is called a microsystem.

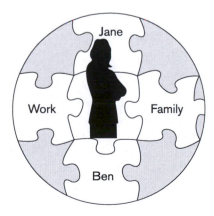

Figure 5.1
Microsystems

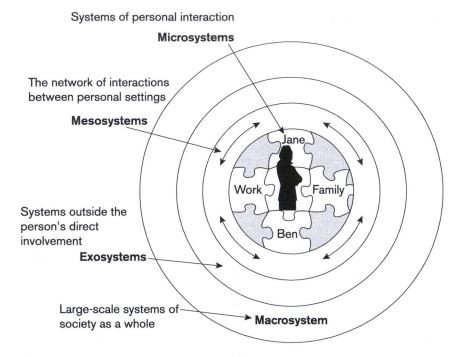

Figure 5.2 Bronfenbrenner's nested ecological model of development

2. Next, consider how the relationships between the microsystems had an effect on you – in the example, perhaps it was a positive factor that the 'family' microsystem had knowledge of what was going on in the microsystem with Ben, or perhaps it was difficult to maintain the link with Jane at the same time as the link with Ben. The relationship between the microsystems is called the mesosystem.

3. Draw a surrounding circle, and in it name some of the systems of interaction which have an effect on your development but which do not directly involve you. For example, for a child, a financial crisis in the father's workplace may have an effect. These are described as exosystems. Finally, the large-scale systems which affect a person – perhaps attitudes towards marriage, expectations of women, availability of jobs – are described as the macrosystem. They influence what happens in all the other systems. See Figure 5.2.

The model is completed by taking account of the chronosystem (from the Greek *chronos* for 'time'), the way in which the systems change over time – perhaps in the 'mesosystem', the relationship with Jane became disrupted because of the link with Ben.

TAKING IT FURTHER

BRONFENBRENNER'S ECOLOGICAL MODEL

Ecological systems

A bee obtains its nectar for nutrition from flowers, and as it does so, it pollinates the flower, enabling it to reproduce. Bee and flower form a *system*, in which each component influences the other. The bee's individual behaviour with the flower is dependent on the organised behaviour of the swarm, so if this is disrupted, the flower is affected. The flower is also dependent on water, and this arrives through a system external to both – it falls as rain, is transported though a river system which irrigates the land as it passes through, flows into the sea where the sun's heat evaporates it into clouds, and atmospheric currents move the clouds over land where they start the cycle again. If this system gets disrupted, deserts form – the bee–flower system is affected by the external water system.

Uri Bronfenbrenner sought to explain clearly how human development was not driven just by internal characteristics of the individual but by a whole range of interacting systems. The bee and flower form an ecological system, and Bronfenbrenner used many ideas from ecology. For example, ecological theory holds that the behaviour of a whole system can never be understood just by listing the properties of each element in the system (in the way that the social behaviour of a person at work could not be predicted just by understanding the biology of each cell in his body); each element in a system is affected by how the others behave. Changes in the system behaviour resulting from the changing behaviour of one element may then go on to change the behaviour of other systems which are interlinked with the first. The model explains how the development of the individual cannot be predicted just from personal characteristics – it is shaped by wide-ranging forces ('systems') in which the individual is not directly involved, as well as patterns of interactions with people in the immediate environment.

Bronfenbrenner's exposition of his model (1979/2006) clearly sets out to be a major new comprehensive model of development. In the course of the work, he defines a set of specially devised technical terms, and identifies fifty hypotheses using these terms. Subtitling this work 'experiments by nature and design', he examines numerous research reports to support or refine his propositions. This essay, however, is not so concerned with the use of his ideas as a detailed **positivist** science that will predict development outcomes, and produce rigorous statements about relationships between variables. Rather, it uses his research as a framework for analysing the situations encountered by social workers. Bronfenbrenner himself saw his work as a challenge to existing theories, including attachment theory. Many researchers, however, were already sympathetic to the importance of social

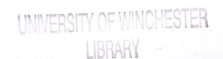

influences, and felt him to have set out a framework which suited their model. Understood in this way, it sheds light on the experience and problems faced by the people who use social work services.

The purpose of this essay is to illustrate how Bronfenbrenner's ecological model of development can be applied to social work situations. An outline is given of the model's application to a relatively straightforward life transition (a young adult leaving home) as a baseline for examining the more conflicted situations of service users who find themselves in a changed environment.

Leaving home – illustrating Bronfenbrenner's analysis

Microsystems

After leaving home, if young people wish a group of friends to form around the use of their house, they have no need to consider the wishes of their parents. The accommodation may perhaps be less comfortable than the homes they have moved from, and it may be in a different type of neighbourhood, but they can give a party all night without negotiating with anyone else. Their routines and meals may change, as they are now responsible for the physical fabric of life. Romantic attachments based at their own accommodation can develop in privacy away from parental influence or supervision. They may be responsible for choosing their work group. These sets of face-to-face interactions, their patterns and environments, roles and activities, are described by Bronfenbrenner as **microsystems**.

So after leaving home, the young adult is likely to be creating their own microsystems to a degree not experienced before. These new microsystems bring new influences, new cultures and beliefs about the world, new challenges to manage money, housing and relationships. In short, as Bronfenbrenner would point out, the changed microsystems bring about development.

Mesosystems

There may equally, of course, be tensions, arguments and disagreements which these young people must now manage much more on their own. A young person at home may not have wished parents to know about, let alone get involved in, any problems they have with their friends. But when living at home, family relationships provide constant alternative microsystems. When they live on their own, these family microsystems may be a long way away, so the friendship microsystem may be the main social context. Disintegration or destructive interaction in that system may leave the young adult isolated in a way that was not the case previously.

This highlights changes in what Bronfenbrenner terms the **mesosystem**. This is defined as the system of relationships between microsystems. In the earlier 'About yourself' section, a fictional suggestion was made that 'perhaps it was difficult to maintain the link with Jane at the same time as the link with Ben'. This is an illustration of the way that the interaction between microsystems has an effect on the individual. For a child, the way the school microsystem relates to the family microsystem (harmoniously, with shared values, or the opposite – with hostility and suspicion) affects individual development – not the home in itself, not the school in itself, but the relation between the two. Making links with the earlier work of Piaget (1950/1997; and see Chapter 3 of this volume) and Lewin (1935), Bronfenbrenner emphasises that the 'microsystem' is not an absolute 'objective' reality, it is what is perceived or *constructed* as the immediate environment (Bronfenbrenner, 1979/2006: 9). In the case of a young adult from a supportive family making a relatively smooth transition to independent living, the newly developing (and, we may hope, often exciting and challenging) microsystems are supported by the stability of older microsystems which remain in the background. These hold varying relationships to experience in the new settings. Being valued, loved, held in good regard and high esteem in the established microsystem is a protective factor for coping with challenges and setbacks in the new one. Security provided in the established systems can make threats to new systems less anxiety-provoking and disturbing. In a similar way, a supportive long-term relationship can provide the resource for an individual to deal with difficulties and challenges at work. Bronfenbrenner (1979/2006: 25, 209– 237) identifies the forms taken by interconnections between microsystems: some of the same people may be active in both; there may be knowledge or ignorance existing in one setting about the other and there may be positive or hostile attitudes from one about the other.

Chapter 3

Exosystems

Bronfenbrenner's **exosystem** refers to systems of which the individual is not a part, but in which changes directly affect the person. In the example on page 143, the parental dyad is an exosystem for the individual concerned (a university student) but changes in that exosystem (the parental relationship) unsettled the student to the extent that they abandoned their university course. Other relevant events in exosystems could be a financial crisis for their new landlord – he may stop properly maintaining their property; or processes in the functioning of the university or business employer (these shape the nature of their studies or employment, or affect their potential for advancement). It may well be the characteristics of 'exosystems' such as neighbourhood gangs or policing policy which determine the physical safety of a young woman or man living away from home.

Macrosystems

The **macrosystem** is the term used by Bronfenbrenner to refer to national and cultural systems – attitudes, social policy and economic climate, for example. Many features of the macrosystem affect the developing experience of the young adult leaving home. Social security policy may treat the individual as more or less an independent adult. Bynner and colleagues (2002), for example, concluded that over the preceding four decades, young adults had been better off in absolute terms but less well off relatively compared with older adults; they remained in education longer than previously, but people from poorer families suffer a 'poverty penalty' related to educational achievement which has got worse over time. The changing economic situation will affect their earning capacity and their ability to own their own home.

Applying Bronfenbrenner's analysis: young people leaving care, and asylum seekers

Bronfenbrenner's model of the different systems which affect development can be applied to care leavers and to asylum seekers.

Like any young adults, care leavers value the greater freedom they have to manage their own 'microsystems'; they enjoy the greater space and privacy they find in their own accommodation, and greater independence (Morgan and Lindsay, 2006: 5). 'You don't have people interfering [social workers]', and one of the ten best things about leaving care was 'not having to ask permission to go places'.

But there are also particular challenges. In the twelve months of Wade and Dixon's sample (2006), a third of young people experienced homelessness. Rainer (2007), an organisation whose work includes supporting care leavers, quotes research that found a third of rough sleepers have spent some time in care as a child. In their own research with 1,244 care leavers, they report that 'in the worst cases, vulnerable young people were placed in housing that was physically unsecured and where they were subjected to harassment and discrimination by other tenants and staff. They could find themselves miles away from work or training and effectively cut off from friends and other support'. The fear of loneliness has already been mentioned, but also in the top ten fears of care leavers is that of being homeless, having nowhere to live. The microsystem, as Bronfenbrenner defines it (1979/2006: 27), includes the 'physical and material characteristics' of the immediate environment as well as the 'pattern of activities, roles and interpersonal relations' experienced in that setting. Compared with the general population there is clearly a greatly increased risk for young adults who have been in care that the 'microsystem' is not positive.

Bronfenbrenner uses what he himself describes as an 'unorthodox' definition of development. He defines it as the person's growing capacity to 'discover, sustain or alter' the properties of the environment, in the light of their 'evolving conception of it and their relation to it' (1979/2006: 9). Like many others features of his model, this seems in general to make more sense when applied to child development, but in relation to asylum seekers or to people in prison, it underlines that there may be barriers or limitations to personal development precisely because central features of their environment are determined for them by other people. Until their refugee status is confirmed, an asylum seeker who has been subject to torture in their own country may have little control over where they live and how they support themselves in their new country, and the decision about whether or not to return to the place of persecution is outside their control.

At the current time, many asylum seekers live with untruths in the relationships within their microsystem. To evade asylum regulations, protect family from vengeance in their country of origin, or hide from pursuers, they keep truths about their past lives hidden, particularly from officials. In his study of social work with thirty-four asylum-seeking children, Kohli (2007: 102) found that their stories reflected those found by Ayotte (2000): about two-thirds, the largest subgroup, were those who had clearly fled from persecution. The next largest groups were those whose stories were similar, but were not believed by investigators. The third group were those thought to be trafficked. Social workers, however, felt that none talked openly about their past lives. Some had been threatened to keep quiet by people in their country of origin; some were too shocked by their experiences to talk; some lied to evade asylum regulations; some wanted to forget their previous lives and put it all behind them. In general, as summarised by a social worker, their concern is with 'the present first, the future next, the past last'. In terms of the microsystem, well-intentioned people intent on their welfare had to relate to them knowing that they were not being told the truth. Kohli points out that there is no clear distinction between the different categorisations – for example, all in a sense were economic migrants because they had come to the UK in order to seek a better life. The Independent Inquiry into Asylum commented that they found the asylum seekers in their study (whether or not their asylum application was accepted) 'were not scroungers and ne'er-do wells, but decent people trying to maintain their dignity in difficult circumstances' (Hobson et al., 2008).

Bronfenbrenner analyses the nature of the links between microsystems. Describing the structure of these links – the mesosystem – again highlights the vulnerability of many care leavers compared with other young adults. 'Shared knowledge between settings' is highlighted by Bronfenbrener (1979/2006: 210) as one positive linkage – but although a care leaver may share some of their recent life experience with other rough sleepers, they may feel that in a conventional work setting, or in other friendship circles, it is a private matter they are reluctant to share. For the general population, new friends may have a degree of interest in each other's family background. Care leavers find the situation easier than when they lived in a children's home, but they may feel that, even if they did reveal it, most people would have little comprehension of the nature of their family life and their subsequent life in care. They face a much more loaded choice than many other young adults in choosing what to keep private and what to share. As already remarked, government initiatives in the UK now require much more involvement from the authorities which had previously been responsible for care.

Similar discontinuities between different microsystems may exist for many asylum seekers. At the time of writing, the term 'asylum seeker' has negative connotations for many of the general public, being closely linked with 'illegal immigrant' or 'street beggar' in widespread public discourse. This is just one aspect to the ignorance they encounter. Most of the people they meet will have little idea of life in their country of origin. A doctor or company director seeking asylum may find themselves treated as ill-educated and undeserving of respect.

Bronfenbrenner considers that, in general, growth is enhanced when there are intermediate structures and people who operate in more than one microsystem of an individual's experience, with a degree of shared knowledge (he acknowledges the value of diverse and cross-cultural experience, but sets this value in the context of well-managed change). He identifies that mesosystems are positive when there is smooth transition between microsystems – positive reasons for the move, careful management, and multiple links between the systems. In these terms, young adults who have left care and refugees and asylum seekers are likely to have experienced poor 'setting transitions' (Bronfenbrenner, 1979/2006: 25, 210).

Bronfenbrenner uses a rarefied, abstract term, but it can accurately be said that in many situations in which social workers intervene, many developmental challenges reside in the 'mesosystem'. There is often discontinuity, conflict, unhelpfulness or misunderstanding between different microsystems. Social workers should be aware of these as part of the problem, their assessments should identify them, and since they are *social* workers – with a routine professional responsibility to get to the bottom of problems and not just apply a palliative sticking-plaster – they have a responsibility to tackle these problems as well as the immediate, individual issues of housing, health or child welfare which may be the tasks identified by their statutory employment. Loneliness does not only arise because of features of the microsystem – it can be generated by the inadequacy of the mesosystem.

It is Bronfenbrenner's thesis that the behaviour of micro- and mesosystems is always affected by exosystems in which the individual plays no direct role. Many such systems are relevant to the development of people whom social workers should be assisting. For example, statistics quoted above indicate how a change in local authority policy caused a fourfold reduction in the number of care leavers who were left without contact with their previous carers. The activity of voluntary organisations directly impacts on the experience of those who are sleeping rough. Asylum seekers are directly affected by policies about their dispersal around the country and separation from other people from their region or culture.

In Bronfenbrenner's account (1979/2006: 258–291), there is a two-way influence between large-scale societal structures (the macrosystem) and different types of exo-, meso- and microsystems. These systems combine to influence the development of the individual. Bronfenbrenner is concerned to emphasise that simply describing subjects or their environment in external descriptive terms – 'British', 'Somali', 'over 85', 'Muslim', 'black British', 'urban', for example – does not convey the characteristics of the macrosystem. He insists (1979/2006: 260) that research attempting to understand developmental influences, processes and outcomes needs to be based on interview, conversation and observation. The same is true of the social work efforts to understand the influence of macrosystems on any individual. Attitudes to rough sleepers, to children in care, to asylum seekers, to Muslims, to gay and lesbian relationships, to African people, to men and women, are important factors in shaping the development of adults or children. It is important that social workers do not ignore the influence of these 'macro-' (cultural) factors. But neither can they think they understand these factors by generalising – they must listen and observe. To simplify is to misunderstand and to stereotype. Within Bronfenbrenner's 'macrosystem' we must now add, to a degree that he perhaps did not, the influence of global structures and cosmopolitan identities. The lives of many people whom social workers assist are caught up in politics and economics that are international in scope; and their identities, sense of belonging or sense of isolation may be linked with cultures, identities and family events thousands of miles from where the social worker meets them.

Finally, in a later addition to his initial presentation, Bronfenbrenner identifies the '**chronosystem**' as the system of elements that involve time – external events such as the political changes which result in a person's exile from their own country, or internal events such as maturational processes affecting their ability to understand and cope with stressors. Clearly, the social worker cannot understand the social problems confronting people in the examples we have cited without taking this time dimension into account. In the case of people with traumatised pasts, the self-narrative which is the 'internalised' chronosystem may be fragmented and contradictory.

Evaluating the use of Bronfenbrenner's ecological model

Bronfenbrenner's model should make intuitive sense to any social worker. It proposes a characteristically *social* perspective on development without denying individuality, personal agency or the importance of interpersonal relationships (some sociological theories, in taking the broader picture, are harder to put into practice). It serves as a reminder to the social worker, busy with day-to-day tasks with the individual, that they may be mis-reading the situation if they do not also take a broader view. Systems theory not only locates the individual at the centre of ever-widening spheres of influence (which is self-evidently accurate), but also draws attention to the importance of links between elements in the wider systems. In acknowledging the mutability of human characteristics in different developmental domains and in different environments and cultures, it offers a more comprehensive view than undifferentiated stage theories. In childhood cognitive development, Bronfenbrenner recognises the work of Piaget in emphasising the child's *perception* of the external world, but draws attention to his lack of reference to social context (1979/2006: 125). He clearly values the work of Vygotsky and later psychologists (see Chapter 3 of this volume).

Bronfenbrenner's work had practical applications in work with children (Bronfenbrenner, 1979/2006; US Department of Health and Social Services,

Chapter 3

2007) and with young people in trouble. It expresses the passionate awareness he demonstrated in his own interventions that the environment of the child, the community setting of the mother or childcare institutions and the political structures within which they are living are all relevant when considering programmes to protect and improve children's development. Most prominently, in UK public policy, the 'ecological' model was described as the underpinning of the *Framework for the Assessment of Children in Need* (Department of Health, 2000). Bronfenbrenner has been a prominent figure who has used his influence to argue that while society has accepted the change to post-industrial conditions in work and finance, it has failed to safeguard the *social* environment, producing hazardous conditions for the rearing of children, and expecting that women should enter the paid workforce without proper respect for the resulting 'social ecology' of their lives and those of their children (Bronfenbrenner, 1990).

However, Bronfenbrenner's ecological model was set out as a specific theoretical research programme. This was intended to determine how different mesosystems produce different microsystems, how the features of macrosystems have a consistent relationship with the mesosystems and the microsystems they then produce, and so on. Although his work has been a vigorous prompt to developmental researchers to take the various systems into account, it is hard to see that there is a body of research creating his 'grand unifying theory'. For the last forty years the UK (as well as the United States and other countries) has been running large-scale cohort studies which attempt to map the development through life of people born on a particular day, and these studies are particularly interested in the effects of various environmental variables. But they have not arisen because of his work, and have not been used to validate or refine the fifty hypotheses he sets out in *The Ecology of Human Development* (1979/2006). His perspective is broad, flexible and comprehensive, but as a **modernist** theory setting out relations between variables (for example, 'Development is enhanced as a direct function of the number of structurally different settings in which the developing person participates in a variety of primary activities and with others, particularly when those others are more mature or experienced'), it has not been especially important. Many of the examples in his work concern children or young people and their families, and are most plausible in relation to them. Although he makes some reference to adult development, the simple relationships proposed in his hypotheses can become impossibly complex (or full of exceptions and counter-qualifications) if applied to the social reality of adult lives such as those of asylum seekers. Perhaps by analogy with the improved mathematical analysis of the chaos and complexity (Elliott and Kiel, 2001) in everyday physical systems, we are now less likely to look for the simple relationship between variables he suggests in human interaction and development.

SUMMARY

This chapter began with information about young people leaving home. It summarised research about gender differences, and illustrated how patterns of 'leaving home' change in different times and cultures by commenting on changes within the UK in the last forty years.

Young people leaving care are particularly vulnerable to bad experiences as they begin to live independently. The chapter looked at statistics, differences in outcomes for young people from different ethnic groups, and drew attention to current policy initiatives to improve the situation.

The chapter then moved on to consider some other life events where social workers are responsible for people who will feel alone with problems. It emphasised that in all fields of work, social workers are likely to deal with people who are or have been refugees and torture victims. It referred to the experiences of parents whose child has died and people who are homeless, and described the experiences of a young man with learning difficulties. For social workers, it will sometimes be possible to tackle the problem of isolation or 'aloneness' by opening up opportunities for social contact, but at other times, the response depends on their own emotional availability and consistency. This is particularly important where they have a statutory duty of care.

Bronfenbrenner's model attempts to classify the various influences on development. After an activity to help understand the application of his 'nested ecological model', the chapter concluded with an essay illustrating its use.

NOTE

1   All the people born in a single week in 1958 have been followed up in the course of their lives by *The National Child Development Study*; a second group, *The British Cohort Study*, follows all the people born in a particular week in 1970 – these are extremely large studies. The cohorts were followed up during their childhood and then at approximately ten-year intervals. *The British Cohort Study* was augmented by including immigrants born in the relevant week for the first three follow-up samples. The website of the Centre for Longitudinal Studies (CLS, 2008) is an invaluable resource about life, development and change. For examples of findings about the comparative development of three generations of people in Britain, see Ferri et al., 2003.

FURTHER READING

About physical, cognitive and social development in early adulthood:

Boyd, D. R. and Bee, H. L. (2015) *Lifespan Development*. Seventh edition. Boston: Pearson/Allyn and Bacon.

About care leavers:

Voice (formerly Voice for the Child in Care or VCC) joined the Coram group of charities and became Coram Voice: www.coramvoice.org.uk.

The Care Leavers Association is a user-led charity run by care leavers for care leavers: www.careleavers.com.

About refugees and torture victims:

Freedom from Torture (formerly the Medical Foundation for the Care of Victims of Torture) is a British charity that provides support and therapy to victims of torture: www.freedomfromtorture.org.

About homelessness:

www.homeless.org.uk – a national membership organisation that works with homeless charities and includes a useful research section.

About the nested ecological model (Bronfenbrenner's model):

Bronfenbrenner, U. (1979/2006) *The Ecology of Human Development: Experiments by Nature and Design.* Cambridge, MA: Harvard University Press.
Boyd, D. R. and Bee, H. L. (2015) *Lifespan Development.* Seventh edition. Boston: Pearson/Allyn and Bacon.

Questions

Based on the text:

1. Is 'leaving home' a characteristic life phase associated with young adulthood in all cultures? What characteristic differences between males and females leaving home did Sneed and colleagues (including Gilligan) refer to?
2. Using an example from social work or from fiction (a novel, film or soap opera), use Bronfenbrenner's ecological model to describe relevant features which have influenced someone's development.

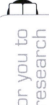

For you to research

Prepare a poster or brief report on one of the following:

■ Erikson's sixth psychosocial stage, 'Intimacy versus isolation'
■ The developmental tasks of adulthood as understood by Daniel Levinson
■ Loneliness and isolation through the life course
■ Women in prison

CHAPTER 6

Sex, love, work and children

In this chapter you will find:

- **Partnership and sex**
- **Biology and psychology**
- **Social aspects of intimate relationships**
- **Gender perspectives**
- **Being a parent**
- **Employment – the effects of unemployment**

INTRODUCTION

This chapter presents some common aspects of being an adult. An initial consideration of sexual relationships and experience broadens out to look at some social features of intimate relationships – changing patterns over time, and the influence of culture. This is followed by a brief review of the influence of gender on adult development. Obviously, for a proportion of the population, 'pair bonding' is closely bound up with the experience of being a parent, and the chapter goes on to look at this in more detail. The place of work (and unemployment) in adult development forms the final subject of the chapter.

As the chapter will point out, there are many dimensions to intimate and romantic partnerships (or to living without them). Many are straightforward, if sensitive, topics for academic discussion. Unlike the other material in this book, however, there may be some parts of the first section of the chapter that are unlikely to be presented to you in lectures and are not necessarily suitable for group discussion – occasionally, as here, a writer (even of a text-book) has the opportunity of 'speaking' to a reader and allowing the reader to 'respond' mentally and privately in a way that is not possible in face-to-face interactions in an institutional setting. A live conversation requires interpersonal confidence and mutual trust between speakers in a way that is not necessary for writer and reader. The material, of course (and your reflections on it), can be a resource which informs your verbal or written presentations, helping to ensure that what is said in an academic or professional setting is rooted in the lived and down-to-earth reality of people's lives. And, paradoxically, although it may be too personally revealing to affirm some of what is presented here, it is entirely possible to comment on it – to criticise it, to disagree with it, or to query the gendered nature of the text – to ponder whether you wish to have these things presented to you by two men. In general, we hope you find that what follows is interesting and useful background to the matters you will discuss about sexuality, intimacy and personal relationships – whether in an academic setting, in supervision, or sometimes with people who need a professional service from you.

PARTNERSHIP AND SEX

Joyous sexual activity is physical and messy. Compared with behaviour in public, it can be undignified. It is the intimate and tender culmination of respect, affection and giving. But in some circumstances it can also be a most indulgent pleasure only tangentially based on relationship, requiring only exuberant chemistry in the present moment. Deep sexual relating, a highly personal – one might say spiritual – engagement, can exist well beyond any erotic contact and entanglement. On the other hand, sex can be an exploitative and destructive physical invasion.

For those who are compatible and relaxed, it may seem like the most natural and unforced activity, but sexual confidence is readily disturbed by early negative experiences, by anxiety, by cultural and religious attitudes – by almost any perturbation in psychological well-being.

One stereotype is of adolescents awakened to the power of sex. For many teenage girls, the subject may be linked with romantic visions, fully persuasive and yet only half-believed, of finding a perfect soulmate; a person who will be reliable and protective in times of stress, but leave them their independence and individuality. For a girl deprived of sufficient caring in her childhood, sexual attention may appear to be a welcome offer of valuing and affection, but may turn out to be exploitation by a predatory male. Some (perhaps many) will consciously focus on being sexy to please boys rather than being sexual for themselves; further exploration, experience and confidence will be needed before they understand their own sexual potential. Developments in social media may only serve to increase a focus on physical appearance and can lead to increased vulnerability.

A young man may have wishes, desires and hunger. He too will have needs for adult comforting, care, reassurance, and affection, but some young men possess as yet only the beginnings of the social skills or experience to create in reality the relationships in which the needs may be met. Some will continue to focus on gratification, and may remain deprived of the satisfactions and pleasures of giving care. Unfortunately, the absence of this satisfaction is likely in turn to be part of a negative cycle – for in men, the experience of giving sensuous care is integral to the overall power of sexual activity to modulate troubled feelings, provide confidence and alleviate distress.

What do people desire in and through sex? There are many aspects, and desire takes many forms. Some are associated narrowly or in a straightforward way with sexual arousal and subsequent satisfaction, and some are not. For most people, over the decades of adulthood there is likely to be a journey of discovery they could not have anticipated.

For more about adolescence and sex, see Chapter 5.

Each generation, of course, discovers good sex for the first time in human history, and even students of human development may need to be reminded to be realistic about the lives of their elders. Some autobiographical notes by the author and playwright Alan Bennett tactfully bring this point home. He recounts a conversation with his mother as she recovered from an illness:

> Dazed by her own illness, and stunned by his, she lay in bed talking about Dad . . . Out of the blue she suddenly said 'He does very well, you know, your Dad.'
> 'Yes,' I said, taking this for a general statement.
> 'No, I mean for a fellow of seventy-one.'
> Again I did not twig.
> 'Why?'
> 'Well, you know when we were in Leeds he had to have that little operation to do with his water. Well most fellers can't carry on much after that. But it didn't make any difference in your Dad. He does very well.'
> Had I known it, the pity was all in the tense, since his doing, however well, was now almost done, and he died a few days later.
>
> (Bennett, 2005: 46)

Intimacy – specifically romantic intimacy – has many dimensions. For one couple, physical comfort, sensuous attention, the gift of giving physically may be at the core of their relationship, whilst for another, erotic engagement may be absent. Affection, attachment, loyalty and commitment can be expressed with varying degrees of physicality.

'When you fall in love, it is a temporary madness', a father tells his daughter in the novel *Captain Corelli's Mandolin* by Louis de Bernières (1994). 'Love is not lying awake at night imagining that he is kissing every part of your body. No, don't blush . . . that is just being in love. Love itself is what is left over, when being in love has burned away.' Some couples will remain deeply in love over the course of their relationship for many years. Others will not. For most, the relationship will contain many elements – of children, finance, surmounting difficulties more or less together, responsibilities for their own parents, enjoyments, pains, disagreements and more or less shared activities and enthusiasms. Sexual relations are dealt with at some length in this section of the chapter, not because they are necessarily experienced as the most important aspect of an intimate relationship, but because they may be one of the least well understood.

Intimate adult relationships (and their absence) are a core aspect of social experience and social distress. Having responsibility for social well-being, competent social workers should be as skilled in supporting people through difficulties in relationships as they are in childcare, health, financial pressures, interpersonal violence or housing. If you glance again at this list of 'practical' difficulties, you will see that they are often closely bound up with the quality of adult relationships.

Chapter 10

Social workers are human, and they are no more immune than anyone else from difficulties in relationships – rejection, violence, betrayal, uncertainty, problems of mental health or drug use. For themselves, they may wonder if satisfactory intimate relationships are ever really possible, or may have made a decision not to share their lives. This is part of what they bring to their work, and it does not in itself impede their ability to help others with relationships. They, too, are entitled to support in their difficulties (and it is probably true that this is the surest way of knowing that there is nothing demeaning in receiving help for personal matters), but they are not diminished by their difficulties. They have to 'hold' their personal experience as a valuable resource, but there are times when they may need to work hard to ensure it is not a filter which distorts their understanding of the experience of others.

Care, affection and attachment

Most studies show that a large majority of people desire a long-term relationship which will provide intimacy, affection and a shared life. This desire seems to persist even in a world in which 42 per cent of marriages end in divorce (ONS, 2017b), and may coexist with personal experience of heartache and hurt of such a relationship. The search for a 'shared life' may remain a hope alongside the conflicting desire for independence, freedom and pleasure which does not have to take account of another person's daily wishes. It may coexist with the experience that the independent life, for all its drawbacks, seems satisfactory and satisfying. Social patterns change and, at the present time, one common outcome of these conflicting wishes and current demographic patterns is '**serial monogamy**' (a series of monogamous relationships that don't last for a whole lifetime, each ending and being replaced by another relationship).

Cindy Hazan and Debra Zeifman (1999: 336–354) set out to see whether adult romantic partnerships should be regarded as 'attachments' in the same sense as infant and childhood attachments. They identify the four characteristics of early attachments as

■ Seeking to maintain closeness (proximity seeking).
■ Showing distress on separation (separation protest).

- Being someone whose presence, reliability and good regard can be taken for granted, and whose physical environment is the base from which the outside world is explored and negotiated (secure base).
- Being someone who can provide comfort, security and protection (safe haven).

They asked questions focusing on these four areas to over a hundred each of young people (children and adolescents) and adults. They found that the target of these 'attachment' functions changes over time from parents to peers. The change occurred progressively from childhood through adolescence to adulthood. The complete switch of the functions occurred in adulthood in relation to romantic relationships of over two years' duration. Their conclusion is that the 'pair bond' is indeed the vehicle of the attachment system. In the 'pair bond' in every culture, they note (following Bowlby) that the physical behaviours of 'mutual gazing, cuddling, nuzzling, suckling, and kissing, in the context of prolonged face-to-face, skin-to-skin, belly-to-belly contact', are found as they are in parent–child behaviours. In a recent follow-up, they concluded that there is mounting evidence to support this hypothesis (Zeifman and Hazan, 2016).

Chapter 2

This suggests that adult affectional relationships are linked with child attachment patterns, but as discussed in Chapter 2, there is no deterministic effect of past experience on later attachment behaviour. The biological basis of attachment is inbuilt; earlier experience provides the foundation on which later attachment is built, but a person's attachment experience is the product of these together with the actual relationships established, both in the past and in the present.

Hazan and Zeifman (1999) went on to explore how the functions of attachment are expressed in adult pair bonds. For example, similar hormones released in physical contact build attachment in both childhood and adulthood, and disruption of the attachment through separation and loss causes similar patterns of behavioural/emotional consequences. The most obvious difference in the functioning of the attachment system in adulthood compared with childhood is that it acts through a *mutual*, not asymmetrical, relationship – in adulthood, each party provides for the attachment needs of the other. Hazan and Zeifman regard the 'pair bond' as the integration of the sexual mating system, the caregiving (parenting) system and the attachment system. Sex, they assert (1999: 340), plays a key role in the transfer of the attachment system from its childhood targets to its adult form.

You may feel that this account says little about the development of care, affection and intimacy in bonds not mediated by sex – such as same- and opposite-sex partnerships that are not physically sexual. Furthermore, to propose this (comparatively) simple model of the function of sex in development is a different matter from understanding the dynamics of sexual experience and relationships.

What social workers need to know about sex

Dunk-West and Hafford-Letchfield (2016) argue that the nature of intimacy and our emotional lives, and how we frame sexual identities for ourselves and others, are central to social work. What do social workers need to know about sexual development and sexual relationships? They need to know that they are capable of empathising with other people's experience, but will not know what that experience is until they have been told. The experience itself, and accompanying attitudes, may be very different from their own, so they need to have open minds. The other person's experience of passion, or sexual frustration, may be very different from their own; they will encounter issues about sexuality in work with children and teenagers, all of whom will have varying amounts of knowledge or misinformation about the subject (see Chapter 4, including the examples of Emma, Lillian and Sue). Social workers also encounter issues of sexuality when working with people with learning difficulties (see 'Donald' in Chapter 5; Truckle, 2000, and the reference to McCarthy's research, 1999, in Chapter 4), adults with mental health problems, people with physical disabilities (see Chapter 4, and Quinn, 1998), parents struggling in their family life, and so on, right through to the final stages of life. As Monroe points out (2004, especially p. 1009, and in her case example, pp. 1012–1013), a woman may appreciate the chance to talk about the impact of breast cancer on her body image, or a couple may value the opportunity to confront the 'elephant in the room' which is the impact a terminal illness can have on their physical intimacy.

Chapters 4, 5

Social workers must demonstrate an openness to hearing about a person's sexual life and sexual development without expecting to be told or seeming prurient. The social worker's professional task is to understand the 'person', in all their diversity, in the 'situation', with all its dilemmas (Perlman, 1957). This is not in conflict with a specific agency remit about housing, justice, health or education – rather, the social worker is often the person in a functionally focused agency who is to bring professional skills about 'social aspects': relationships, emotions, housing, employment and finance. This social 'context' is comprised of both individual personal development and social relations. Social workers must allow 'space' for areas about which they do not know any detail, and take account of it in their mental model of the social situation.

In the early stages of your career, there will be occasions when you should ideally be asked to understand this aspect of development for one person at a time, with others (other workers, a supervisor, various planning structures) taking responsibility for the other people in the situation. There will be a number of occasions when this is not appropriate, and, unfortunately, agency practice may militate against it even when it is desirable. But ultimately, as a social worker, you often need to understand simultaneously the developmental experience of several people in a situation – for example, the nature and effects of sexual abuse and the sexual motivation and needs of the abuser, or the person in an intimate relationship who feels sexually deprived and their partner who feels put under sexual pressure.

There are specific areas of sexual life in which social workers may have responsibility. These require them to build on a more general understanding, and include:

- Promoting sexual health.
- Sexual abuse involving children, including that between young people.
- Other sexual violence – in institutions, within adult relationships, or from strangers.
- Sexual identity and uncertainty.
- Imparting sexual knowledge.
- Sexual satisfaction and enjoyment in relationships – for example, in relation to learning or physical disabilities, or the effects of childbirth, illness or surgery on sexuality.

These areas, of course, overlap. For example, Kristensen Whitaker et al. (2006) found that boys who were sexually violent or abusive had lower levels of sexual knowledge. Like David Thompson's emphasis on 'erotic education' for men and women with learning difficulties (Chapter 4), Jenny Higgins and Jennifer Hirsch (2007) emphasise the need in all these subjects, especially 'sex education', for constant attention to the specifics and variety of sexual pleasures (and desires) of all the individuals concerned. The aim of sexual support and education is, as these authors put it, 'to maximise sexual enjoyment and minimise sexual harm'.

Chapter 4

A social worker will sometimes be unsure about whether a client conversation should have been more explicit about sex or less intrusive. Sooner or later, if this subject is raised, the social worker is likely to experience either sexual attraction and fantasy, or alternatively distaste, in relation to their clients (in psychoanalytic terms – Chapter 2 and 'Essential background', section 4 – these are aspects of countertransference). The hazards are to deny these feelings on the one hand, or on the other to behave unprofessionally. One measure of social worker's competence is their own self-awareness about sexuality – and social workers are as likely as anyone else to have had difficult sexual experiences and relationships and will have to face questions which they find difficult to answer. Adequate supervision and support should allow these matters to be discussed.

Chapters 2, EB4

Social workers must have an educated awareness of the basic processes in sexual relations and in reproduction. But they also need to be comfortable (if sometimes curious) about the fact that there are many things about sex and sexuality that they, like everyone else, do not understand. If all goes well, the social worker is likely to discover that there are people whose attitudes, knowledge and experience can assist their understanding. There is no one, however, who 'has all the answers'. There are many questions about sex, about what is common and what is unusual, to which no one has the answers.

Biology and psychology

The hormones released in affectionate stroking and in orgasm, particularly for women, are the same as those (oxytocin and prostaglandin) released in mother and child during breastfeeding. They focus attention inwards, away from outside stressors, and are thought to reduce the fight/flight response (Huber et al., 2005; Taylor et al., 2000). They also have the effect of building attachment – whether in child or adult relationships. Testosterone is a major factor in sexual readiness and sexual activity, and this hormone circulates in both the female and the male body (Bales and Carter, 2009). Although its level fluctuates, women generally have greater quantities of testosterone than the 'female' hormones oestrogen and progesterone. In men, a minimum level of testosterone is required to maintain sexual drive, but above that minimum, higher levels do not increase it. Testosterone is also produced in women during cuddling and intercourse, and it appears (van Anders and Watson, 2007; van Anders et al., 2007a, 2007b) that regular sexual activity in women tends to increase sexual desire – 'sex is the best aphrodisiac' – probably through maintaining levels of testosterone.

Clearly, sex is part of a biological imperative to reproduce, but this should not be interpreted simplistically – as in other animals, and sometimes to a greater degree, sexual activity may be homosexual or masturbatory or occur in other contexts in which it is not directly linked to reproduction. And a preference for a sexualised link (for example between same-sex partners) which is not reproductive does not mean there is no drive to reproduce – a woman in a same-sex relationship may feel the drive to have children as strongly as anyone else. This should hardly need empirical justification, but if sought, it can be found in Morrow and Messinger (2006; see also Siegenthaler and Bigner, 2000).

No one is born with knowledge about the biology of intercourse and reproduction. Curiosity, peer conversations and information from books, television and the internet dispel that ignorance for many, but social workers are particularly likely to be dealing with a proportion of the population that has gaps in essential knowledge, either while they are young or later on. Van den Akker and her colleagues (1999) found in their survey of 212 UK teenagers that boys were less informed than girls. Beyond the most unsophisticated awareness of their own physical responses, males in general are unlikely to understand the physiology of their arousal and reproductivity until there is a physical problem (such as erectile dysfunction, infertility or prostate trouble) which requires them to do so. One of the more obvious differences between same-sex and opposite-sex relationships is that opposite-sex partners are likely to interact with less knowledge of each other's biological nature and experience.

The *psychological* experience of desire and attachment takes us into a very different domain from the biological. Lust, disgust, love and hatred are familiar to everyone. They may drive the most satisfying and important relationships in life, or result in the most destructive of behaviour. Classical Freudian theory regards the unfolding of psychological life as essentially the history of the individual's struggle with an underlying drive (*life force*) related to all these emotions. According to this view, the fantasies and behaviours associated with adult sexuality – of union, of possession and devouring, of pain as well as pleasure, of giving and receiving, of 'wickedness', transgression and punishment, of feeding and contentment – are linked with fantasies of the body which predate adult knowledge by many years. To use the terms introduced in Chapter 2, the relevant 'states of mind' in adult sexual encounters have evolved out of these earlier states of mind.

Chapter 2

Fluidity and variability

Sexual intimacy is a complex interplay of biology, psychology and society. Objective, sensitive and reliable data about the subject are difficult, if not impossible, to achieve. What is clear is that there are patterns of difference as well as similarity between male and female sexual response. The 'standard' model for both sexes, originally proposed by Masters and Johnson, is of excitement/arousal proceeding to plateau, orgasm and resolution. Kaplan added a phase of 'desire' to this and adjusted the phases to produce a simple three-stage model – sexual desire leads in chosen circumstances to arousal and later orgasm. In fact this seems more typical of men, and the minor adjustments allowed for women still leave it unsatisfactory as a model (Basson, 2005; Kaplan, 1979; Masters and Johnson, 1966).

In reality, a woman's sexuality varies considerably over her lifespan, and is affected by factors such as pregnancy, the menopause, self-image, previous negative sexual experiences and especially the relational context. Arousal may well precede desire or be independent of it (unlike men, women may be subjectively unaware or subjectively unaroused when experiencing physiological sexual arousal – Basson, 2005). The (American) Association of Reproductive Health Professionals (ARH) (2005) views women's sexual desire as more volitional and responsive than men's. Desire proceeds from numerous sources as well as the 'sexual hunger' which is described by men (for example, the desire for intimacy, overtures from a partner, commitment to the continuance of a relationship, or the wish to please). Sexual desire – in the form of sexual thoughts or fantasies – experienced when seeking a partner or in a new relationship may disappear from the experience of women in established relationships, who may infrequently think of sex. The goal of sexual relations for women is often described as personal satisfaction, which can be a variable combination of physical satisfaction and emotional satisfaction (intimacy and closeness). This goal is vulnerable to being derailed by a wide range of psychosocial or practical concerns. Women are likely to be interested in and concerned about their sexual response and that of their male or female partner, but do not necessarily feel distress when they lose interest in sex. This creates ambiguity because for some women the loss of sexual desire may be wrongly understood to be a sign of 'sexual dysfunction', while for others, lessened sexual appetite may be incorrectly accepted as unproblematic.

Lisa Diamond (2008) interviewed 100 women over a period of ten years, talking regularly with each of them over this period about their sexual desires and sexual relationships. She describes about three-quarters as 'sexual minority' women, but her findings and their relation to existing literature led her to the view that her constructs are likely to be relevant to women in general. She concludes that it is important to distinguish *sexual orientation* (which, although open to different definitions, she found to be relatively stable and located on a scale of entirely lesbian to entirely heterosexual) from three other factors – sexual behaviour, sexual desire and loving/romantic attachment. Each can vary independently of the others. The last she found to be aligned with personal, relationship and situational factors rather than gender. She describes this as *sexual fluidity*, and concludes it is characteristic of women in a way that it is not of men.

Like Basson, she quotes studies showing that whereas men's bodies respond physiologically according to their orientation to the sexual attractiveness of males or females, 'women do not appear to be sensitive to these categories'. Although they may express same- or opposite-sex attraction, and 'may subjectively prefer one sex over the other, their bodies respond to both'. (Chivers et al. (2007), whilst confirming this general statement, also report differences between lesbians and other women.) Men's physiological responses, sexual behaviours and emotional attachments tend to follow their sexual orientation far more predictably. For example, 30 per cent of lesbian women had full-blown romantic relationships with men in the course of Diamond's study, but did not necessarily feel that this had changed their sexual orientation, although it caused some ideological friction with friends. Two-thirds of her sample of sexual minority women changed their 'identification' over the period – not, she believes, because their sexuality was changed or misjudged, but because the categorisations did not fit the nature of female sexual fluidity. To summarise a complex work, she sees women's romantic behaviour as highly specific to the partner (independent of gender and sexual orientation), and located in the situation and social influences in a way that men's is not, their physical sexual behaviour being much more tied to their sexual orientation.

About 10 per cent of men describe some level of same-sex attraction. Estimates for women are varied, and depend significantly on the criteria used – for example, whether the attraction was an isolated incident; the frequency or intensity of attraction; or whether the woman's behaviour was affected by it.

Sexual experience within enduring relationships is likely to change over time. Laumann (Diamond, 2008: 140) found in a large-scale study of American women that 30 per cent reported low or non-existent sexual desires, and Diamond believes this too should be linked with the fluidity of female sexuality to biology, environment, situation and relationship, quoting some clinicians' suggestion that 'low sexual desire' should be reframed as 'desire discrepancy' between partners. Klusmann, studying 2,000 people in Germany, is one of a number of researchers who found that when settled in a stable relationship, a much greater proportion of women than men no longer expressed the sexual hunger they expressed when seeking a partner or when their current partner was absent from home (Klusmann, 2002, 2006; Wellings et al., 1994). This is in keeping with the model of Basson and the ARH (2005) mentioned above that, particularly when in a relationship, women's erogenous sexuality tends to contrast with men's in having a responsive motivation. This did not mean that sexual contact necessarily discontinued. But women described their motivation as different – it might be out of affection for their partner, out of the pleasure that arose, out of a responsiveness to sexual interest shown by their partner or out of negative motivations like fear, threats, or money. This should not be described as a 'lessening' of sexuality, although it would appear to indicate that its expression has changed. Nor does it mean that some men (the numbers are unclear) do not lose sexual drive, sometimes to the distress of their female partner. As discussed in Chapter 8, a significant proportion of couples in long-term relationships report that sex continues into their seventies, discontinuing when interrupted by events such as the hospitalisation of one partner.

Chapter 8

Giarusso, Feng and Bengtson (2005) describe marriages in later life as being less based on romance and more on loyalty, cohesion and solidarity with the wider family. Their analysis of bonds within the family draws on research which shows older partners experiencing less friction and resolving conflicts with less negativity.

What do you understand by 'sexuality'? (It is unlikely that you will find a simple answer!)

The expression of sexuality is very diverse. Researchers differ in the degree to which they regard human sexuality as socially constructed, and where they place the limits of variability. Having said that:

- What aspects of their own sexuality might people find troublesome? . . . How does this apply to men? . . . And to women?
- What aspects of male sexuality may women find troublesome?
- What aspects of female sexuality may men find troublesome?

Reflective thinking

The ending of relationships

Intimate relationships eventually come to an end, but the majority of marriages still last until the death of one of the partners. The Office for National Statistics calculates that for marriages since 2000, the divorce rate is about 42 per cent, with around half of these divorces expected to occur in the first ten years of marriage (ONS, 2017f). Figures for the disruption of non-marriage relationships are obviously difficult to establish – one related snapshot is that 80 per cent of children live in two-parent families (including 6 per cent who live in stepfamilies), 18 per cent live with lone mothers and 2 per cent with lone fathers (Smallwood and Wilson, 2007). In a classic work, Holmes and Rahe (1967) asked participants to rate the stressfulness of various life events. Top of their scale came death of a spouse, followed by divorce and then marital separation (fourth was being sent to jail). In this textbook, we have referred to various models that chart responses to transitions – Chapter 4 introduced Hopson's model of transitions, and Chapter 9 will refer to models that have been put forward in relation to dying and bereavement. Before either of these were formulated, the anthropologist Bohannan (1970) analysed what he called six 'stations' on the route of relationship separation.

Chapters 4, 9

Bohannan's work referred to this specifically as divorce, but aspects of it apply equally to separation of other intimate relationships. This separation is complex, he says, partly because the following different aspects of separation occur simultaneously. The first phase of 'emotional divorce' occurs as the couple grow apart, the relationship deteriorates and there is increasing tension. The 'legal divorce' requires the transformation of (only partly understood) subtle and intangible reasons into concrete legal terms. Extensions of the 'legal divorce' are the third and fourth 'stations' – 'economic' and 'co-parenting' divorce. In these, property and care of children are settled, and bad feeling in various other aspects may contaminate attempts to resolve these issues, both at the time of the separation and later. The 'community' divorce involves changes in friends and community for the two people, and tackling the resulting loneliness. Emotional ties to the other person may persist (even in hostile relationships) long after the practical separation, and Bohannan regards the final 'psychic divorce' as the most difficult of all.

Hazan and Zeifman (1999: 343), like Parkes and colleagues (1991), understand the distress and other reactions which follow the loss of a partner as expressions of separation from an attachment figure. They note that these reactions can end either in emotional detachment from that person or in emotional reorganisation in which the attachment figure is 'relocated'. This is discussed again in Chapter 9, which considers the subject of loss and bereavement. They describe the patterns, which in grieving include anxiety, searching, and depression, as 'the norm among adults separated from their long-term partner', and yet not the normal reaction to the breaking of other social ties.

Chapter 9

Reflective thinking

Think back to Chapter 5, about living alone.

Weiss, who was quoted there, found that loneliness takes two different forms – one associated with absence of an intimate companion, and another caused by lack of friends. Hazan and Shaver refer to this work, and point out that further research has confirmed that the two forms of loneliness have different origins and different outcomes. Social support in the form of friendship does not alleviate the loneliness arising from the loss of an intimate companion. However, the renewal of relationships with parental attachment figures was found to be helpful.

Thinking about social work situations, are there implications about the way social workers should understand what they need to offer or arrange?

Chapter 5

Social aspects of intimate relationships

The reference to divorce illustrates the link to the *social* influences on love, sexual behaviour and partnerships. In 1971, 90 in 1,000 single adults over the age of 16 got married. In 2004, this figure was 28. Figure 6.1 illustrates the change in young women's experience. It shows the proportion of women who experienced various events before they were aged 25 – categorised by how old they are now.

This data from the Office for National Statistics shows, for example, that for women who are in the 25–29 age group now, 21 per cent lived with a partner ('cohabited') before they were 25, but of women who are 55–59 now, only one-twentieth of that figure – 1 per cent – had done so (follow the downwards path of the broken line marked 'cohabitation' in the graph). Around a quarter of women aged 25–29 now had married before they were 25. But about three-quarters of women now aged 55–59 had married before they were 25 (follow the unbroken line marked 'marriage' upwards from just above 20 to nearly 80). Similarly, less than a third of the younger women today had given birth to a child before they were 25, compared with over a half for women who are now in their late fifties.

In 1955, many women stayed at home until they married, at which point they set up a joint home with their husband. Today, a much larger proportion of women live independently of their parents and create their own home or one shared with friends before setting up a shared family household with a partner. Similarly, in 1955, men would generally need to secure income for a whole household before marrying, and this part of their culturally created role has been a valued if burdensome part of personal identity for many men. Even now, some men might find the prospect of forming a partnership without the ability to financially support a household through paid employment undesirable, as though it implies a loss of place in the world. Changing patterns of adult intimate relationships imply emotional and social changes

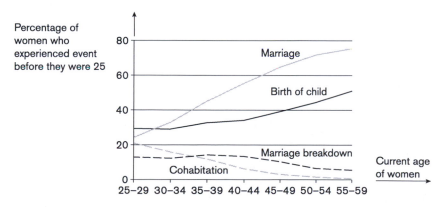

Figure 6.1 Experience of family events before the age of 25: comparison of different generations

Source: ONS/Smallwood and Wilson 2007, figure 1.13.

in other areas – for example, fathers face an increasing risk of losing touch with their children, with severe emotional and social consequences for both.

Until 1967 (1980 in Scotland), male homosexual activity was illegal in England, so a gay lifestyle was inherently countercultural. Hicks (2000) analyses lesbians' discourse about the relation between their chosen partnerships and traditional family relationships (in the context of their applications to become foster carers or adoptive parents). He distinguishes two contrasting ways in which the 'lesbian family' is presented. On the one hand, lesbians are at pains to emphasise that loving and consistent care for children meets the essential needs of childhood as they have always been understood – the gender of the parent is not relevant to the child's well-being. And on the other, he analyses the way in which they present gay and lesbian relationships as breaking new ground, challenging repressive, taken for granted aspects of 'traditional' marital and family structures.

So social and cultural factors impact as strongly as biological and psychological factors on behaviour within partnerships, and there are changes in sociocultural influences over time. Sexual behaviour and thoughts seem to be a specific target for those who tell others how they ought to behave – from traditional Judaic prescriptions about when to have sex, through Christian or Islamic prohibitions of masturbation or homosexual acts (and thoughts), through to some feminist polemicists. This does not mean that intimate behaviour will conform to the dictats of respected figures in a culture – the published speakers of a culture may be strident in proclaiming what is 'approved' precisely because behaviour is known to be different. At the time of writing, official Catholic orthodoxy states that contraception other than 'natural' methods is immoral, as are homosexual and lesbian relations. But the majority of Catholic couples in the UK use conventional contraception, and gay and lesbian Catholics find no contradiction between their life and their religion (Sullivan, 2002). Homosexual acts may have been illegal until 1967 but diaries of ordinary people, such as 'Barry Charles' in Garfield's (2005) collection *Our Hidden Lives*, indicate how individual private lives varied from 'official' culture. Public attitudes made some partnerships (permanent publicly recognised households) difficult, but enabled the development of countercultural attitudes. Similarly, the stigma relating to sex before marriage, or sex with multiple partners, created both external problems (prejudice and disapproval) as well as internal pain (guilt and confusion) for some women – but this didn't stop it happening. Social factors influence private behaviour, but do not necessarily produce conformity. In general, sexual desire and expression are targets for social and religious condemnation, resulting in shame or guilt.

In this context, there are three mechanisms through which development may be negatively affected, and the social worker has to adopt different strategies in relation to each. First, non-conformity may realistically result in penalties. As in the case of a woman ostracised by her family (and facing violence) for leaving an arranged marriage, these may be severe. Second, the social attitudes become internalised so that external threats are no longer needed. Ino's mother and aunties (Chapter 5 above) may well have believed

Chapter 5

Chapter 4

that it was necessary to cut her clitoris or she would be unable to be sexually faithful; no one spoke to Donald (Chapter 4) about erections, masturbation, and sexual relations because they had internal barriers to talking about such things; many boys have felt guilty or ashamed about masturbation; girls feel they ought to look pretty or form a self-valuation based on a peer-measured idea of attractiveness to boys; the young Muslim quoted in Chapter 4 knew the nature of his sexual attraction, but thought this was the work of the devil and that he would go to hell. Rogers' ideas of the 'false self' and Woodmansey's of the 'punitive superego' (pages 119, 94) are attempts to describe this 'internalisation'. And thirdly, we can only use the words of a language to communicate, and these derive their meaning from a host of related concepts and their social connotations. So 'promiscuous' is typically used of females, not males, and carries a host of value judgements with it. 'Childless', 'impotent', 'barren', 'queer', 'wanker' are words which each connect with a whole range of social ideas. Although the three processes – external consequences, internal guilt, and cultural construction – require the worker to be alert to different remedies required, they are often interlinked in any given problem.

In relation to cultures other than your own, it is important to have two complementary views. On the one hand, to recognise that another culture is more or less strange, remote and different, and that ideas (such as child abuse, romantic love, marriage) may have genuinely different meanings which are embedded in a whole network of other experiences you will not understand. But also to recognise the likely common understanding which arises from your shared humanity. Many (perhaps all) cultures have aspects which are oppressive or restrictive in relation to intimate relationships. However, with all its irrationalities and injustices, culture always plays a crucial role in supporting sexual development and social relationships. Individual experience can never be predicted from summaries of cultural attitudes and practices, although the elements of an individual's life always take meaning within a specific culture. This can be particularly paradoxical in relation to those beliefs which you will want to say are absolute (for example, that genital mutilation is wrong) – these beliefs will nevertheless always be expressed within the terms of a particular culture.

Marriage is a remarkably widespread institution across human societies, but, notwithstanding this, the forms and expectations of marriage vary considerably across cultures. Buss and colleagues (1990) examined the views of married people around the world to find out how different marriage arrangements and cultures affected what qualities are valued in partner selection. In their sample of nearly 10,000 people, they found agreement across cultures, across marriage procedures, and between men and women that the most important factors are love and mutual attraction, with very little variation from the recognition of dependability, emotional stability, kindness, and understanding as key qualities being sought. The research by Hazan and Zeifman (1999) into attachment and pair bonding also makes reference to this finding. Many Westerners, particularly modern feminists with an individualist outlook, regard the possibility of satisfaction in arranged marriages with elements of curiosity, questioning and disbelief. Factual cross-cultural findings are ambiguous. Myers and colleagues (2005) quote Shachar (1991) as finding minimal differences in marital satisfaction in an Israeli sample of 206 married couples between arranged and autonomous marriages. Yelsma and Athappilly (1988), in a study of eighty-four couples, found higher marital satisfaction scores for those in arranged marriages; whilst Xu and Whyte (1990) found, among 586 married women in China, higher satisfaction for free-choice marriages. In their own study, Myers and her colleagues reported that they found no difference in reported satisfaction with marriage between arranged and free-choice marriages.

GENDER PERSPECTIVES

'Sex' and 'gender'

When do you use the word 'sex', and when the word 'gender'?

When she's pregnant, Nicola may be asked, 'Do you know what sex the baby is?' But the application form Tia fills in might have spaces for name, address, date of birth, and boxes to select for 'gender: m ❑ . . . f ❑'. As you will have found with many of the terms in this book, there is no single definition, but a range of overlapping ways in which the words may be used, overlapping concepts to which they may refer:

■ 'Sex' can refer to the biological characteristics of the body, and used in this way, the great majority of people (but not all) can be allocated into one of two categories, 'male' or 'female'.
■ 'Sex' can also refer to sexual activity, and with its adjective 'sexual' this can be associated with other matters – 'sexual instruction', 'sexual initiation' and so on.
■ 'Sex' and its adjective 'sexy' can have even more specific reference to subjectively erotic subjects.

Using the same word can lead to the second and third uses being seen incorrectly as the defining feature of the first (that is, that what makes a woman female is her 'sexual function' whether romantically or in relation to childbearing). To avoid double meanings, and probably also sometimes out of an English-speaking squeamishness about using the word 'sex' in certain conversations, people sometimes use the word 'gender' instead of 'sex' in the first meaning:

Chapters
3, 8

■ 'Gender' refers principally to masculine and feminine (not male and female). 'Gender' is used particularly to indicate the social constructions and consequences associated with being male or female. The finding (see Chapter 8) that more women than men over 65 live in poverty, and the patterns of educational achievement described in Chapter 3, are examples of gendered features of society.

- More specifically, 'gender expression' refers to socially constructed ways of behaving that have a link with sex – for example, wearing skirts in modern European dress.
- Finally, as explained below, there is the complex argument that 'gender' is the essential fact, and the categories 'woman' or 'man' are socially created within this context.

In relation to the second of these, the term has significance because some cultural constructions wrongly emphasised an intrinsic link with biological sex (that men were more suited to intellectual work and women to domestic work, for example; or that a man dressing in a skirt or a woman in trousers is 'unnatural'). Once these expressions of gender are understood to be created by society, they are less bound to the idea of the biological sex of a particular individual. There can be a wide range of gender expression which has no deterministic link to the two sexes. At one stage in her life, a girl may like rough physical activities and taking physical risks, mainly in the company of boys, and describe herself as disliking pink and 'girlie' things, but at another she may enjoy courtship and romance that has many traditional heterosexual features. A man may sense that his own 'gender expression' challenges oppressive traditional norms. Because conventional gender expression has been so bound up with sexual orientation, there are many respects in which gay men and lesbians are conscious of creating their own gender expression. Later in the chapter you will see the words of Helen Hill who was born intersex, and brought up as a boy, but feels more comfortable and integrated now that she is a woman.

So you can often think of 'sex' as referring to physical characteristics and 'gender' to social features. But the previous paragraphs remind you that this is not the only way the terms are used, and the third bullet point above indicates one final analytical approach which specifically questions it. Recognising this physical/social dichotomy between the two terms, Butler argued that we need to revise them: it is not that physical sex is the basic fact, and gender is built socially on it. Sex is not 'a bodily given on which the construct of gender is artificially imposed, but . . . a cultural norm which governs the materialisation of bodies' (Butler, 1993). Any reference to bodies, she argues, will always be expressed in cultural terms, which have a strongly gendered basis. As Jackson and Scott put it, 'women' as a social category needs explanation independently of the biological: 'If sex, as well as gender, is a construct, it follows that the body does not have a pre-given essential sex' (2002: 19, commenting on Butler).

Gender and society

Gender has an enormous influence on development through the life course. It seems to be one universal basis through which societies organise themselves, codify expectations of individuals and groups and allocate work, power and resources. Feminists not only seek equality between men and women; many also believe that all women are oppressed by men (Abbott et al., 2005: 38), that there are 'patriarchal' structures which have to be dismantled or challenged to achieve this equality, and that any gender divisions in society are always organised the world over so as to oppress and exploit women (Humm, 1992: 1).

The influence of gender on the experience of life is illustrated in every chapter of this book. In this section, three topics are chosen: gender expression, health and violence. As in so many areas to which this book is an introduction, there are further resources, including specialist journals (some geared specifically towards social workers), devoted to exploring the facts, analysing the processes, and describing social action initiatives relating to the topic.

Gender expression

Chapter 7

For many people, ways of expressing that dimension of their identity we call 'gender' are largely hidden, because it is so much taken for granted as part of their everyday interaction. There is a long sociological tradition (Goffman, 1959/2008; Butler, 1990) which sees social roles as 'performance' rather than innate identity, and examines the stigma which results when this 'performance' is unacceptable to others (see Chapter 7). People whose 'performance' is not intuitively or comfortably within the approved range have cause to become self-consciously aware of the processes involved. The details/specifics of gender expression vary from micro-culture to micro-culture, from relationship to relationship and from setting to setting. A woman may enjoy a pole dancing class as part of her 'hen night' as an expression of something quite different from that of her usual behaviour in mixed-sex evenings out. 'Gender expression' being largely hidden (because taken for granted), it can take an unusual experience to highlight what is involved. Here are the words of Helen Hill and the response from 'Gerda', another correspondent, in an online discussion sponsored by the BBC. Helen is a therapist who was born hermaphrodite/intersex, and was brought up unhappily as a boy, and then settled as a woman when she became an adult. Helen and Gerda are telling personal accounts which highlight 'gender' as a learned feature of social presentation:

> I find this topic fascinating, as I have had to learn a lot really, really fast so that I can stay safe, and present my body as it was meant to be without being ashamed of it . . .
>
> It was really hard to learn in a few quick years (five now) what other women have learned 'from the ground up'. It was also really hard to learn to be safe. Not that I didn't know I was now in a vulnerable position. Knew that one really well. But I didn't realise how QUICKLY I would be put in compromising, vulnerable and threatening positions! . . .
>
> So my education as Helen has been quite an eye-opener. I never fit in as a guy anyway, being hermaphrodite/intersex. But the immersion

into the world of women was baptism by fire. And the matter of sexualisation seems to be a catch-22.

[. . .]

'Gerda' replies: Well put, Helen! I had a harrowing few years when
I lost a lot of weight. Previously, as a 'fat lass', I had not been preyed on
socially as much as other girls, and as a punk/biker I felt safe walking
at night because I was wearing big boots and a leather jacket (and nice
sharp keys in my pocket) – but suddenly I was 'in scope' and I had not
developed those protective tactics either.

(BBC, 2007)

Both go on to comment on how the change in what we can call 'gender
expression' led to violence and unwanted approaches from men (the double
bind, of course, is that for a woman to present in a way that is not conventionally 'feminine' may also provoke male complaints and disparagement). Helen's
experience gives an adult's self-aware view of what girls learn by trial and
error without the conceptual sophistication possessed by adults, although
they may be intuitively aware. Norah Vincent (2006), a lesbian woman who,
for an experiment, lived for a year as a man, was often surprised by the gendered behaviour of women towards her as a man. She found women less
tolerant of varied gender behaviour than men, and in romantic encounters
(dates and approaches for dates), more rejecting and hostile towards their
partners. She describes men's gendered behaviour in romantic relationships
as forged in the crucible of the risk and reality of rejection by women, a rejection that she was shocked to experience, and felt that her life as a lesbian
had not prepared her for. Social workers often deal with men who are least
equipped to manage this challenge, and also with women who have been
most exposed to the destructive effects of sexual intrusion.

'Gender expression' is a mediating factor in the power of women's sexuality over men (and vice versa); it is bound up with sexual orientation, and is
subject to wide variations in different cultures. It is inextricably bound up with
sexuality in all its aspects, but more importantly, serves as a marker in many
areas in which society organises itself through gender.

Health

The experience of health is strongly linked with sex and gender. Physical
wellness is experienced in a sexed body, patterns of health and its maintenance are gendered, and working in health provision is gendered. Other
matters related to health, such as disability and ageing, have strongly
gendered aspects.

A man's life, on average, is likely to be shorter than a woman's, and men
are more likely to suffer from a chronic illness (Smith et al., 2008). Some 72
per cent of (female) breast cancers are successfully treated but the rate is
only about 53 per cent for (male) prostate cancer (ONS, 2006); as discussed
in Chapter 7, women are more likely to be diagnosed with depression, and

Chapter 7

men with schizophrenia. In general, women make more use of the health service. In many of these areas, there are different explanations: at the biological level, at the level of individual behaviour and experience, at the level of organisation and policy, and at the level of society and social organisation. Particularly at the level of social theory, the explanations may be contrasting and disputed.

In the UK, health provision is clearly gendered. Health practitioners – in the National Health Service or in self-employed complementary health activity – are predominantly female, and health management is also predominantly female, although in both, the proportion of men increases as the jobs become more highly paid.

Family care – of children or dependent parents – is disproportionately undertaken by women, and this means that they are also far more involved in negotiating with the health service and health practitioners on behalf of others.

Chapter 7

Gender and violence

Violence is considered at greater length in Chapter 7, but it is impossible to provide even a short overview of gendered aspects of development without referring to it. Violent offences are overwhelmingly committed by men. Figures for the extent of violence in intimate relationships vary, partly because of definitions and research methods used. The Office for National Statistics (ONS) (2017d) estimated that there were 1.9 million adults aged 16 to 59 years who experienced domestic abuse in the previous year. Of this 1.9 million, there were an estimated 1.2 million female victims and 713,000 male victims. The majority (70 per cent) of victims of domestic homicides recorded between April 2013 and March 2016 were females (ONS, 2017d).

These references to gender and violence in intimate relationships prompt a return to the theme with which this chapter began – the development of sexual relationships. One's understanding of what is involved develops through experience. For most, this picture is influenced by the experience of managing conflict and difference. For some men and women – and social workers may often be in contact with them – violence, inflicted or received, will be a significant part of their developing understanding about what is involved in 'intimacy'. Once again, biology, psychology and culture interact with specific situations to produce the problems of violence with which social workers must contend.

Reflective thinking

Are there occasions in your work or placement when your professional responsibility is to influence human growth and development?

BEING A PARENT

The subject of this book is growth and development. Being a parent – living life as a mother or father – involves personal development and change on an unprecedented scale. For reasons of space, Chapter 1 made only the briefest reference to the dramatic physical changes experienced by Nicola, Naoko or Tia during their nine months of pregnancy. Many women after birth feel their bodies are never the same again, though that change is different for women of different ages – the effects on a 16-year-old are different from those on a 42-year-old. The chapter referred to the complex social lives in which these changes were set. We quoted Donald Winnicott's words: 'There is no such thing as a baby, only a mother-and-baby' – and certainly, for most, the experience of constantly having to care not just for oneself but also for another, totally vulnerable person is a dramatically different life experience. This is the beginning of many such revelations over the coming years. With the arrival of the first baby, a woman may well feel her social position changes – as one writer put it, she has 'joined the matriarchy'. This of course may partly be reflected in the actual composition of her immediate social circle and topics of conversation, as well as the marketing group in which her shopping habits and interests now place her.

Commonly, after nine months inside her, the newborn baby preoccupies the mind of the mother. Although this will lessen as the years go by, many mothers will be generally aware of what their children are doing at any stage of the day, and planning the hours ahead even when they are not physically with them. As ever, every woman's experience is different – for many, birth brings the experience of falling in love, of closeness and protectiveness – and Nancy Chodorow (1999) claimed that women are more likely than men to have 'powerful experiences of connectedness'. But equally, there may be feelings of being overwhelmed at the responsibility for another person, or of disappointment at the lack of a bond, or, indeed, birth may bring with it protracted desolate feelings, of recognised or unrecognised depression.

In Holland, the *Kraamzorg* (approximately, 'midwife') may live with the parents for the first week after the birth to give practical help with many domestic matters and to assist the parents with their care of the new baby. In a radio discussion (BBC Radio 4, *Woman's Hour*, 17 June 2008), a *Kraamzorg* explained the satisfaction of her work – 'You're there at the birth of a new baby, but also at the birth of a mother.' A father commented on what he learnt from her – 'I learnt from her how to give support to a mother, what she needed me to do.'

Looking Closer

Basing her work on interviews with over 200 parents, Ellen Galinsky (1982) described how adults develop through interaction with their children. She worked within Erikson's framework and identified six stages of development, starting with a 'parental image' stage, in which the man and woman start to form an image of themselves as parents, and progressing through constant changes to a 'departure stage'.

Chapter
EB3

For the moment, continue to think about the mother–child dyad, one of the different evolving 'microsystems' (in Bronfenbrenner's terms – 'Essential background', section 3). The constant awareness of someone else and their state of mind will in time be fitted in alongside other external concerns, whether domestic (washing, cleaning, cooking, shopping and social contact) or work- and career-related. Later, a dramatic change in this physical awareness is no doubt one reason why many women feel a great loss and a major transition ('empty nest' syndrome) as children leave home.

The experience of motherhood, its place in life, varies considerably between different cultures and historical periods. It is different if it begins during or immediately after adolescence, compared with its beginning when a woman is in her late thirties or early forties. The likelihood of its happening at one age rather than another reflects social and historical trends as well as personal choices, as illustrated in Figure 6.1. The Office for National Statistics (ONS, 2017e) gave mothers' average age of first birth in 2001 as 29 compared with the age of 21 thirty years earlier. Compared with the past, women are more likely to have an established career before motherhood becomes part of their experience. Later childbearing is associated with significantly more difficulty in getting pregnant, and women are not always aware of this, or of the stress and invasiveness of IVF treatment. Some are acutely aware, though, and struggle with competing demands – the urge to have a child, the lifestyle associated with work and career, and pressures about partnership. Compared with thirty years ago (but not ninety years ago, when the massive killings of the First World War were still felt and there were 1.7 million women surplus over men – GBHGIS, 2008), women are more likely to be child-free. Women who are single now have greater social freedom and more practical options about becoming mothers, and more women are choosing to be child-free. The 'pathways' to being child-free appear to differ between men and women. In a study of 6,000 men and women, Keizer and colleagues (2008) found that both educational attainment and a stable career increase the likelihood of remaining childless among women, but, on the contrary, increase the likelihood of becoming a father for men. For men more than women, spending years without a partner, or having multiple partnerships, are associated with childlessness.

Many fathers are in full-time work. For them, the transition to parenthood will be different from that experienced by a mother. For a proportion of women, the length of time they stay away from work is affected by public policy on maternity leave. Many would like to stay out of paid work longer, and current regulations allow that to happen for a year after giving birth. Similarly, depending on the extent of take-up, increases in the parental leave entitlement for fathers will change the situation for them. Michael Lamb's research (2004) has been influential in examining the role of fathers in child development, and in (opposite-sex) families, he found that the relationship between the mother and father was a significant variable in affecting the attachment and interaction between the father and child. Research findings are fairly reliable that the warmer and richer the relationship between the mother and father, the better the relationship between father and child. This leads Lamb to emphasise that child development is influenced by 'family climate' as well as by individual relationships with caregivers. He found that in the early stages of development, the father's attachment has similar functions to the mother's: a secure bond helping the child to be confident in social relationships and exploration. Subsequently, in a number of countries (but not all), fathers show a more active physical interaction with their children than mothers (see also Boyd and Bee, 2015). Lamb suggests that this may have led some researchers using mother-centred measures to underestimate the attachment of children to fathers. More notably, he reliably found that there is a long-term effect as the child grows older: in two-parent families, a strong relationship between father and child at the ages of 7 and 11 was associated with more mature romantic relationships in adolescence, better examination results at 16, and no criminal record at age 21. His main explanation for this is that the earlier strong relationship probably continues through the years of adolescence.

Susan Golombok's studies of same-sex parents (particularly lesbian parents) 'tend to show that children . . . are no [more] disadvantaged in terms of their emotional well-being or other aspects of development than children in comparable heterosexual families, which leads to the conclusion that it is really the second parent that is most important . . . the relationship is more important than the gender of that parent' (UK Parliament, 2007).

It is not only that the child as an outside object of concern preoccupies the mind of the mother to a greater or lesser degree. 'Mind-mindedness' in a responsive parent involves the flexible ability to attune to the mind of the child. This requires the adult adapting to cognitions, emotional needs and responses which are very different from their own. Sometimes very fast-moving, sometimes unreasonable by adult expectations, sometimes fantasy-laden or rooted in cognitive errors, the child's mind, as discussed in the earlier chapters, requires active adaptation as well as stimulation from the mind of a caring adult. This may be experienced as fascinating, extremely tiring, frustrating, infuriating or mind-numbingly boring. Along with the physical work which childcare entails, this effort is undervalued in much contemporary society. The child's mind, too, is constantly exercised as it engages with all the different people in its life. The two parents have different personalities and approaches to giving comfort or behaviour management. In sharing the tasks of parenting, more or less harmoniously, each parent's developing attitudes, expectations and behaviours will be influenced by the other's. When grown up, the children will no doubt find that they have taken different qualities, beliefs and skills from each parent.

There is give and take in parenting. Sometimes the wishes and demands in the mind of the child can be met, and sometimes they cannot. But, in general, enjoying parenthood involves sacrificing some self-regarding wishes. This is a real demand, a real loss, but many parents in the long term achieve a special satisfaction because of the exchange they have been prepared to make. Both mother and father are likely to grow in maturity as they have the new experience of dealing with a potential battle of wills – an experience which they resolve not by imposing their will, nor by retaliating, nor by allowing the other will to win because they 'ought to' submit, but because it makes sense for them out of a higher drive (the child's well-being) to put their own needs on hold. The hazards in this are, on the one hand, that a parent (typically a mother) submerges herself in the task to the extent that she experiences a loss of 'self', and feels that her identity is entirely bound up with that of her child; or, on the other hand, that parents are unable to put their own feelings and impulses on hold in order to attend to children's needs. At each stage, from infancy to adolescence, the child's emotions are likely to evoke comparable feelings in the caregiver – whether of calmness and satisfaction, of murderous frustration or rebellion against external control.

All parents need support and recognition in their experience of these tasks and challenges, and directly or indirectly this is often what a second parent provides; for parents – men or women – who are limited in their ability to cope with these feelings, social workers or other social care staff have an important role in becoming part of the developmental experience of the parent. The experiences of a child evoke age-appropriate related feelings in a parent. It is much easier when they have someone who cares; someone who comforts and supports them, lessens stress, takes care of some of the practical matters, and supports self-esteem and mutual learning about behaviour management. For many, but not all, this comes from intimate or 'extended' family relationships, as well as naturally evolving social networks. But in modern society, social workers, school supports and organised family services are part of the networks created to meet this need.

One component of this family support relates back to the parental relationship, the subject of the earlier part of this chapter. Problems with children can pull this relationship apart, and strain between parents certainly has an impact on children. Social workers have an important function when they enable parents to maintain their relationship, to recover respect and care for each other. Sometimes separation seems unavoidable, and the parents collaborate effectively in the continuing lives of the children. On other occasions, though, in the words of a UK government report, 'parental separation often has a traumatic effect on children' (DCFS/DfES, 2004). Data from the Office for National Statistics show that, on average, the effect of parental separation is negative on each aspect of a child's life – educational attainment, emotional and social well-being (Smallwood and Wilson, 2007). The chances of adverse outcomes in these areas are doubled after separation or divorce (the evidence also shows that children's emotional difficulties precipitated by divorce are counteracted after a period of years). Obviously, separation does not necessarily reduce the parental conflict which children report as harmful to their happiness, or propel parents into cooperating in the care of their children. In addition, the effect on at least one of the parents is often destructive. Social workers also have a role in understanding the child's experience of loss and in enabling – or arranging for – mediation with the aim of collaboration and shared care. Principles and practical guidance for parents and others involved are given in a resource from the Children and Family Court Advisory and Support Service (Cafcass, 2018).

The loss of children

Social workers are particularly likely to be working with parents separated from their children. This may be because their child has died, or is fostered, or is cared for only by the other parent. Fathers who are estranged from their child's mother, or who are in prison, are especially likely to lose relationships with their children. Dunn and Layard (2009) quote statistics which show that 28 per cent of children (about 1.6 million) whose parents have separated have no contact with their father, a situation they regard as a major cause for concern.

Many people would describe the relationship with their children as the most important in their lives, and the loss of a child is perhaps the most grievous that anyone will suffer. Each person experiences it differently, but most will tell you that it is not something that can be resolved. The death of a child has its own way of marking a parent thereafter. So too does the experience of a loss which seems just as final (through adoption, for example) but which has to exist irreconcilably with the knowledge that somewhere the child is growing, developing, being happy or unhappy. As the mothers in Charlton's study describe the adoption of their children, 'It's like a death', and decades later they describe themselves as 'still screaming', thinking about their children 'most days' or 'most weeks' (Charlton et al., 1998; see also Howe et al., 1992).

> What is harder is having kids, knowing they live quite nearby but now being separated. They are withheld from you by the mother – that is a kind of torture, especially when you are powerless to do anything about it.
> (contribution in an online discussion, BBC Radio 4, 2 June 2008)

Although development after this parent–child separation is a central social work concern, and an important dimension to be aware of in any assessment, you will often find that it is not drawn to your attention in procedural guidance or assessment forms. In care proceedings it is the child who is the focus of official work, not the future needs of the mother. After its medical function has ended because a child dies, the Health Trust management may not understand that the social worker involved still has a professional task in relation to someone they have been helping daily, but who has never been the patient. The court service, in preparing reports about child custody, does not allocate any 'aftercare' responsibility. In family support services, the emotional needs of a father who is problematic in the immediate situation may not be appropriately understood – his childcare incompetence in the present family, aggressive resentment of anyone threatening to take 'his' children, might need to be seen in the context of his earlier experiences involving loss of children. In all of these situations, however, it is the social worker's responsibility to make an assessment of the needs of each person and to appraise realistically and holistically how the function of their agency relates to those identified needs.

The impact of losing a child is also discussed in Chapters 5 and 9.

Constant development

In summary, changes in the parental experience occur all the time as children grow and new babies are born into the family. A child reaching adolescence is a particular point of change as the child expects new levels of responsibility and autonomy, as are the transitions when a child leaves to live on their own. Some 60 per cent of marriages around the world are arranged, so at this stage in their children's lives the parents are actively engaged in negotiating with their children and seeking spouses for them.

Moving on again, the parents have new experiences as the 'children', now adults, take responsibility for them in everyday ways (such as paying for meals out, which may seem like a reversal of roles!). Children thrust new learning upon their parents as they marry or settle in partnerships, bestowing the new role of 'in-laws'. Later, a further phase for the parent is created if the child cares for them, possibly with the parent being behaviourally difficult or resentful and intellectually deluded about the relationship (as in dementia). This is discussed further in Chapter 8, about old age. In this phase, the parent is adjusting to the psychological dynamic of *placing* burdens on their children (not removing them). The 'child' is highly likely to be a woman in middle age, with children of her own and a job – as Brody and Saperstein (2006) say, a 'woman in the middle'. In the introduction to their book, the family care of older people by women is described as a 'normative phase' in family life. As a stage in life, it has not received the 'normative' attention (and support and recognition) it deserves. It has, perhaps, been understood non-developmentally by ideological perspectives on women's experience, and sidelined in policy formation about public provision.

Chapter 8

?

Reflective thinking

Discuss the development that takes place in parents, *as parents*, after their children's school days are over.

WORK

Adults who are in full-time paid employment spend a large proportion of their waking hours at work. It is the setting of much of their physical, intellectual and emotional activity. At its best, it is the setting for intellectual stimulation and learning. For social workers, for example, it is a place of learning about the world of organisations and social policy, but also of learning about emotions and people, about human need, and the management of conflict; it forces continuing reflection about what, in the long term, is of value in human life. The majority of social contact may take place through work – when people retire from full-time work, their level of social contact may drop dramatically. At its worst, work is a cause of injury, early death, or a source of constant stress (Walsh et al., 2005).

In a classic text, Jahoda (1982) described obtaining income as the 'manifest' (openly visible) function of work, and identified a further six 'latent' (concealed, or dormant) functions. This scheme is summarised in the box below.

Employment can provide:

- a source of income;
- a form of activity;
- a structure for time;
- a source of creativity and mastery;
- an opportunity for social interaction, a source of identity;
- a sense of purpose.

Warr (2002) built on this work to develop a ten-factor model of work. This can be used not only to analyse different work experiences but also to understand the effects of unemployment. For example, one of their factors is 'opportunity for control'. Workplaces differ in the degree to which they give the worker autonomy and responsibility to control their own work and to participate in decisions which affect it; greater control is associated with greater satisfaction at work and better mental health. Unemployment and dependency on welfare tend in general to restrict environmental options and decrease opportunities for making life decisions. Work provides finance, one of the most obvious of Warr's (2002) categories, and they write of unemployment: 'Studies of unemployed people consistently indicate that shortage of money is viewed as the greatest source of personal and family problems. Poverty bears down not only upon basic needs for food and physical protection, but also prevents activity and reduces one's sense of personal control.' Rogers and Pilgrim (2003: 117) point out that unemployment correlates with higher psychiatric diagnosis, and re-employment is consistently shown to reduce diagnosis of psychiatric disorder. They discuss the factors involved in this statistical link. These include the question of whether unemployment causes the mental health problem or the reverse, the different effects of voluntarily or involuntarily leaving the workforce, the difference between secure and insecure employment status, and the level of financial pressure caused by lack of work.

Chapter 7

Poverty has a major influence on development throughout life, and is one of the subjects in Chapter 7. It is a prime example of a problem which social workers are constantly dealing with, and in which they cannot professionally just deal with the personal – to act with integrity, they must also be concerned with societal causes.

The social psychologist Bales introduced the terms '**expressive**' and '**instrumental**' (originally about social roles) to distinguish between activities whose value lies mainly in personal and interpersonal expression, and activities whose value lies strongly in practical outcome (you have an expressive relationship with a love partner, but a purely instrumental relationship with the people who keep the electricity supply working). For many, work is closely bound up with social identity and has an expressive function. While this may be true to a degree for many parents with a career, they are equally likely to be in the category of people whose work has a purely instrumental value – it needs to be trouble-free, leave them energy for their children, and pay them reliably – although social relations within work, as distinct from the formal work itself, may have an important expressive function in their lives.

Emotions in work

Some work obviously involves hard physical labour and requires physical strength. Arlie Hochschild devised the term 'emotional labour' to describe work which involves working with emotions. The value to the employer is the effect the employee has on the customer's feelings. Her classic study was of flight attendants, who at the time were usually female (previously called 'air hostesses' – 'from trolley dolly to emotions manager' as one reviewer put it). Some parts of their job involved physical labour – managing the food and physical space in the aircraft. In addition, however, they also were expected to keep the atmosphere calm; soothe passengers' emotions, leave them feeling contented, relaxed, attended to, and even pampered. Many features of the job – appearance, uniform, demeanour, constant and even-tempered presentation – were related to this. Hochschild saw this emotional labour as an economic exploitation. It violated the integrity of workers by getting them to display pseudo-emotion, not as deliberate acting (as in the theatre), but as if it was truly felt. It devalued genuine human contact by mimicking it for profit motives.

To be practised effectively, social work also involves demanding emotional work (Howe, 2008; Sudbery and Bradley, 1996; Whittaker, 2011). This is skilled, it is sometimes wearing, it can be stressful, and it is the source of much of the satisfaction in effective social work. To be helpful when dealing over a period of time with a volatile (or dangerous) teenager who clashes with his parents and others in authority, requires considerable emotional invest-ment. Intense feelings are involved in working out the best course of action when dealing with a baby who has been severely injured by his parents, or, as in the example in Chapter 9, helping a dying person when the practicalities of what you can offer turn out to be inadequate. In all these cases, good work-ing practice requires that the worker finds and uses someone helpful and reliable to support their heightened feelings. It is a sign of maturity, not inad-equacy, to be able to use a senior or more experienced person for emotional support.

Chapter 9

At the moment, men's earning power reaches a peak about the age of 45. The work prospects (including pay) of childless women are similar to those of single men (Waldfogel, 1998), but in many other respects, women's lifetime experience of work is often very different from men's. They are more likely to find that being a parent, a partner and an employee creates con-flicting demands and priorities – women are actively mothers (and 'wives') while they are at work, but men are more likely to experience their roles as sequential – 'workers' at work and 'fathers/partners' in separate periods during the day (Boyd and Bee, 2015). Women tend to judge themselves about how well they manage relationships (as mother and partner) as much as their performance as an employee. At the moment, the degree to which the boundaries around work time can be penetrated by other responsibilities seems to be different for men and women.

Write down some of the ways in which, from your observation or experi-ence, emotions at work are an important part of social work.

(Think of the team and organisational setting; the demands of the task; the sort of understanding required of social workers; the impact of the work; the effect of non-work life on work performance.)

Reflective thinking

Most women move in and out of the world of external work at least once, and often many times. In 2017, almost three-quarters of mothers with dependent children were now in full- or part-time work (ONS, 2017g), mark-ing a social change, as in 1974 the figure was 47 per cent (Iacovou, 2004b). Women who are in continuous paid work earn more than those whose work pattern is not continuous (Boyd and Bee, 2015, quoting Drobnic et al., 1999). Hersch and Stratton (2002) found that time spent in housework (not necessarily including childcare, and for both men and women) explained a significant amount of the income differential in paid employment – the effect is strongest for housework that occurs daily and this tends to be undertaken by women. On average, women earn less than men. The gap between what male and female workers earn fell to 9.1 per cent in 2017, compared to 17.4 per cent in 1997 when the ONS first collected the data (ONS, 2017h), but there is still much work to do to close the pay gap.

ARE THERE DEVELOPMENTAL STAGES IN ADULTHOOD?

You can probably identify various stages to your life as an adult. Different attempts have been made to describe general developmental stages, such as the schemes to divide childhood and adolescence. These have the merit of continuing developmental study into adulthood, but there are many difficulties with such attempts.

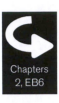

Chapters 2, EB6

In describing adulthood, many authors make outline use of three stages – early adulthood, described as the period from about 20 to 40; middle adulthood from 40 to 60; and older age from 60 onwards. Older age in turn is often described using the terms 'young old' (about 60 to 75), old old (about 75 to 85) and the oldest old (85 and older). Erikson's scheme (Chapter 2 and 'Essential background', section 6) places emphasis in early adulthood on the formation of close personal arrangements – the characteristic 'crisis' he identifies is intimacy versus isolation. As with all his stages, he understands the positive development of identity in the previous stage as a springboard for relinquishing it in the next. In the case of the transition between adolescence and early adulthood, he suggests that the person who has successfully avoided identity confusion or foreclosure in the earlier stage will have sufficient confidence in a secure adult identity to relinquish some of it without damage in order to form a close intimate relationship. In the next stage – middle adulthood, aged 40 or so to 60 – Erikson places issues to do with 'generativity'; doing something of value for the world, leaving something creative behind. It is in this stage that he places parenthood. Although this might seem rather late, and is an aspect which has sometimes been criticised over the decades since he wrote *Childhood and Society*, perhaps it is placed appropriately for many people today, as more women have their children later. However, parenthood is only one form of generativity, which is a broad term and refers to the production of things and ideas through work as well as the next generation, e.g., through social work, education and other activities that involve showing care for others. Boyd and Bee (2015) summarise later empirical evidence which backs up or critiques this analysis by Erikson.

Daniel Levinson devised a stage model of adult life. He regarded the totality of a person's roles, relationships, responsibilities, conflicts and so on as forming a '**life structure**'. Basing his research on forty men (1978) and forty-five women (1986), he examined a wide range of factors in people's lives – biological, economic, work-based, and psychosocial. He concluded that life structures are formed and dissolve during adulthood in fairly predictable ways. So there are periods of structure-building (entering early adulthood, entering middle adulthood, and entering late-life) and periods of structure-changing (the early adulthood transition, mid-life transition and late adult transition). Like Erikson, he regarded these changes as presenting the person with a life crisis as they adjust and transform (as Erikson is responsible for 'identity crisis' entering common language, Levinson is responsible for the phrase 'mid-life crisis'). Once again, the concept of crisis here does not mean something which is avoidable and unwanted, but something inherent in human development.

Lifespan theory (the framework behind Sugarman's textbook (2009) and Boyd and Bee's (2014, 2015)) is less focused on finding universal 'stages' in life development. Those working within this framework regard human development as always the outcome of a specific culture and a particular historical period, 'so it becomes less relevant to search for predictive theories which hold across cultures and across generations' (Sugarman, 2009: 3). This approach is used as a summary framework in Chapter 10.

Chapter 10

SUMMARY

Sexual behaviour is shaped by biological, psychological and social influences. Social workers have to build on a general understanding in order to deal appropriately with specific areas of responsibility such as promoting sexual health and preventing or dealing with the aftermath of sexual abuse or sexual assault.

As a category word, 'sex' is generally used to refer to bodily characteristics, while 'gender' refers to expression, behaviour, expectations and social outcomes which have some link with sex.

Biological influences on sex include the drive to reproduce and immediate factors related to hormones. It appears that sexual orientation, sexual behaviour and romantic attraction can vary independently of each other in different ways for men and women. Circumstances and personal psychological history affect sexual relationships, as do cultural and historical factors.

Parenthood is a major influence on development for many adults. Galinsky described a six-stage development, from forming an image of being a parent through to 'departure'. The experience of parenthood has both universal elements and elements strongly affected by culture (such as average age for becoming a parent). Many people describe their relationship with their children as the most important in their lives, and social workers are particularly likely to be working with parents separated from their children.

Work has both an explicit function and a number of other latent functions, including that it can provide a source of identity and a sense of purpose. Some work, such as social work, involves genuine emotional investment. The great majority of women move in and out of the workforce at least once and often many times; being a parent, a partner, and an employee is likely to inflict more incompatible demands and a clash of priorities for women. Patterns of men's and women's work change over time and culture. Social workers are likely to deal both with the practical financial effects of unemployment and the reduced well-being (including the increased rate of psychiatric disorder) which it brings.

FURTHER READING

Adult relationships:

Boyd, D. R. and Bee, H. L. (2015) *Lifespan Development.* Seventh edition. Boston: Pearson/Allyn and Bacon.
Stewart, I. and Vaitilingam, R. (2004) *Seven Ages of Man and Woman.* London: ESRC, ch. 3, pp. 16–19 (maps relationships in modern Britain).

Fathers and mothers – their influences on children's attachment:

Howes, C. and Spieker, S. (2016) Attachment relationships in the context of multiple caregivers. In J. Cassidy and P. Shaver (eds) *Handbook of Attachment: Theory, Research and Clinical Applications.* Third edition. New York: Guilford Press.

Social work and emotions:

Howe, D. (2008) *The Emotionally Intelligent Social Worker.* Basingstoke: Palgrave Macmillan.

RESOURCES FOR PARENTS

About parental separation and responsibilities:

My Family's Changing (leaflet for children from Cafcass – version for younger children contains pictures, games and extra stories).
Cafcass (2018) *The Parenting Plan. Putting Your Children First: A Guide for Separating Parents.* London: TSO. A booklet with a wealth of accessible advice, help and suggestions, covering legal, emotional, financial and social matters.
All are available free from Cafcass or from The Stationery Office, London, or downloadable from www.cafcass.gov.uk (click the link 'publications').

There are many websites offering relevant information and advice, such as that of Relate: www.relate.org.uk/

Questions

1. 'Mother–father–child (one year old)'. This triad, which may exist in varied living arrangements, contains both adult–adult and adult–child relationships. What are some of the influences (on the experience and development of the three people) highlighted by attachment theory and by Bronfenbrenner's ecological model?

    In your answer, you may refer either to a single illustrative example or to a variety of possible family arrangements; you may wish to vary the question title to include same-sex parents.

2. Choosing one of the topics introduced in this chapter (adult sexual relationships, gender, parenting, work), discuss the application of Bandura's model of social learning.

Prepare a poster or brief report on one of the following:

- Postnatal depression
- The ending of intimate relationships
- Warr's analysis of the function of work and the effects of unemployment
- Gender in work

For you to research

CHAPTER 7

Maturity and some of its hazards

In this chapter you will find:

- **Poverty**
- **Violence; violence in intimate relationships**
- **Mental health**
- **Stigma**
- **Social influences on the development of people with learning disabilities**

POVERTY

The last chapter ended with a reference to the poverty caused by unemployment. In fact, about half of people in poverty live in households where at least one adult is in paid work. Poverty is one of four factors which negatively affect the development considered in this chapter. The others are mental health difficulties, violence, and the influence of social prejudice and stigma.

Poverty is defined in official UK statistics as having less than 60 per cent of average income. In 2015/16, one in five children lived in poverty and just under two-thirds of individuals had a household income less than the national mean average (DWP, 2017). There is a problem of poverty associated with all the different groups of people with whom social workers are concerned – families in need of support, children and adults with physical disabilities, people with learning difficulties, people with mental health problems, and older people. After discussing the experience of poverty, this section discusses the extent of poverty and some of its effects. Poverty research has often in the past been carried out and presented by people who are financially secure writing about others. This following section makes particular use of work carried out and presented by people experiencing poverty themselves.

The experience of poverty

When the Child Poverty Action Group presented their book, *Poverty First Hand: Poor People Speak for Themselves*, they noted that 'poverty . . . affects young and old, respectable old and disrespectful young; people conventionally included in the middle class as well as working class' (Beresford and CPAG, 1999: 47).

As a social worker, you have to make a 'social assessment' of a situation, either as formal procedure or as a non-formalised basis for deciding how to act. At the core of the assessment must be your understanding of people's day-to-day experience and (in Bronfenbrenner's terms, see Chapter 5) the different microsystems which frame their reality. A large proportion of people who use your service will be in poverty. Users of the service frequently criticise social workers for not taking sufficient account of this and not realising that their main problem is to do with finance.

Chapter 5

The most basic experience of poverty is going to bed hungry – mothers going without food for themselves because they have spent on their children, or feeling too worried to eat properly. Particularly for an older person, it may mean choosing between eating or keeping warm.

For many people, being poor creates a sense of being locked in: 'You've got no money and you can't see any way out of it.' It is 'a lack of choice . . . I enrolled on a college course which had the fees paid for me. I could have continued with the course but I looked at my piece of paper and worked out my expenses and I couldn't afford the bus fare in and out, and I couldn't have afforded food, so I could not go on that course . . . maybe in the future I could think of going back to college, but not at the moment' (Beresford and CPAG, 1999: 61).

Money does not create happiness, but poverty can create unhappiness: 'It creates disharmony in the family – because if you've got a teenager who can't get a job and they've got no income coming in, you've got to keep them here . . . 16- or 17-year-olds – they can't even buy clothes. They'll not be able to go out anywhere for a night out to the pictures – any money to go with their friends. I think it could put them in a depression. It can lead to them feeling useless and hopeless' (Beresford and CPAG, 1999: 81). About half of the participants in the CPAG discussion groups thought that poverty causes depression. It makes people anxious, frightened and miserable; 'it causes fear, humiliation, rejection, stress . . . constantly worrying, twenty-four hours a day, about money and having to manage for the rest of the week, month, year, whatever.' Poverty does not 'cause' bad treatment of children, but money makes it much easier to keep level-headed when a child comes home having torn his new pullover or kicked the toes through a new pair of trainers.

'Poverty', says one of the participants in the CPAG study, 'strips your dignity'. How do you go to the supermarket, she asks, and then go home and tell your children you haven't bought enough food?

There's nowt as cruel as kids, is there? I mean, they that get free clothing – you can tell. So you have to go out and buy a uniform and while they're wearing that one you have to save up and get another one because it's changing.

On benefits I don't think any allowance is made for brushing your teeth, or buying loo rolls or soap or the odd bubble bath . . . luxuries for people in benefits are, 'Do I buy toothpaste this week or soap? . . . Buy toilet rolls, toothpaste, scouring powder, washing powder, washing up liquid, and you can double just what you pay for your food bill.

(quoted in Beresford and CPAG, 1999: 51, 55)

Research shows that adolescents who are poor are more likely than others to be ashamed of themselves, or to think they are no good (Iacovou, 2004a). Roker's account (1998) of the experiences of sixty young people on low incomes identified that one common theme was having to take early and significant family responsibilities.

The extent of poverty

Analysing poverty is inescapably a political issue. Statistics change according to the state of the economy and the implementation of public policy. These are some core statistics about poverty in the UK in 2016 (JRF, 2016):

- In total, about 13.5 million people were in low income households.
- There were 3.9 million children in poverty.
- Over a third (35 per cent) of children living in poverty lived in a lone-parent family.
- Two-thirds (66 per cent) of working-age households in poverty had someone doing paid work.
- Almost one in four households in poverty had a family member who was disabled.

There is much academic analysis about different ways of specifying and understanding poverty. Many people on low incomes say that they cannot afford selected essential items or activities – but so do quite a lot of people on average incomes. A classic definition of poverty was given by Peter Townsend, a major campaigner and researcher: people are in poverty when they 'lack the resources to obtain the type of diet, participate in the activities and have the living conditions which are customary in the societies to which they belong' (Beresford and CPAG, 1999, quoting Townsend, 1979: 31). Note two particular points about this. It is a *relative* definition of poverty, like the government's own measure – it relates to the income and living standards of the society in which people live. This means, for example, that in periods of prosperity when average incomes rise, poverty is deemed to increase (because the level at which an income counts as in poverty rises). Second, the definition does not refer just to income and wealth. Living in a damp, unpleasant and dangerous house without proper services is poverty, as well as income poverty; a child is impoverished by a lack of access to education and a healthy, safe environment with opportunities to play and explore.

The first sentence of this section states that 'analysing poverty is inescapably a political issue'. In the light of the text above, or other arguments, in what sense is this true?

Two relevant areas:

1. Some politicians, concerned about inequality and how people experience their lives in relation to others, will accept the relative definitions of poverty, even though this means that in periods of prosperity, measured levels of poverty may rise. Other politicians may be scornful, arguing that poverty must be about not having food, clothing, or heating.
2. Political debates will be concerned about causes of poverty, and take different views about the balance of responsibility of the individual and of social factors (the economy, the level of benefits) in causing poverty. These different views about cause imply different political remedies for the problems of poverty and inequality.

Pensioner poverty

In 2016, about 14 per cent of pensioners lived in poverty, a marked decline since 1997 (JRF, 2016). The risk of living in poverty increases with age, and is greater for people over 75 than for younger pensioners. Women on their own over pensionable age are more likely to live in poverty than couples. For any specific single pensioner, the risk of low income does not rise with age, but the proportion of single pensioners rises with age, and in general single pensioners are more likely to be poor. For a pensioner couple the risk of low income does rise with age. The lower wealth of older pensioners is partly a 'cohort' effect rather than a pure 'ageing' effect – as time has passed, a greater proportion of the population have owned their own house, so fewer older pensioners than younger pensioners have this investment (JRF, 2016).

As is the case with so many factors considered in this book, the experience of life is not determined by poverty or other social circumstances – a full understanding has to include the influence of culture, individual makeup and individual 'agency'. But to think that these override the importance of social factors is to misunderstand human experience.

Effects of poverty

Poverty has both immediate and long-term effects. Childhood poverty is associated with lower educational achievement and leaving home early. Young women are more likely to have children early. When they grow up, children from poorer families are more likely to be out of work and to have children with similar disadvantages to those which they suffered (Stewart and Vaitilingam, 2004: 15; Smallwood and Wilson, 2007). Pensioner income 'is highly reflective of *financial* circumstances earlier in life'. Poor people die younger, enjoy poorer health and make less use of health services than richer people.

VIOLENCE

Violence is a significant feature in the experience of many people who use social work services. This may be because they have had to live with violence or because they themselves are violent and dangerous. It may be because they have been involved in war or communal violence, in which one section of a population seeks to harm or exterminate another.

Violence in intimate relationships – across the lifespan

Violence instils fear, it evokes the urge to retaliate, and it damages self-esteem. Thus, in the first place, children subjected to abuse by adult caregivers are made frightened of the very person who should provide comfort when they are threatened. Second, they may either fight back at the time, often putting themselves in further danger, or they may suppress the anger they feel, turning it on themselves or letting it out in other settings (they may come to have an expectation of criticism or harshness from other adult figures). And third, they may internalise the message that their feelings are disposable, or that there is something wrong about them – perhaps that they must always control their feelings for fear of being hurt and despised, that it is safest to be subservient and unassertive. The experience of violence is a risk factor for adult mental health problems (Rogers and Pilgrim, 2003: 113). It is perhaps worth emphasising that for most of the childhood victims of attack met by social workers, the violence is not a one-off event, or even a series of events, but one manifestation of a lack of care about the child – the opposite of mind-mindedness, attunement. So research about later effects cannot disentangle the two.

There is a discussion of child abuse in Chapter 3, and intimate violence in Chapter 6.

The many forms of destructiveness in close relationships are interlinked and while different terms have their merits – 'domestic abuse', 'violence against women', 'emotional abuse', 'child abuse', 'sexual or physical abuse' – they can sometimes be misleading by identifying a situation by one component only, or by focusing the hearer's attention in a selective way. Words used to characterise the people concerned can create similar problems – 'perpetrator', 'victim', 'abused child' can partialise a person's qualities and experience and homogenise them with other people who are very different. Chapter 6 referred to statistics about the extent of domestic abuse.

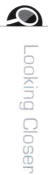

Definitions of 'abuse' are used for different purposes:

- for research;
- for criminal investigations and convictions;
- for statutory data collection;
- for social work practice and educational discussions.

The different purposes can produce different statistics about the prevalence of abuse. Why might definitions used for research and for criminal investigations be different, and why would they produce different indications of the prevalence of abuse?

Response: Criminal investigations are based on the exact wording and purpose of the law. Statistics require victims to have come forward to the police, but the threat of further abuse and dependence of the victim on the abuser may make this impossible. Research, on the other hand, will use the definitions appropriate for its study – it may be seeking to establish if there is abuse which is not defined as a crime by the law; it may be using anonymous self-reports by victims or abusers to investigate the extent of abuse which is not reported. For these and other reasons it will produce different results from crime figures.

Domestic violence and abuse is currently defined by the UK government as 'any incident or pattern of incidents of controlling, coercive, threatening behaviour, violence or abuse between those aged 16 or over who are, or have been, intimate partners or family members regardless of gender or sexuality' (Home Office, 2016). The five main forms of abuse are psychological, physical, sexual, financial and emotional abuse.

Violence committed by a perpetrator towards a partner's children is likely to be intrinsically damaging. This violence hurts the partner emotionally, and has the effect of putting her or him in an impossible psychological position, in which self-respect as a parent is compromised.

From a child's point of view, violence towards their parent is intrinsically hurtful. As child protection guidance (DfE, 2015c) points out, it should also

Reflective thinking

- What might be the impact on an individual if their partner beats their child?
- Why might they stay with the partner?

Chapter 6

alert workers to the possibility that there may be direct violence towards the child. Attempts by a child to intervene to protect the mother increase the child's risk of injury (Rogers and Pilgrim, 2003: 146).

In Chapter 6, the gendered nature of domestic abuse was discussed. It is a social problem of enormous proportions. Over 100 women are likely to be killed by their partners in the UK each year (Brennan, 2016). Besides the physical damage and pain it causes, domestic abuse brings misery to all members of a family. Approximately one in five children (18 per cent) have been exposed to domestic and family violence by the time they are 18 years old (Radford et al., 2011).

In adult intimate relationships, it is abuse towards women in hetero-sexual partnerships that has traditionally received the most attention, but there is growing evidence of abuse experienced by other groups. Stonewall, the organisation for lesbian, gay, bi and trans people, state that their research found that one in four lesbian and bisexual women have experienced domestic abuse in a relationship (Stonewall, 2018). Two-thirds of those say the perpetrator was a woman, a third a man. Almost half (49 per cent) of all gay and bisexual men have experienced at least one incident of domestic abuse from a family member or partner since the age of 16 (Stonewall, 2018).

In a survey conducted by the Scottish Transgender Alliance (2010), 80 per cent of respondents stated that they had experienced emotionally, sexually, or physically abusive behaviour by a partner or ex-partner. They conclude that this would suggest a prevalence rate of domestic abuse that is higher than among any other section of the population.

Older people

The issue of violence towards older people by their caregivers has received more attention in the last couple of decades. Overall prevalence studies indicate that approximately 6 per cent of older persons in the community are likely to have experienced significant abuse in the last month (Cooper et al., 2008). A systematic review of forty-nine studies of elder abuse (Johannesen and Logiudice, 2013) identified the following risk factors:

- Elder person: cognitive impairment, behavioural problems, psychiatric illness or psychological problems, functional dependency, poor physical health or frailty, low income or wealth, trauma or past abuse, and ethnicity.

■ Perpetrator: caregiver burden or stress, and psychiatric illness or psychological problems.
■ Relationship: family disharmony, poor or conflictual relationships.
■ Environment: low social support, and living with others.

War and communal violence

At the other end of the social range from domestic abuse is the public violence experienced in war. Civilian populations through the ages have feared war, but in the twentieth century the terrorisation of civilians became a systematic strategy, an industrialisation of killing and bodily damage which reached into a large proportion of homes on the planet. This experience, either directly (as in the case of young people such as 'Vivian' in Chapter 4, or the current users of older people's services) or indirectly through relatives, will have touched the lives of many users of social work services.

Chapter 4

In any population, the 'cohort effect' of the experience of war is strong. In the UK, some 870,000 British men died in the First World War, and in the 1921 census there was a surplus of 1.7 million women over men. In 1945, as the result of two bombs alone which brought the war to an end, Pilgrim and Rogers quote that over a third of a million people died in Japan, some of them dying lingering deaths. In Northern Ireland's sectarian conflicts, or in Uganda's ethnic cleansing, generations of children have grown up with violent death, barbaric retribution, and hatred between communities as part of the public landscape. This picture seems remarkably widespread in human society. The more far-reaching effects of public violence last long after the immediate physical damage.

When traumatising violence ends, one possible self-preserving human response is to emotionally lock the experience away, and avoid recollections that bring back the unmanageable memories. This can apply both to children who were abused and to soldiers in battle situations. Years later, in order to feel understood, the person may wish to raise this part of their life without going into detail, or may need to talk much more specifically, sometimes graphically. This can arise particularly when these experiences are reawakened by later, deeply emotional events (such as the illness of a child or the death of a partner).

In these circumstances, social workers need the skill to be able to listen without prying, and to respond therapeutically at the level needed by the individual. This response will sometimes be a dispassionate but concerned and attentive listening. At other times it may involve an overtly emotional interaction. The response may be appropriately contained within a single meeting, or may require further contact in order to be handled in a developmentally helpful way. It may combine practical help, social intervention and emotional support. It is similar to other activities in which the social worker explicitly offers a relationship to attend to the after-effects of earlier trauma (Howe, 2008; Sudbery, 2002). This is sometimes described as using 'counselling skills' but is more appropriately understood as 'therapeutic social work', a psychosocial intervention with a long tradition.

?

This section has focused on the destructive effect of violence. A female university graduate, now a professional 'cage fighter', said reflectively in a radio interview that she thinks there is an intrinsic human pleasure in inflicting violence. This may be a very frightening, disturbing thought for you.

Do you agree? What are some of the sources of human violence and destructiveness as you understand them?

MENTAL HEALTH

To understand development is to understand the unfolding sequence of a person's life – of biological expression, of cognitions, emotions and other components of states of mind, and of external social experience. Problems in adult mental health require a range of factors to be taken into account.

■ *Social construction:* societies and groups within society interpret the issues in different ways.
■ *Genetics:* there is good evidence that one factor in a number of mental health problems is the unfolding of genetic makeup.
■ *Other biological factors* may be at work which are not known to have a specific genetic origin. For example, Alzheimer's disease is a form of dementia found mainly in older people and is caused by problems in neural pathways in the brain, resulting in the death of brain cells. Epilepsy similarly has a biological cause, and illustrates how conditions may be described at different times as the province of psychiatry or of neurology, both disciplines which are concerned with the functioning of the brain (see Corr, 2006: chs 14–16).
■ Often, as is thought to be the case with schizophrenia, a problem in mental health arises when a raised genetic risk combines with predisposing environmental experience in earlier life (adversity such as poverty or abuse) and a present-day precipitating factor (such as domestic abuse or other social stress).
■ *Childhood suffering* and the experience of neglect, abuse or other adversity increase the likelihood of some kinds of mental distress in adulthood.
■ *Other aspects of early experience:* behaviourists (Chapter 3 and 'Essential background', section 8) believe that some forms of disorder are accounted for by early conditioning – the forms of behaviour and thought patterns that have been reinforced; attachment theorists refer aspects of adult experience back to aspects of early attachment relationships or their absence (Chapter 2 and 'Essential background', section 2); and psychoanalytic thinkers place an emphasis on early relational processes as underlying later psychological experience (Chapter 2 and 'Essential background', section 4).

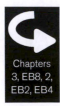

Chapters
3, EB8, 2,
EB2, EB4

■ *Victimisation and trauma:* first formulated as 'shell shock' affecting soldiers in the First World War, much more is now understood about post-traumatic stress disorder (PTSD). Also, many of the 'symptoms' typical of institutionalised patients in long-stay institutions such as psychiatric hospitals and asylums are the responses to oppressive institutional regimes ('institutional neurosis').

The experience of mental distress and mental disorder

To some degree, everyone experiences emotional disturbances such as anxiety, anger or depression. Sometimes, you may feel the emotional response is relatively appropriate – anxiety about a court appearance; depression following a loss or separation; or anger at being attacked. At other times, in retrospect (or observing similar emotions in someone else) the emotions will seem out of proportion to the external reality – though not, of course, to the internal reality of the individual. The anxiety may turn out to be 'all over nothing'; anxiety when there was no real cause to be fearful. Anger may be 'misplaced' and out of proportion to the precipitating event. Depression may just 'arrive', seeming to have no particular 'cause'. These are all universal experiences.

Psychiatry is the medical discipline concerned with the origins and treatment of emotional disorder and 'abnormal states of mind'. A distinction you will come across, though it is somewhat dated, is that between **neuroses** and **psychoses**.

The distinction is not clear-cut and professionals from different disciplines (psychiatry, sociology, psychology, social work and philosophy) have very different understanding about what is being described when psychiatrists make a diagnosis. However, in a rough and ready way neuroses may be thought of as exaggerated versions of the universal emotions described above – anxiety which persistently interferes with normal day-to-day life; depression that doesn't lift (interfering with sleep, appetite and sex drive); or the excessive, repetitive need to perform rituals and check, clean, or wash in order to keep anxiety at bay (Horrobin, 2002: 157; Corr, 2006: 405; Rogers and Pilgrim, 2003). We can all understand these as extreme versions of familiar feelings. Psychoses, on the other hand, using the same broad definition, involve experiences that do not seem continuous with everyday worries. Schizophrenia is an example of psychosis. Its active phase may include delusions, hallucinations, speech and thought disorder, and feelings of persecution (American Psychiatric Association, 2013).

This distinction does not minimise the suffering experienced in neurosis, which may disable people in their day-to-day life. 'The onset of my neurosis was marked by levels of physical anxiety that I would not have thought possible', wrote a professor of psychology. 'If one is involved in a road accident, there is a delay of a second or two and then the pit of the stomach seems to fall out and one's legs go like jelly. It was this feeling multiplied a hundredfold that seized me all hours of the day and night' (Sutherland, 1998: 2, quoted in Corr, 2006: 413).

The *Schizophrenia Bulletin* is a research journal that sometimes carries personal accounts. Here David Zelt, a regular scientific contributor to the journal, gives his own account of a psychotic episode, written in the third person to convey a sense of psychological distance:

> A drama that profoundly transformed David Zelt began at a conference on human psychology. David respected the speakers as scholars and wanted their approval of a paper he had written about telepathy . . . David knew that the paper, in reflecting engagement with an esoteric subject, was a signpost of his growing retreat from mundane reality.
>
> David's paper was viewed as a monumental contribution to the conference and potentially to psychology in general . . . his concept of telepathy might have as much influence as the basic ideas of Darwin and Freud.
>
> Each speaker focused on David. By using allusions and non-verbal communications that included pointing and glancing, each illuminated different aspects of David's contribution. Although his name was never mentioned, the speakers enticed David into feeling that he had accomplished something supernatural with his paper . . .
>
> David was described as having a halo around his head, and the second coming was announced as forthcoming. Messianic feelings took hold of him. His mission would be to aid the poor and needy, especially in underdeveloped countries . . .
>
> Several hundred people at the conference were talking about David. He was the subject of enormous mystery, profound in his silence . . . [Over the next few weeks] it dawned on David that the CIA was listening to most of his thoughts wherever he went, even sometimes during sleep . . . Because his thoughts were broadcast around him, David often felt that his consciousness was controlled from outside himself.
>
> (1981, quoted in Horrobin, 2002: 138)

Sometimes, mental health problems involve one aspect which is diagnosed by psychiatrists as a medical condition, and another which is not. Some people who are diagnosed with neurotic or psychotic mental illness, for example, are also misusing alcohol or drugs. Studies quoted by Rogers and Pilgrim (2003: 151–155) show that these people are more likely than others to be involved in violence after discharge from mental health services. These situations are commonly referred to as 'dual diagnosis'. Mental health services may also be responsible for services to people who misuse drugs but have no mental illness. The services are also concerned (particularly in relation to control rather than treatment) with people who are deemed to have mental disorders such as antisocial personality disorder (psychopathic personality) which are not regarded by psychiatrists as treatable illnesses.

The term 'dual diagnosis' is also used in relation to people with learning disabilities who have mental health problems. A learning disability does not, in itself, cause mental distress or personality disorder. Nor does it 'get better'; it is not an illness. People with learning disabilities can experience difficulties in understanding new or complex information, and take longer to learn than other people. As discussed later in the chapter, the term 'learning difficulty' is currently the term preferred by many service users. 'Learning difficulty' is also, however, the term used by people who have no intellectual impairment but have specific difficulties in learning (such as dyslexia). The 'Taking it further' section of this chapter analyses how many of the difficulties experienced by people with learning disabilities are the product of social arrangements. It is estimated that the prevalence of mental health problems amongst adults with a learning disability is approximately 40 per cent (McCarron et al., 2011).

Social features of mental distress

The personal accounts given above were both written by professional people. We do not know their personal histories. But a large number of people with psychiatric diagnoses have not had access to further or higher education, face current social adversity, and have experienced trauma during their childhood (Rogers and Pilgrim, 2003: 18, 25, see also 108–167).

There is a paradox about the sociology of mental illness compared with the sociology of physical illness. There has been extensive examination of the question whether mental health problems reflect social processes or medical conditions; nevertheless, the understanding of how social class and social causes relate to physical illness is in fact much more advanced (Rogers and Pilgrim, 2003: 24). Research does not fully resolve the resulting debates in relation to mental health, but has led to an ever-increasing body of findings and analysis allowing for complex and competing interpretations. At its simplest, the statistical association of mental illness with social adversity – with poverty and social exclusion, for example – can be described as having three explanations.

The first explanation is that mental ill health may be caused by poverty, stress, poor environment and housing. One important implication, if this is correct, is that ameliorating the stressful conditions, or preventing the occurrence of stress in childhood, will lower the incidence of mental health problems in the population.

The second, almost opposite, explanation is that people with mental health problems are more likely to be found in poor and stressful environments because that is where their difficulties cause them to live. If this is so, there may be other reasons to improve such conditions, but it will not necessarily reduce the occurrence of mental illness.

And third, there may be an independent factor that is associated both with areas of poverty and deprivation and with mental health. Contentiously, genes have been suggested, or cultural behaviours alleged to be associated with communities in poverty (such as poor antenatal care, or rigid emotional behaviour and outlook).

A moment's thought will tell you that these explanations can be associated with particular political ideas – the first is emphasised by those concerned about the adverse effects of exclusion and deprivation, and by people who emphasise how life is shaped by social forces beyond the control of the individual. Those who emphasise that people's position in society is related to their individual qualities and behaviours will be drawn to the second and third, as will those right-wing political philosophies which believe that some people and groups are superior to others.

Another aspect of social debate concerns the rates of 'service' among different groups of people. Higher rates of diagnosis and treatment are not always interpreted as signs of better health provision and social inclusion. This is because, unlike in most areas of physical medicine, there is what Rogers and Pilgrim describe as a 'treatment-coercion gradient' in mental health. High rates of attention to postnatal depression in prosperous suburbs may imply good attention to the well-being of new mothers, but high rates of schizophrenia diagnoses in an inner-city black population may imply greater levels of state control and coercion, because schizophrenia is associated with compulsory removal of freedom and enforced medication. One concern of those who contest the medical model of psychiatry is that different rates of diagnosis between different social groups (men and women, or African Caribbean and white European men) reflect differences in how social behaviour is interpreted rather than differences in mental disturbance.

Services offered – and experiences following the diagnosis of a mental disorder

Many people diagnosed with anxiety or depression find that these problems spontaneously lessen (Andrews, 2001). In a medical model, this does not necessarily mean that the problem has been 'cured' – Andrews argues that it should potentially be assessed as 'in remission'. Neither does it mean that there is no need for assistance during the episode.

Chapter 3

The largest proportion of people diagnosed with a mental disorder will receive service from '**primary healthcare**' such as their family doctor and the related provision (Rippon, 2004). They may receive a prescribed course of drugs or services such as counselling or CBT – cognitive behavioural therapy (see Chapter 3). They will continue living at home, and experience only small disruption to their lifestyle.

Those seen by the specialist mental health services (initially by a psychiatrist) are more likely to experience marked changes in their social and life circumstances. A significant number will take part in self-help groups or use activities and services provided by voluntary organisations (such as Mind or facilities for specific ethnic groups) – sometimes, since these are user-led, becoming a service provider as well as a service user. Staff from the mainstream services will value and support these opportunities, but voluntary organisations are frequently critical of the services provided by national and local government. Bamber (2004) discusses the range of service-user organisations, their relationship with state psychiatric services and their role in raising debates about the nature and treatment of mental health problems.

After being diagnosed by a psychiatrist, people should find that the facilities to be made available to them are organised under the Care Programme Approach (CPA). This sets out where they are likely to be seen and by whom; which hospital inpatient or outpatient or community-based services are offered and who will be involved.

For people with severe conditions, an episode in hospital may at first be frightening. Sometimes it becomes a place they can trust, or they may continue to be alarmed at the variety of people they meet, the lack of control, the unpredictability of other people's behaviour and the difficulties of sharing accommodation with other patients. Bamber (2004: 184) points out that many people in the service-user movement prefer the term 'survivor'. This is not only because they regard themselves as survivors of acute mental distress, but also 'because it acknowledges the ordeal they have experienced with services'.

For many, maintaining a positive life in the community (that is, not in hospital) depends on taking regular medication, and having this checked at regular intervals. Patients are likely to have mixed feelings about their medication. Although medication enables them to 'get by', they often dislike its side effects or the sense that their feelings, their 'self', are controlled by drugs. Some, particularly in the service-user movements, may regard it as part of the inappropriate pathologising and medicalisation of life problems.

For some, their life may feel (and be regarded by others) like a deterioration, a part of destruction and decline. But many others will feel that, although unwished for, their difficulties have enriched their understanding of life and of themselves. They can take pride in overcoming something that many other people do not have to:

> My perception of myself and the world around me has almost completely reversed. I have abilities now that as far as I was concerned those years ago did not exist. I have uncovered creative thinking and abilities that I did not have or were buried . . . I can say, and do, that Manic Depression is not an illness, on the contrary it was for me a fundamental part of my growth process.
>
> (Myerscough 1981: 134, as quoted in Allott, 2004)

At the opposite end of the spectrum to these comments about the enriching effects of mental illness on life, for approximately 5,500 people aged 15 and over in the UK each year, the mental distress ends in suicide (ONS, 2017). Of these, around three-quarters of all suicides are male and suicide is the most common cause of death for young men. This is a changing picture, as suicide rates generally fell between 1981 and 2007 and then increased to a peak in 2013. However, the 2013 peak was substantially less than the rates in the 1980s and 1990s (ONS, 2017a).

In this area, as in all others, social workers deal not just with the individual experience of mental distress, but with its causes and effects in the social network. These require a perspective of what has happened before the social worker's involvement and sensitivity to the need for continuing tactful attention afterwards. In an appeal leaflet, the Mental Health Foundation quotes the words of a 12-year-old boy:

> I was nine when it happened. I'd been at a sleepover and I still remember the terrible atmosphere in the house when I walked in. My mum told me dad had taken a lot of tablets in the night to try and kill himself.
>
> (Mental Health Foundation, undated)

Some mental health problems are caused by brain deterioration and (at the moment) are irreversible. Alzheimer's disease and other dementias may involve a progressive loss of self in older people – as painful for those around them as for the person themselves. This is a fictionalised version of the words of a woman who spoke to me about an incident involving her husband:

> We had our ups and downs like any couple, but I had shared decades of my life with him, and we loved each other. As his dementia developed, the man I had loved was taken away from me in a confusing and disturbing way. When it became too much, I gave up my work as a social worker to care for him. After he went into [a home], I put myself out to make sure I visited him constantly, with all that entailed. Then one time the staff told me (I think they thought it was amusing) that he had taken a fancy to another resident, Clare. I had given up my life for him and I saw him fawning over her, being sweet and charming and flirtatious, and he didn't even acknowledge me. I felt murderous hatred, that he should take me so for granted, show me no feeling, and offer his affections to another woman in front of me after all I did for him and all we had together.

Chapter 8

Equally, however, many problems in cognitive functioning and mood in later life – such as depression, which affects one in five older people (Mental Health Foundation, 2016) – are responsive to drug treatment or nutrition, to psychological techniques such as memory training, or to attention to social problems. This is discussed more in Chapter 8.

The 2014 Adult Psychiatric Morbidity Survey highlights that every week, one in six adults experiences symptoms of a mental health problem (McManus et al., 2016). Mental health statistics contain many ambiguities as they attempt to reduce problems in social life to numbers, but you are certain to encounter the issues for individuals and families in your work. There are constant developments in the field, and areas about which you will discover more detail in your specialist studies and continuing practice are:

■ Psychiatric perspectives, the medical approach to diagnosis and treat-ment (in more detail appropriate to your work or level of study).
■ More details about the debates relating to mental health – the oppos-ing accounts of what mental illness is, differing views on its causation, including the social origins of mental distress, and the place of social inequality (Wilson et al., 2011).
■ The service-user movement and organisations.

- The role of the social worker in providing an emotionally therapeutic and developmental experience (Firth et al., 2004; Howe, 2008; Sudbery, 2002; Wilson et al., 2011).
- Policy development as it affects social workers.
- Assessment and other practice procedures in mental health – attending to needs, rights and risks.

When someone reveals that they are receiving psychiatric treatment, they have to deal with many prejudices and inaccurate expectations. Even when they do not experience direct discrimination, the fear of discrimination can be distressing for people experiencing mental health difficulties (Green et al., 2003). In some contexts it will raise questions about whether they are 'normal', whether they are safe to be near children, or whether they are violent. One way of describing this is to say their social identity has been 'spoilt'. To have a 'spoilt identity' has many consequences. It exposes the individual to prejudice (essentially the same word as 'prejudgement') and it may mean the individual has to deal with fear, discrimination in practical and financial matters, and physical attack. The next section of this chapter is concerned with 'spoilt identity'.

IDENTITY, PREJUDICE AND STIGMA

Everyone is entitled to be proud of themselves. They have a right to a self-image which reflects their actual abilities, potential and value – their value as a human being. This view of themselves should include their feelings and aspirations, valuing their good points and their special individual worth. It should leave them secure in their entitlement to the same rights as everyone else.

But you will have realised in reading this book that for many people, social attitudes, prejudgements, ideas of what is 'good', 'moral' or 'normal' make this hard to achieve.

Identity – different approaches

In the social work literature, you will find the term 'identity' used in two ways. The personal 'sense of identity' is something psychological, enabling the individual to have a clear view of themselves independently of, and sometimes in opposition to, outside forces. A 'social identity', on the other hand, is created from the outside, by conventional, cultural and historical expectations and divisions. In using the term, most people will recognise that both meanings are relevant.

When a newly qualified person says, 'I'm still coming to terms with my identity as a social worker', both aspects are in play. The two aspects interact; people can place themselves deliberately into a particular social identity, as when a gay man decides to be out to his family, friends and colleagues, or a social worker from an Asian family can decide before going to court whether to wear a business suit and accessories which will blend in, 'pass' with 'white' colleagues, or to wear a sari, hairstyle and make-up which will identify her socially as 'Asian'. Equally, the 'psychological' aspect of identity is heavily influenced by the social attributions from others. Cooley (1902) coined the phrase 'looking-glass self' to describe the way in which the sense of self is created out of the 'reflections' received from others. Bilton quotes G. H. Mead's concept of the 'I' and the 'me' to represent respectively the impulse to act socially and the social identity that is formed through social action. Individuals differ in the degree to which they are influenced by others' attributions, and there are profound disagreements between theorists about the relationship between the social and the individual (see Bilton, 2002: 501–506, 528–531).

Among those who emphasise the social creation of the self are 'role theorists' (Biddle, 1979; Goffman, 1959/2008) who point out that a person's identity is always structured by their relations to those around them – parents, siblings, partners, employers, social 'location'. A 'role' is defined as a 'set of mutual expectations', and 'role conflict' occurs when the expectations of different roles are incompatible. For example, it was suggested in the last chapter that the roles of parent, partner and employee are likely to contain more contradictory expectations for women than for men. The usefulness of role theory is illustrated by the way it describes the effect on men of becoming unemployed (they lose a major role in their life) or of a woman becoming a mother (she gains a new role and a new identity). The criticisms come from those (such as Raffel, 1999) who argue that some of the major role theorists leave no room for the 'self' at all; it is as if they see the person as solely created by the social roles they enact.

'**Postmodernists**' also emphasise the social creation of the 'self'. They regard 'personal identity' as much more flexible and fluid than previous theorists acknowledged: 'There is no self behind the mask'; the individual is the sum of their performances. Earlier generations might have looked upon a stable and consistent sense of self as a sign of maturity, with qualities similar to those listed by Maslow as characterising the 'fully achieving person' (see Chapter 5). A person with a changing identity might perhaps have been seen as 'still trying to find himself', but this strand of 'postmodern' thinking sees personal and social identity as always open to transformation and personal redefinition – there is no such thing as a core 'self', and a consistent sense of identity is largely an illusion. One positive effect of this view is to undermine the rigidity of certain identities that are couched in terms of binary opposites – hetero-/homosexual, sane/mad, indigenous/foreign – which have always been troublesome for those who do not fit the social categories.

Chapter 5

Prejudice – examples

Some people have a harder task than others dealing with social expectations directed at them. There are numerous 'out-groups' who are subject to the threat of a negative social identity. The discrimination they face may be subtle or hidden in some areas and open, even directly dangerous, in others. The following paragraphs refer to some of the issues in relation to ethnicity, sexual orientation and learning disabilities.

Tajfel (with Turner, 1982) argues that people form identities by means of the membership of a social group. They exaggerate differences with those in the 'out-group'. They gain positive self-concept by valuing the in-group and devaluing the out-group (forming hostile expectations of them). Ward and colleagues (2001) argue that in relation to ethnicity, this process takes place within both the majority and minority group. However, the impact bears more heavily on the out-group since members will be constantly negotiating with the power of the majority.

Phinney's research about the experiences of African American and Native American teenagers (Phinney and Rosenthal, 1992) led her to suggest a model of stages through which people form an identity as a member of a minority ethnic grouping. The first stage is an *unexamined ethnic identity*, during which they may unquestioningly take views which are explicit or implicit in surrounding culture – that black men are sporty, UK politicians are white, and so on. To the degree that these are negative they may not realise they are part of the negative group, or there may be disconnects between different aspects. Issues come more into conscious focus with the greater cognitive ability in adolescence: 'the young African American may learn as a child that black is beautiful, but conclude as an adolescent that white is powerful' (Spencer and Dornbusch, 1990: 131, as quoted by Boyd and Bee, 2015). The second stage is of *ethnic identity search*, often triggered by some experience which makes thought about perceived ethnicity unavoidable – perhaps an experience of abuse or discrimination. Finally, Phinney identified that men and women in minority ethnic groups achieve *secure ethnic identity*. For some, this is an ability to live in a bicultural way, which her research found to characterise high achievers with high self-esteem and good interpersonal relations. For others it may be a strong single cultural identification, even if this means some practical losses because the person excludes themselves from the dominant culture and proclaims an identity which attracts discrimination and hostility.

'Sexual identity' and 'sexual orientation' are conceptualised in many different ways. We have discussed the work of Freud (Chapter 6 and 'Essential background', section 4), which has left a legacy of seeing sexuality as a central aspect of ourselves. This legacy was criticised by feminist scholars in the 1970s for depicting masculine traits as being overwhelmingly dominant over women's (Dunk-West and Hafford-Letchfield, 2016). The work of the French philosopher Michel Foucault has been influential in scholarly thinking about sexuality along with others within queer theory (Butler, 1990, 1993). Whilst Foucault focused upon the wider social level, Butler argues that it is within individual boundaries that we subvert and re-make the categories of gender and sexuality that may seem 'innate' (Dunk-West and Hafford-Letchfield, 2016).

Chapter 6

Morrow and Messinger (2006: 4), in a volume intended for social workers, state that 'sexual orientation' is a preferred term to 'sexual preference' because the latter implies too much of a willed choice, in contrast to what is experienced as the 'innate essence of their affectional nature'. They describe that the choice available is whether to embrace or reject their essential orientation. As discussed in Chapter 6, Lisa Diamond's ten-year longitudinal study (2008) led her to conclude that 'sexual orientation' does not feel 'chosen' by women, does not feel like a decision. But she also concluded that, in contrast to typical male experience, it does not determine specific sexual desire, affectional impulses and sexual behaviour, which arise out of strongly situational and interpersonal factors rather than gender categories. In a social world of 'compulsory heterosexuality', in a context 'of cultural denial, distorted stereotypes, rejection, neglect, harassment, and sometimes outright victimisation and abuse' which complicates attachment relationships (Tharinger and Wells, 2000: 159, quoted in Morrow and Messinger, 2006), different people face different challenges in establishing a sexual identity.

In forming an identity as a gay man or lesbian, a person confronts some people's expectations of 'normality'. What is experienced differs between individuals, between men and women, and between decades and cultures. There are issues at the interpersonal level, issues to do with cultural views which colour anonymous interactions and dealings with organisations, there are practical issues of finance and personal safety, and there are issues which have mainly to be addressed at the political level. Examples of the first include managing conversations with friends and family members. The second includes dealing with false expectations, ignorance or prejudice in work encounters, or dealing with other organisations such as health services. Practical issues include gaining adequate rights as 'next of kin' to a partner, or pensions, or issues of personal safety from attack. And all people who have a classification which gives them a 'spoiled identity' are ultimately involved in problems which require a political remedy, ensuring rights, protection and equality. In Chapter 4, we discussed the prejudice and discrimination experienced by transgender people whose gender identity differs from what is normative for their biological sex in a particular time and culture.

As you might expect, researchers have proposed stage models of how a gay, lesbian, bisexual or transgender identity develops. Some regard the word 'phase' as more appropriate because it does not suggest some universal sequence. In discussing the developmental pathways in becoming a lesbian parent, Morningstar (1999) refers to 'components' of a process rather than 'stages'. Morrow and Messinger (2006: 86, 96) summarise a total of ten models in diagrammatic form. Morrow concentrates particularly on Cass's six-stage model which incorporates pressures from both outside society and internal dynamics. She portrays a movement of *identity change* (starting with 'identity confusion') in which a previously held view of sexual identity based on surrounding social messages about the universal self has to be replaced by a clear homosexual identity. The model is based on the idea that development occurs when the self-experience is made to be congruent with the environment. In this view a homosexual identity has to involve 'the presentation of a homosexual self-image to both homosexual and heterosexual others' (Morrow and Messinger, 2006: 24, quoting Cass, 1984). For

Healy (1999), the issue is less clear-cut – she takes it as given that every day there are conscious or unconscious decisions about concealment or self-disclosure.

Morrow and Messinger propose guidelines for good practice throughout their book, including work related to the ongoing process of identity formation throughout the life course, and work with older gay and lesbian people. In relation to adults they list risk factors such as emotional distress, isolation, depression, violence, suicide and family conflict (several studies found that one of the most distressing experiences of gay and lesbian identity formation is loss of parental affection and support). Protective factors include positive and supportive family relationships, strong self-esteem, stable intellectual functioning, special talent (for example, musical or athletic) and supportive friendships – and in adolescents, supportive school relationships.

Spoiled identity

Erving Goffman (1959/2008) studied how people's identity can be defined by those with power over them, and how the individual's actions are then interpreted through this definition of their identity. He paid particular attention to people in prison and mental hospitals, noting how the inmates acquired a despised and low status identity in society. He used the phrase 'spoilt identity' to describe this. This research tradition did not look at these aspects of life from the point of view of those in power who ascribe the identity (the psychiatrist diagnosing the 'mental illness' or the court convicting a 'criminal') but from the point of view of those who find themselves on the receiving end of the judgements.

To a degree, as Goffman points out (1963/1990: 152), social interaction always involves managing aspects of spoilt identity. Everyone has to form an identity in the face of social disapproval from significant cultural groups about some of their qualities and attributes. This section has singled out a few examples for comment, because it is in the nature of social work that most service users experience these issues intensively – as children in care, parents of children in care, adults with learning disability, older people, and so on.

Goffman described several ways in which people cope with the dangers that come with being allocated a 'spoilt identity' in society. Some *conceal* the qualities which give rise to it. For example, during racist segregation in the USA, a large number of adults defined by the state as 'negro' achieved entry to legal and other professions by 'passing' as white people, often claiming Mediterranean ancestry; gay and lesbian young people may find it safer to pass as 'straight'. Others respond with defiance and challenge, and others with irony, as in the self-attribution of 'nigger' and 'queer'. The chosen name of a campaigning mental health group, 'Mad Women' (Ryan and Pritchard, 2004: 198), combines irony with defiance. Tajfel and Turner (1982) reported a similar range of strategies individuals use to combat threats to their identity, but also included 'leaving the group'. They highlight the importance of group strategies, where a group changes its social identity. These can be positive, as when it challenges the negative valuation and asserts its members' pride in themselves. On the other hand, they can have further negative effects – as when the 'out-group' chooses a different, more disadvantaged group for comparison, and gains positive valuation by disparaging this more vulnerable group. An example occurs when people with milder learning disability gain status in an institution by devaluing those with severe disability. Goffman highlights that a secure reference group is important in supporting identity formation in the face of cultural condemnation.

Within each of the examples there are wide differences in social experiences depending on age, gender, social context and generation – in most cases, there is no single pattern that applies across individuals, or to both sexes, or in different decades, even though in an intellectual way we can abstract some common features.

The next chapter looks at the experience of older people. One distinctive feature of the management of spoilt identity in relation to older people is that the individual is entering an identity towards which they themselves have been prejudiced in the past. The chapter will refer to research which shows that this complicates the process of positive identity formation and has negative physical and psychological implications.

In summary, for the purposes of understanding development through the life course, we can identify four areas in which a social worker has to understand the implications of stigma and spoiled identity:

■ Identity development and identity change through the life course – a perspective on the evolution and modification of a person's social and psychological identity.
■ The management of that identity in personal interactions – the constant pressures of what Goffman describes as 'information management' and 'image management'.
■ The practical implications for finance, safety and freedom.
■ The role of social and political action which is necessary to change the social value assigned to the group.

The anti-oppressive value base of social work makes it a responsibility not only to understand these issues, but also to be active in undermining the stigma and prejudice with which they are associated.

?

Reflective thinking

Consider yourself or someone to whom you provide service in order to discuss:

■ In what ways has it been hard to form a positive social identity because of negative attitudes, misinformation or negative views spread by opinion formers?

- In what ways is this 'same' prejudice different for people brought up in a different decade or in a different culture/nationality?
- In what ways does this person have privilege compared with others? (What stigma do they not have to cope with, and are there any ways in which they contribute to the stigma of others?)

It is relevant to the subject itself, as well as being necessary for personal comfort, to note that some aspects of what is relevant to this discussion have to remain private.

PEOPLE WITH LEARNING DISABILITIES

The concluding section of this chapter, 'Taking it further', is about people with learning disabilities. They may face a particular challenge in forming a personal identity which matches the label and categorisation applied to them:

'I won't think of meself as a learning disability. But I have.'

These were the words of a member of a self-advocacy group which campaigns for rights and recognition for people with learning disabilities. They are quoted by Suzie Beart (Beart et al., 2004, see also Beart, 2005). They illustrate how difficult it is for someone to identify themselves as having a learning disability. She quotes Davies and Jenkins' research (1997) which found that only 28 per cent accepted it as applying to themselves, while 30 per cent gave a definition which specifically excluded themselves. When Beart discussed people's reactions to being asked whether they had learning disabilities, one respondent put it like this: 'It would upset them and they would feel scared.' People First, a self-advocacy organisation which acts as adviser and research partner for official bodies, describes its members as experiencing 'learning difficulties' compared with other people, and adopts this as a description.

People with a learning disability may understand that they live in a house for people with learning disabilities, but not identify themselves as within that classification. According to Beart's study, they may understand at the level of lived experience that they experience discrimination, need assistance to do certain things that others do unaided, and take longer to learn, but do not identify themselves as part of the group of people described as having a learning disability. Some resolve this by identifying themselves as having a learning difficulty, but others feel they are advocating for a group with which they do not identify.

The final section of the chapter moves on from issues about personal identity and self-description to a broader look at the social influences on the development of people with learning disabilities. The subject illustrates how, in anti-discriminatory practice, the personal, the organisational and the political are closely connected.

- What do you understand by the term 'learning disability'?
- What words have you heard used to describe people with a learning disability?
- What is the source of those words as you understand it?

TAKING IT FURTHER

SOME SOCIAL INFLUENCES ON THE DEVELOPMENT OF PEOPLE WITH LEARNING DISABILITIES

Introduction

Learning disability refers to an impaired social ability linked to reduced intellectual ability. Since it refers not just to 'low IQ', it is not surprising that the life of a person with learning disability is profoundly affected by social factors. This section of the chapter reviews the impact of some of these factors.

The experience and development of people with learning disability vary considerably depending on social attitudes and arrangements about the label which is applied to them. In every area of social care, staff will meet and have responsibilities for people with learning disability. What follows considers dimensions of development such as health, education, presence in the community and self-determination.

Terminology

A discussion earlier in this chapter referred to the challenges to identity faced by people to whom this description or label is applied. People First prefers the term 'learning difficulties', which describes what its members experience in comparison with other people, and emphasises their motivation to learn. Service organisations in the UK usually refer to 'learning disability'. The World Health Organization recommends the use of the term 'intellectual impairment'. The term often used in the USA is 'mental retardation'. This is regarded as a pejorative label in the UK, and the situation is further complicated because American usage specifically separates this from 'learning disability', which is used to mean a specific disability (such as dyslexia), usually manifest in people of otherwise average intellectual ability or above.

Background

There is no accurate statement of the numbers of people described as having learning disability, and this statistic would vary according to the definition. Emerson and Hatton (2008) estimated that about 3 per cent of children and 2 per cent of adults in the UK are described as having a learning disability – they based their work on data from local councils, the Department of Health, the Department of Education and the census. This indicates about 1.5 million people, of whom 1.2 million are described as having mild disability and 210,000 as having severe or profound disability. About 5 per cent of people with learning disability have Down's syndrome, which is caused by a single genetic abnormality (an extra chromosome 21 – see Corr, 2006: 57, and 'Essential background', section 1). A specific physiological cause is known for a further small proportion who suffered brain trauma during birth, and there are a large number of very specific syndromes which affect extremely small numbers of people. Race (2007), however, points out that in total, physiological explanations are known only for a small minority of people.

Chapter EB1

The experience and development of people with learning disabilities in the UK is shaped by class, income, ethnic community and urban or other geographic differences; it is obviously affected by living in institutions. Michael (2008: 14) reports that severe and profound learning disabilities occur independently of class and income, while moderate learning difficulties are related to poverty and deprivation and occur more frequently in cities. Rates are also higher in people in prison. Emerson and colleagues (1997) found that rates occurred in some South Asian communities at about three times those of other families.

There are differences within the population of people who have learning disabilities. For example, the major survey by Emerson and colleagues (2005) found that: 'Men were more likely to have less privacy, see friends who have learning difficulties less often, be a victim of crime and smoke. Women were more likely to be unemployed, have been bullied at school, attend a day centre, not exercise, feel sad or worried.' Younger people were more likely to live in unsuitable accommodation, have less privacy at home, be bullied, be poor, be a victim of crime, and feel unhappy, sad or worried, left out or unconfident.

Factors affecting health and life expectancy

The most basic question is whether a person gets born at all. David Race (2007) and his son Adam, who has Down's syndrome, visited seven different countries and reported how Adam's life would have been in the different societies. The likelihood of Adam being born varied considerably. In England 92 per cent of women who receive an antenatal diagnosis of Down's syndrome take the decision to terminate their pregnancy (Morris and Alberman, 2009). This represents about 58 per cent of all pregnancies of a child with the chromosome abnormality. The emphasis on a positive test as the gateway to entitlement and advance establishment of the necessary social support is much weaker. In Sweden, by contrast, the expectation is much more that the person with Down's syndrome should be a routine member of society. This is backed by social policy and provision. Although screening is available, it is not normally expected that the pregnancy will be terminated. The positive result of the screen would simply trigger the necessary supports and entitlements for a family which includes a member with Down's syndrome. The Down's Syndrome Association does not believe that a diagnosis of Down's syndrome is a reason for termination of pregnancy.

This discussion, of course, gains some of its vehemence from twentieth-century history. In Nazi Germany, people with intellectual impairment were systematically sterilised or killed in an attempt to remove the 'inheritance of defect' and 'improve' the breeding stock. Race's account (2007: 25–26ff.) indicates that none of the seven countries from which he reports have been immune from eugenics policies, which have strongly affected attitudes towards 'inferior' people with learning disabilities. Indeed, he thinks that Sweden's current positive arrangements are partly a response to the horror experienced when the population realised there had been compulsory sterilisations of people with learning disabilities as late as 1975.

Life expectancy for people with learning disabilities is significantly lower than that for the general population. A person with learning disabilities is sixty times more likely to die before they are 60 (Michael, 2008: 15). Much of this is as a result of biological factors – people with Down's syndrome, for example, are far more likely to have heart problems and to suffer Alzheimer's disease or cancer. However, even here, social as well as biological factors have to be recognised. Mencap (2007) investigated five people with learning disabilities who had died while in the care of the NHS, and found that their deaths were preventable and not associated biologically with their disability – 'death by indifference' as the report described them. This was the prompt for an independent inquiry by Sir Jonathan Michael (2008) into healthcare for people with learning disabilities. He found widespread discrimination and poor practice in the medical treatment of people with learning disabilities; his report details 'convincing evidence' that in general medical matters they received less effective treatment than others. He gives many examples, including one woman who had repeat prescriptions from her GP for twenty years without once being seen; and a systematic pattern of inadequate provision of pain relief or palliative care. He recorded evidence (2008: 16) from the Welsh Centre for Learning Disabilities that over half had an unmet medical need.

On the other hand, many changes in healthcare have had dramatic positive effects. These have steeply increased the average life expectancy of people with Down's syndrome to around 60 years (only a few decades ago, parents might have expected their child to die before the age of 20). Even here, however, the significance of social factors must be understood. Eyman and Call (1991) found that the life expectancy of people with Down's syndrome did not vary according to the severity of their medical conditions, but according to the competence of their self-help skills.

Education

Education services have a major impact. For people with learning disabilities, they have varied substantially over time and between social systems. The 1944 Education Act in the UK can be seen as part of the founding of the welfare state. At the same time as it set up a 'universal' system of free education, however, it enshrined in law that some children were 'ineducable'. These children, with what would now be called learning disabilities, were often left in medically run institutions. If parents chose to raise them at home, there was no school for them to attend. Race (2007: 194–196) refers to the series of scandals about life (and abuse) in the institutions which have led to new social policies and to the expectation of a more open life for people with learning disabilities in the last forty years.

There are approximately 200,000 children of school age in the UK who have a learning disability (Mencap, 2018). Children and young people with learning disabilities are usually assessed as having special educational needs (SEN), but this covers more than just learning disability, and not all children and young people with SEN have a learning disability. In England in 2015, 8 per cent of pupils with SEN attended special schools (DfE, 2015b).

Family support and involvement

As Bronfenbrenner's model (1979/2006) emphasises, a child's development is shaped by a whole network of systems that affect the family. This has already been illustrated with reference to services before birth. It continues through childhood and is of great significance when the individual is an adult. In the UK, a child with learning disabilities is automatically regarded in law as a 'child in need' (Children Act 1989, section 17). This entitles the child and the family to services to promote his or her well-being. Many parents with a disabled child, however, feel in reality that obtaining entitlements is a constant battle with education, social and health services. Financial implications for public authorities, or disputes concerning whose budget is responsible, may be experienced as constantly interfering with the content of assessments and the services required to give them effect. The services involved include counselling and personal support, short-break care, care at home, adaptations to accommodation, education, and leisure-time activities such as holiday play schemes.

Having a son or daughter (as a child or an adult) who requires intensive support reduces the parents' earning capacity while creating additional financial costs (Emerson et al., 2005). It makes an enormous difference to the quality of life of a family – the person with the disability, parents and siblings – if the state expects to make allowance for this additional cost as part of its commitment to ensuring equal citizens' rights for all. Race (2007: 37) lists the non-educational services specified as entitlements in Swedish law for people with intellectual or other impairments. He cautions that, in all systems, official policies do not necessarily describe the reality 'on the ground', but states that the culture of Swedish society combines with the enforceable nature of these legal rights to ensure that the policies are largely put into operation. A society that ensures that the relevant services are provided for each individual – including finance and personal assistance – automatically allows the life of that individual, and those of other family members, to be 'normalised'.

In different societies, services may recognise the significance of family members more or less effectively, both in childhood and in adulthood. The official inquiry *Healthcare for All* (Michael, 2008: 20) found many examples of good practice. However, it also heard many statements such as the following: 'My daughter needs 24/7 care and when she is in hospital I or another person who knows her well have to stay with her . . . I often have to sleep in her wheelchair, or the seat by her bed, or a mattress on the floor if I am lucky. I am not offered a drink or food, or access to a toilet for myself.' The report describes as totally unacceptable this situation in which relatives who were 'reluctant to leave a vulnerable and possibly confused patient . . . sometimes spent long hours without a drink or food on the ward; indeed, they were sometimes explicitly barred from access to these basics.'

Social presence and an independent voice

The ways in which social attitudes affect the independent voice of people with learning difficulties can be dramatically illustrated by reference to the UK. *Healthcare for All* made use of an expert panel of researchers who themselves had learning disabilities, and the National Statistics survey *Adults with Learning Difficulties in England 2003/4* (Emerson et al., 2005) was carried out by a research team whose members included people with learning disabilities. Both final reports were published in forms accessible to people with learning disabilities. The experts on learning difficulties are those people who experience them, and on social work courses, the lecturers in this subject are sometimes disabled themselves (Citizens as Trainers Group et al., 2004). There is always a possibility of 'tokenism' in such participation, but nevertheless the situation shows different social attitudes and outcomes from those in a society where many people with learning disabilities live in institutions and have been deemed 'uneducable'.

For society to listen to the voice of people with learning disabilities requires that social structures and staff make 'reasonable adaptations' (Disability Discrimination Act 2005), and expect the routine presence of people with learning disabilities, both in everyday situations and in policy development. It requires open attitudes to their participation, and a recognition of the importance of advocacy services.

Current thinking in learning disabilities services is influenced by a scandal at Winterbourne View, a private care home in South Gloucestershire for adults with profound learning disabilities or autism. Six staff members were given prison terms for 'cruel, callous and degrading' abuse of patients with disabilities after being secretly recorded by a reporter for the BBC's *Panorama* programme.

Finance, poverty and deprivation

Money is a fundamental requirement for participation in society. To investigate the level of poverty experienced by people with learning difficulties, Emerson and colleagues' survey (2005: 60) adapted nine items from the Millennium Poverty and Social Exclusion Survey (Gordon et al., 2000). The box below shows the percentage of people who could not afford the item listed.

A holiday (26%)
Going to a pub or club (18%)
A hobby or sport (17%)
Going out (16%)
New clothes (16%)
New shoes (15%)
Telephoning friends and family (10%)
Food (5%)
Heating (4%)

Source: Emerson et al., 2005.

In general, people living in private households (with family, partner or alone) were most likely to be unable to afford one or more of these items. Emerson classified someone who cannot afford two or more items on the list as 'poor' and on that basis identified 23 per cent, nearly a quarter, as 'poor' (the impact of poverty is considered further earlier in this chapter).

However, control over money is as important as the amount of money people receive. Emerson and colleagues (2005: 7) report that 'just over half of the people we asked (54 per cent) said someone else decided how much money they could spend each week, and just over one in ten (12 per cent) said that someone else decided what they could spend their money on'. They summarise their findings under the heading 'People with learning difficulties often have little control over their lives'.

Social attitudes – discriminatory or affirmative

Social attitudes and structures can be positive or negative towards people with learning disabilities. As reported above, Race describes how the Swedish antenatal system, like the Norwegian, is generally oriented towards encouraging the birth of children with Down's syndrome, 'differing, in my view, from most of the industrialised world', where screening out is common (2007: 35). Abortion is available on demand up to eighteen weeks, and screening is available to all. However, a multidisciplinary 'habilitation team' operates with the family from before the birth if the diagnosis is known, and the different members are active as appropriate before and after the birth. If it is known that the child has learning disabilities, the family has access both to the Swedish universal childcare arrangements and also to more specialist childcare. Swedish law provides entitlement to a range of assistance, financial and personal (such as a 'companion service'), for people with impairments and their families. The philosophy behind this is broadly that the state must provide facilities which enable all citizens to have equal access to the way of life considered normal for people in the country. Thus, David Race describes a person, evidently with Down's syndrome, leaving her own flat in the apartment block where he was staying, every morning, off to her business about town.

Current policy in Britain is also directed towards ensuring that people with learning disabilities have the right to be 'full members of the society in which they live, to choose where they live and what they do and to be as independent as they wish to be' (Department of Health, 2001: para. 1.2). However, the inquiries by the Parliamentary Joint Committee on Human Rights into the rights of people with learning difficulties (UK Parliament, 2008), and by Sir Jonathan Michael (2008) into their healthcare, found that despite much progress in the last thirty years, there are 'appalling examples of discrimination, abuse and neglect across the range of health services', 'discrimination is active in access to and outcomes from services' (Michael, 2008: 7, 21), and that 'it is still necessary to emphasise that adults with learning disabilities have the same human rights as everyone else . . . stronger leadership is urgently needed to create a more positive culture of respect for human rights in the United Kingdom' (UK Parliament, 2008: 6). The parliamentary inquiry found concerns about basic human rights in relation to residential care, childcare services, and the criminal justice system.

The social changes that Michael recommends include those directed at the implementation of equal healthcare for all. He concludes that staff often interpret the NHS standard of 'equal healthcare' to mean 'the same healthcare', and points out that in fact it has different implications. In relation to people with learning disabilities, it means that staff need to understand how the person communicates and absorbs information, and that signs, for example, should include easy-to-understand pictorial information. Some staff tend to stereotype people with learning disabilities, not taking the time to see their individuality, or to understand their specific form of communication. He analyses 'diagnostic overshadowing' as a significant problem. This is the term used when illness symptoms and behaviour are wrongly attributed to the general learning disability. He found the problem to be particularly acute in relation to pain relief: 'One parent described vividly how symptoms of severe pain that she could see in her daughter were denied by staff because they mistakenly attributed them to her learning disability. There is also some evidence that staff believe people with learning disabilities have higher pain thresholds' (Michael, 2008: 17).

Mir and colleagues (2001) investigated the experience of people with learning disabilities from minority ethnic communities. Compounding the factors just described, they and their families may face stereotyping or prejudgements. There are likely to be failures of communication or understanding about cultural factors that are relevant. As for all people with learning disabilities, access to advocacy is important, but for British South Asian cultures the European emphasis on individuality may be experienced as running 'counter to the values of collectivism and close family relationships that exist in some communities. The roles of family and community networks need to be taken into account when planning services for individuals' (Mir et al., 2001: 3). In Mir et al.'s view, racism is involved, based on power structures rather than just cultural difference, and these can be expressed either through culturally specific services or generalist services (2001: 8, 9). Sensitive services have to be able to tackle prejudice faced by people with learning disabilities from within family and community structures.

The effect of the label 'learning disability' can be to stress what people can't do, to conceal recognition of their special gifts, to engender low expectations, to create an identity which is dominated by the role of client, and often to restrict meaningful interaction to other people with the same label. This is likely to create a cycle in which low expectations are confirmed by the person's behaviour and performance and go on to confirm the stereotype, fostering greater disability.

It is important to adopt a capability approach – recognising risks, but building on relationships, social skills and competence. O'Brien (1989) summarises the attitudes which assist people with learning disabilities, along with their families and friends, to discover and move towards a desirable personal future as part of ordinary community life (see Table 7.1).

Table 7.1 Characteristics of positive social systems and services for people with learning disability (based on O'Brien, 1989)

Systems which focus on a desirable future will:	
move away from system-centred perspectives of:	*move towards:*
congregating people with disabilities together for service purposes	expressing visions of desirable personal futures, even for people who have very limited experiences or great difficulty communicating, and even if these involve major changes in policy
a primary focus on people's deficiencies; attention to specific negative behaviours to change; emphasis on treatments; awareness of professional–client interaction	alliances with people with disabilities, their families, and friends
buildings owned and operated by health and social care services	better incorporating necessary, skilled help with health, mobility, communication, learning, and self-control into the routines of ordinary settings
organising support around agency administration; around policies and procedures; around occupational identities and boundaries	personalising support to match individual needs

CONCLUSION

Race uses the framework of Social Role Valorisation to analyse experience in the seven countries he compares. He quotes (2007: 31) Nirje's formulation, which embeds principles in the standards of a society: that society acts correctly, it states, when it makes available to all persons with intellectual or other impairments:

1. A normal rhythm to the day.
2. A normal rhythm of the week.
3. A normal rhythm of the year.
4. The normal experience of the life cycle.
5. Normal respect for the individual and the right to self-determination.
6. The normal sexual patterns of their culture.
7. The normal economic patterns and rights of their society.
8. The normal environmental patterns and standards in their community (Nirje, 1999).

This section of the book has briefly reviewed a few of the social factors – including health, education, family services, finance and social attitudes – which affect the development of people with learning disabilities. Using Bronfenbrenner's words (1979/2006), it has concentrated on the systems beyond the microsystem. Other equally important dimensions to explore include housing, sexual relationships, the justice system and parenting. Any consideration of this area of disability which concentrates only on psychological, 'learning', or medical dimensions will neglect major factors in development.

SUMMARY

This chapter focused initially on three painful and difficult aspects of development – poverty, violence and mental health difficulties. It then turned your attention to the effect of stigma on identity formation. This involves an understanding of the effect of cultural forces on individual psychology.

About 13.5 million people in the UK were defined as in poverty in 2016. Poverty affects all areas of family life and well-being, from infant mortality to adult life expectancy. The effects of childhood poverty last throughout life.

Social workers deal with violence or its after-effects in relation to children, adults in intimate relationships, street violence, and public violence such as war. They have responsibilities to influence subsequent developments in positive ways: by intervening, for example to ensure that children are safe from violence, by advocacy, by undoing the after-effects of violence, and by working with the violent person.

Every week, one in six adults experiences symptoms of a mental health problem. Causal factors involved in mental health difficulties can include genetic makeup; stress factors in earlier life, including abuse; current stress; relational factors in childhood; and the after-effects of trauma or victimisation. The chapter included brief accounts of the experience of mental health difficulties and the distinction you may encounter in the historical division between 'neurosis' and 'psychosis'. Different accounts are given of the association between mental health difficulties and social adversity, including the view that the core issue is the diagnosis and treatment of mental illness, a social process in which certain problems in living are defined as medical problems. Mental illness in the form of anxiety or depression can sometimes lessen spontaneously. After longer-standing mental illness, some people experience a sense of renewed personal growth, as well as damaging effects. Some forms of organic brain deterioration, like Alzheimer's disease, are at the moment irreversible. For about 5,500 individuals each year, the outcome of mental illness will be suicide; this figure has varied over recent decades, and the government has targets to reduce it.

Social forces create difficulties for some people in forming a positive identity. This poses a psychological challenge for them in their development; it has to be managed in personal and business interactions; and socially it leaves them disregarded and exposed to practical discrimination. The chapter picked out three illustrations: in relation to ethnicity, Phinney's model of identity development; the example of gay and lesbian people who have to form integrated identities in the face of elements of social (even family) disapproval; and in relation to people with learning disabilities who, unlike members of other self-advocacy groups, may not see the label as applying to themselves. Although there is a sociological logic in identifying 'spoilt identity' in different situations, the operation of social forces is profoundly different for different people, different sexes, different cultural settings and different periods of history.

The chapter concluded by analysing how the development of people with learning disabilities is fundamentally affected by social factors and attitudes – in health, education, social presence, and finance. To remove these barriers involves focusing on what people *can* do rather than on what they cannot do.

FURTHER READING

Poverty statistics; links with health and education:

The Poverty Site: www.poverty.org.uk.
Crowley, A. and Vulliamy, C. (2007) *Listen Up! Children and Young People Talk: About Poverty.* London/Cardiff: Save the Children Fund. Available online: www.savethechildren.org.uk/en/docs/wales_lu_pov.pdf.

About social work and mental health:

Golightley, M. (2017) *Social Work and Mental Health.* Sixth edition. London: Sage.
Wilson, K., Ruch, G., Lymbery, M. and Cooper, A. (eds) (2011) *Social Work: An Introduction to Contemporary Practice.* Second edition. Harlow: Pearson.

About learning difficulties:

Williams, P. and Evans, M. (2013) *Social Work with People with Learning Difficulties.* Third edition. London: Sage.

RESOURCES FOR PEOPLE AFFECTED BY ISSUES DISCUSSED IN THIS CHAPTER

Resources for people affected by domestic violence:

Women's Aid have a range of information sheets available at www.womensaid.org.uk/ information-support/downloads-and-resources/

Resources for people affected by mental health problems:

Both Mind (www.mind.org.uk) and the Mental Health Foundation (www.mentalhealth. org.uk) offer free fact-sheets and booklets for people with mental health problems and their families. A wide range of subjects are covered by both, from statistics and suicide rates to crisis intervention teams and drugs. Most are also available for free download.

Resources for people with learning disabilities and their families:

Mencap: www.mencap.org.uk. Mencap describes itself as 'the voice of learning disability'. The Down's Syndrome Association: www.downs-syndrome.org.uk/for-people-with-downs-syndrome/information/

Questions

1. What is meant by 'relative poverty'? Discuss some of the short- and long-term effects of poverty.
2. What are some of the contexts in which social workers deal with problems of violence? What developmental knowledge is relevant to understanding the problems?
3. What are some of the insights given about problems of violence by (a) attachment theory, (b) psychodynamic models, (c) Bandura's social learning theory, (d) Bronfenbrenner's ecological model of development?
4. What are some of the contexts in which social workers need to understand problems of mental health? What challenges might these situations present to a social worker?

For you to research

Prepare a poster or brief report on one of the following:

■ Socioeconomic circumstances of families with a child with a disability
■ The potential effects of domestic abuse on victims
■ The service user movement in mental health
■ Parents with learning disabilities

CHAPTER 8

Adulthood and ageing

In this chapter you will find:

■ **Body and mind in later adulthood**

■ **Theories of ageing: disengagement theory, activity theory and feminist perspectives**

■ **Political and social influences: social policy, social exchange theory and political economy**

■ **The mature imagination**

INTRODUCTION

'I didn't know I'd fall for him', said Nicola's mother, Ann, about her grandson. 'It's hard to explain if you haven't experienced it. You look into his eyes and there's something . . . you just fall totally and deeply in love. They haven't come from your body, but when you see them, the feeling of love is overwhelming, instantaneous. It's quite extraordinary, holding your daughter's baby.'

By contrast, Bob didn't know that at 49 he had become a grandfather, a year after he and his daughter Bella had parted so acrimoniously. He didn't know anything about the lives of his daughter and granddaughter, could only fill in the gaps with (incorrect) imagination and worry. He did not know that twelve years later his granddaughter Tia was in care, or that when she was 17 her baby was born. Eight years after the birth of Tia's baby, he is 74. He had kept his job in the plastics factory until two years before he was due to retire, and then emphysema had caused him to stop work. His arthritis made movement difficult, and he seldom got out of the house even to see the friends he used to meet at the pub.

Naoko's grandfather, Yasuyoshi, 70, lives in a small village called Yomogita in Japan. His daughter had recently gone to work in Toyko and his granddaughter, Naoko, had moved to England. He read an article in the paper this morning which said that the proportion of people aged over 65 years in Japan is the highest in the world, almost one in four people. The article said that there are almost 8 million people who are still working after 65 years, stressing that this shows how valuable older people are in society as they contribute towards the economy. The article went on to say that older people command a respect born of the Confucian tradition, unlike the West where older people tend to be marginalised and treated as unproductive members of society. Indeed, Japanese researchers are arguing that health and life expectancy gains mean that the current definition of old age as over 65 years is out of date and should become over 75 years. Like many older people in Japan, Yasuyoshi is worried that this may mean that the government will delay state pensions until later.

However, the article also stated that more older people are worried about not being looked after by their families, saying this was linked with more women entering work. Yasuyoshi is proud of his daughter and granddaughter, but also fears having to go to a nursing home. When he grew up, they were seen as only for people who had been abandoned by uncaring relatives, and he remembers that a Japanese term *oyasute* ('parents dumped on the mountain') was used to refer to people looked after outside their family.

This chapter will describe some aspects of the later phases of adult life. As throughout the book, it has several aims:

■ First, to encourage you in the flexibility of imagination which is required in order to enter into the lives of people at different ages and to see the world from their point of view.
■ Second, to highlight a few relevant biological aspects of human ageing.
■ Third, to comment on some of the lifespan theories with which researchers have tried to make sense of development in later life.

The topics affect people from those in their forties to those over 100. Since a common preconception might be that somewhere there is a body of knowledge about 'older people', we need to start with clear messages about diversity. Any treatment of late adulthood, 'older age', is covering a wide age span; a moment's thought will assure you that this group is no more likely to be uniform than any other group whose ages cover a span of forty or fifty years. Furthermore, research about any particular subgroup finds that the most striking feature is diversity and difference.

This emphasis is important because people of all ages hold stereotypes about 'old people'. As a social worker, it is important that you are aware of these stereotypes, in order to understand the social contexts in which older people are trying to create their lives, and that you have some facts to replace the stereotypes.

In relation to older people, it can be as if a stooped frame and cautious gait, white, thinning hair and fragile bones somehow convey a 'thinner', less vigorous self. Referring back for a moment to the discussion in Chapter 7 about 'identity', this social identity may be wildly at odds with the reality of a person whose sense of self is undiminished. Their vital sense of identity may be felt just as strongly, and perhaps more so as they have more experience to draw upon. The practice in hospitals of displaying photographs of their older patients which show them in earlier adulthood may be a helpful prompt to younger staff members.

Chapter 7

> Open your eyes . . .
> Look beyond my leg
> Look beyond my illness
> Look into my world . . .
> Open your eyes
> And see me.

(from a poem by Madeleine Alston)

To be competent in understanding people in the later decades of their life (as in understanding anyone) requires the social worker to have the imagination to enter into the current chapter of the 'narrative' of the person they are talking with.

Problems of terminology

Problems of terminology are more prominent here than in most of the other chapters. In part, this is because 'ageing' means the process of growing older but has attached connotations of decline (the difference between what some philosophers call the 'denotation' of a word and its connotations). Specifically, however, the difficulty is that 'ageing' in relation to cell biology actually means ('denotes') the process of deterioration. There is a constant danger that 'ageing' (the process of living during the second half or so of life, the process of adding age to a younger organism) is taken to mean the process of decline, damage or deterioration.

Gerontologists refer to the characteristic profile of the 'young old' (about 60 to 75), old old (about 75–85) and the oldest old (85 and older). The lives of the young old (60 to 75) may include caring responsibilities for grandchildren or for their own parents, and also the enjoyment of active leisure pursuits previously squeezed out by paid employment. Adults who suffer from a chronic condition at 65 are less likely to do well, cognitively and physically. The oldest old (85 and older) are more likely to suffer from disability, but people who survive longer seem actually to be constitutionally and cognitively more robust than younger people who die earlier (ONS, 2005; Boyd and Bee, 2015).

What does 'old' mean?

Imagine you are 88 and about to move into residential care, a move prompted in part by severe problems with your short-term memory. You are having a chat with a granddaughter of whom you are very fond, and you recognise her well. You have met some of the residents and share with your granddaughter that some of them really are, sadly, pretty out of touch with reality.

In a somewhat sad and wistful mood, you talk with your granddaughter about what 'old' meant to you at different ages in your life. Write down what you say.

Perhaps begin: 'When I was 2 I didn't know what "old" meant. Though I remember my mum saying that it didn't matter if that towel got dirty because it was old. When I was 5, "old" meant anyone over the age of . . .'

Perhaps after going through views at different ages, end 'and what does "old" mean to me now? "Old" means . . .'

BODY AND MIND IN LATER ADULTHOOD

The older you become, the longer you can expect to live. The average life expectancy of a 65-year-old male in 2010–2012 was a further eighteen years, to live until 83; but the life expectancy of an 85-year-old was six years, to live until they were 91; and life expectancy continues to rise, for both men and women, as they grow older. This can be seen clearly in the life expectancy tables from the Office for National Statistics (2013). It can also be seen from these tables that at the present time, a woman has to be several years over 100 before reaching the age at which a half of her contemporaries will no longer be alive at the end of the coming year. In general it appears that older people may be constitutionally fitter than younger people who die earlier. People at the age of 100 tend to have the cognitive ability typical of people in their sixties, and examination after death finds their brains are similar to those of these younger people.

The mortality statistics quoted in the previous paragraph are based on rates of death at different ages at the present time. In addition to this are changes brought about by improvements in future health or social care, which cannot be statistically predicted (see ONS, 2007a, 2007b). In the last hundred years these have consistently operated to increase lifespan. So the chances are that the 65-year-old male will on average live to be older than 83.

Bodily experience at different ages is affected by which decade you were born in. As Professor Tom Kirkwood put it in his distinguished BBC Reith Lecture of 2001, people in their seventies today are in the same physical condition as people in their sixties were when he started practising medicine (Kirkwood, 2001). Heredity is an important influence in ageing, but so is environment, earlier disease and so on.

Loss of function, as well as life expectancy, is related to social, cognitive and emotional factors in interaction with physical change. The emotional and cognitive features may be out of awareness, as illustrated in an experiment by Hausdorff and colleagues (1999). Walking speed is a common indicator of physical fitness, and has been found in American studies to correlate with nursing home admission and with death. In the work of Hausdorff, forty-seven men and women aged between 60 and 85 played a computer game about the interaction of their physical and mental skills. For one group, negative words about age, such as 'senile' and 'dependent', were flashed up for a few thousandths of a second. This is long enough for the brain to decode the word-image, but not long enough for it to enter conscious awareness (the images are 'subliminal'). For the other group, the words used were positive, such as 'wise' and 'accomplished'. The researchers were themselves surprised to find that the foot-speed of the 'positive message' group increased by just under 10 per cent, a substantial change equivalent to gains found in older people after months of rigorous physical training. The researchers went on in other experiments to find that unconscious positive stereotyping had a similar effect on memory performance. It seems likely that positive self-image (taking it for granted that one is competent, effective and has a functioning memory) has a direct effect on performance. Older people who apologise for their memory and expect to be less sharp then their younger colleagues, become so.

As you would expect, the processes involved are thought to be linked to the stereotyping effects referred to in Chapter 7. In relation to ethnicity, Levy and Banaji (2006) refer to research that showed that simply asking students to note their ethnicity was sufficient to diminish the cognitive scores of African American boys. They point out that in relation to prejudice about 'race', gender or sexuality, there is a large difference between strong, consciously held views and unconscious negative bias – intellectual beliefs and conscious anti-discriminatory attitudes can override subconscious bias. By contrast, explicit attitudes about 'old age' appear to have less potency to override negative bias. In implicit attitudes about 'old people', the negative bias is stronger (than against other 'out-groups') and the difference between explicit and implicit attitudes is smaller than in relation to other groups. In relation to ageing stereotypes, the negative implicit stereotypes do not diminish as the person enters that group themselves. Unlike membership of other stereotyped groups, all younger people eventually become part of this stereotyped group themselves, and both the conscious and unconscious stereotypes remain unabated. In addition to other implications, this ensures a feedback mechanism for the perpetuation of negative stereotypes. Levy and Banaji (2006), in their survey of 660 adults, found that people with positive stereotypes of ageing (measured up to twenty-three years before they died) lived on average 7.5 years longer than those with negative stereotypes. This was the measure of the effect after allowance was made for functional health, and gender, and other relevant socioeconomic factors were taken into account. As Levy and Banaji comment (2006: 60), 'with friends like oneself, who needs enemies?'

Chapter 7

In addition to biological and psychological factors, social arrangements clearly have an effect on functional independence – family, friendships and community involvement as well as social policy play a large part in determining whether a person with a degree of physical limitation has an engaged or dependent life.

SOCIAL AND PSYCHOLOGICAL ASPECTS OF STEREOTYPING

What are some of the different images of ageing that are presented in the mass media? Check some television schedules, television programmes and newspapers and see if they bear out your answer.

Explicit stereotypes and attitudes can be measured by self-report studies.

Implicit stereotypes and attitudes, as described by Levy and Banaji (2006: 51), 'operate without conscious awareness, intention or control', so they cannot be measured by self-report. The authors describe some of the methods used to assess the strength of implicit stereotypes and attitudes (2006: 53–54).

They found that implicit negative attitudes towards older people are stronger than those of other prejudices – 'based on 64,000 tests, it remains one of the largest negative implicit attitudes we have observed, consistently larger than the anti-black implicit attitudes amongst white Americans' (2006: 54). Explicit attitudes were closer to implicit attitudes than in other prejudices.

Bodily development – living with change

Sexual system

The ovaries of most women stop producing eggs some time between the ages of 45 and 55. 'Menopause' is technically defined as occurring after a year in which there has been no menstruation, and it occurs at an average age of 51 (Boyd and Bee, 2015). The impact of the associated hormonal changes varies considerably. For some women, the transition is clear and brief; for others it may be irregular and extended. It may be accompanied by physical symptoms such as hot flushes (the rush of heat from chest to head), night sweats, vaginal dryness, sleep disturbance and mood swings or heightened emotional variability, which are experienced as intrusive and uncomfortable.

As in other ages of life, specific reliable information about physical sexual activity and its relation to cultural and historic circumstances is unlikely to be established. Some women gain a new energy in their sexual lives, perhaps because of a general lack of concern about periods or the risk of getting pregnant (see, for example, Purnine and Carey, 1998). Others, whether living on their own or in heterosexual or lesbian relationships, end physical sexual activity before or during the menopause. Some of these nevertheless experience their feminine sexuality as undiminished, not considering erogenous stimulation as central to their sexuality; some derive great satisfaction from touching and other physical contact; and some are less clear about their sexuality or consider it is no longer an important part of themselves. Bartlik and Goldstein (2000, 2001) found that 70 per cent of heterosexual couples were sexually active at the age of 70. For these couples, it seems to be usually an episode such as separation or illness which breaks the pattern and leads to the discontinuation of physical sexual activity. The vagina is essentially a (lubricated) muscle and although regular use maintains muscle tone and lubrication, hormonal changes after the menopause precipitate loss of muscle tone (atrophy). This is reversible. For women, these changes mark the beginning of the second half of life.

The decline in male hormones occurs more gradually. It is very variable in healthy men, and effects are rarely evident in those under 60 (although levels have usually been changing since the age of about 45). When they occur, changes in testosterone levels may be associated with a decline in the experienced level of sexual desire. Until this decline occurs, any loss of erectile function is unlikely to be caused by hormonal changes. The loss of sexual desire or hunger will mean different things for different men, reflecting the variety of earlier experience. By the age of 80, about half have low testosterone, and many will still not notice the effects (Mayo Clinic, 2018; Sternbach, 1998). In men, variations in sex hormones appear to be linked with cognitive functioning – Boyd and Bee (2015) quote findings that lower levels of testosterone caused by prostate cancer treatment had reduced cognitive functioning and this returned to normal when hormone levels were restored. Sternbach (1998) summarises that testosterone decline or deficiency in men is not analogous to the female menopause.

Joints and movement

The joints between bones are kept mobile by tough, slippery material (cartilage) and lubricant. With constant use, this cartilage eventually wears down and compresses. When, as a result, bones grind against each other, they cause damage and pain, known as arthritis. In 2006, 115 women and 72 men in 1,000 people aged between 65 and 74 were likely to have suffered from arthritis (ONS, 2008a). Many arthritis sufferers have movement which is slower, stiffer and more painful.

Muscle strength and skin tone

In general, muscle strength declines with age, and skin elasticity diminishes, causing wrinkles.

Strokes

A stroke (cerebrovascular accident) occurs when a blood vessel bleeds inside the brain. If this results in damage, it can involve immediate loss of function, potentially followed by recovery as the brain recreates new pathways for achieving the function previously carried out in the damaged part of the brain. A stroke can vary in severity from something which is barely noticed, to being a cause of sudden death. Strokes occur more frequently in later life. When Olsen and colleagues (2007) studied all 40,000 stroke sufferers in Denmark from 2001 to 2007, they found that women had fewer but more severe strokes than men, and were more likely to survive them.

Dementia and confusion

Dementia is a decline in cognitive functions such as thinking, reasoning, memory, language and speech. Confusion and memory loss may be accompanied by changed personality, aggression and physical inability. These are the possible outcomes of various physical conditions affecting the brain, including Alzheimer's disease, multi-infarct (or vascular) dementia, Parkinson's disease or Huntington's disease.

In Alzheimer's disease, areas of the brain become coated with a sticky 'plaque'. Recently, for the first time, brain scans have been able to show these deposits, holding out the promise of making diagnosis more reliable (at the moment, diagnosis is made through a subtle process of judging patterns of memory loss). Its cause is not well understood. Both Parkinson's and Huntington's disease involve a loss of nerve cells in (different) parts of the brain. Huntington's disease is a hereditary condition caused by a variation in one specific gene; Parkinson's has a large hereditary component involving various genes which have not been fully identified, but it is also the result of environmental factors. Multi-infarct dementia is the result of blockages in the blood flow to parts of the brain (because of deposits in the arteries) and is responsible for 40 per cent of cases of dementia (Sergo, 2008).

Cognitive functioning

Short-term memory and working memory decline with age. Working memory is a short-term memory store which is deleted after use, so that its contents are not transferred to long-term memory. Working memory is used when, for example, you hold the overall requirements of a ten-minute task in your head while performing a sub-task that takes one minute. The decline is kept at bay by activities such as crosswords, sudoku or general intellectual activities. There is, however, some evidence that these only delay its onset, the rate of subsequent deterioration being faster for these people. There have been similar discoveries in relation to education. Higher levels of education delay the onset of dementia, but it appears that this factor only 'holds it at bay', perhaps by unconscious compensation for physical deterioration. Once the symptoms show, the condition progresses more rapidly, one suggestion being that this is because the brain decay is already at a more advanced state (Goudarzi, 2008). There is some evidence that skills which depend on social intelligence improve with increasing age (Hakamies-Blomqvist, 2006; Henry et al., 2004).

The philosophy of healthcare

It is understandable that younger people sometimes wonder whether striving to tackle and prevent illnesses in later life is not self-defeating – might it not simply lead to a prolongation of sickness and pain-ridden existence with an ever-increasing number of people needing treatment? This is not the way to understand ageing and health; the aim is to make the 'healthspan' equivalent to the lifespan. The end of life will then come with a comparatively short, life-ending illness, after preventable and treatable conditions have consistently been dealt with. The majority of older people assess their health as 'good' or 'very good', and illnesses should not be left untreated as if 'it's just your age' (Boyd and Bee, 2015; Soule et al., 2005: 42; Vincent, 2003: 136). Additional research information about patterns of decline in competence for daily living activities currently found among older people in the period leading up to their death is provided by Lunney and colleagues (2003).

> Interview someone over retirement age. Ask them what they find rewarding about growing older, and what they dislike.

Reflective thinking

THEORIES OF AGEING

As with other areas of life, there are many lenses through which we can view full adult maturity. Each brings into focus different aspects of life. The biggest gap in the literature is probably firsthand articulated accounts by people who are themselves in late old age; reflective accounts which explore the experience in its richness and ambiguity. 'The young [the author means anyone who is not old] know nothing directly about old age, and their enquiries of the subject must be done blind . . . the condition for [most writers and research-ers] must in a sense be a closed book to them . . . those who have had actual experience of old age are likely to be dead or very tired or just reluctant to discuss the matter with young interlocutors.' Thus wrote Frank Kermode at the age of 88, reviewing *The Long Life* by Helen Small (Kermode, 2007; Small, 2007).

It has proved difficult to create theory which reliably combines all the different factors in later life. Such a theory must recognise both similarity and variation in psychological development. It must account accurately for biologi-cal influences and the effect of illness. It must not over-generalise cohort effects which affect only people born in a particular time. It is required to identify and explain the specific impacts of economics, culture, social policy and social stratification. The theory must give a convincing account of change and continuity in 'identity', and in general must establish both the extent of variability and the limits on variability. The lifespan approach, which will be discussed in Chapter 10, has paid particular attention to these features in later life, but nevertheless Bass (2006) regards this synthesis as still 'the holy grail' of theory about old age – something everyone searches for but no one has found.

Chapter 10

Disengagement theory

The first comprehensive multidisciplinary theory of ageing was proposed by Cumming and Henry (1961). They moved away from purely psychological, biological or sociological approaches and emphasised that ageing cannot be understood separately from the characteristics of the social system in which it takes place. Based on a study of 279 men and women between the ages of 50 and 90, they identified 'social disengagement' as a characteristic process of older people which benefited both the individual and the social systems of which they are a part. Cumming (1975) proposed three factors in the age-ing process: shrinkage of life space, increased individuality, and acceptance of these changes. First, older people experience a shrinkage in their life space as they interact with fewer and fewer others and fill fewer and fewer roles. Secondly, they experience increased individuality because, in the roles and relationships that remain, the older individual is much less governed by strict rules or expectations. Thirdly, the older adult embraces these changes, actively disengaging from roles and relationships, turning increasingly inward and away from interactions with others.

The implication (or assumption?) of disengagement theory is that because of inevitable biological and intellectual changes, older people become decreasingly active within the external world and increasingly preoc-cupied with their inner lives. Cumming and Henry understood disengagement to be a functional aspect of social order and continuity because it allowed the systems in place in a society to be handed on from one generation to the next, as older people withdraw and pass power and influence to the younger.

Disengagement was viewed as an adaptive behaviour because it allowed older people to maintain a sense of self-worth while adjusting to the loss of earlier social roles. This process was seen to have a positive function and positive qualities, in contrast to activity theory (outlined next) which assumed older people needed to be 'busy' and 'engaged' to remain well-adjusted.

Criticisms of disengagement theory

Despite claims to take account of social systems, critics argue that disengagement theory is based on an abstract analysis of social systems, not the diverse realities of different societies, the different societal position of men and women, and so on.

In present-day wealthy industrial societies, for example, many people remain socially and economically active well after they have retired from paid work roles. Research by Afshar and colleagues (2002) finds large differences in disengagement between different subcultures in the same area of Britain. Older people's parenting role may change from its earlier physical manifestation and yet still be highly significant. It may involve a closely coordinated sharing of the daytime (or overnight) care of grandchildren, and involve a substantial financial element as well as continuing emotional interaction. The level of daily physical activity may change, but the amount they travel may increase and their leisure activities, their cultural and social engagement, may become more evident.

In general, the theory is criticised (Bengtson and Achenbaum, 1994) for failing to take account of:

- individual choice;
- individual personality dimensions;
- different economic and environmental opportunities;
- different sociocultural characteristics.

Nevertheless, despite these criticisms, many people, old and young, recognise an element of realism in the analysis which Cumming and Henry made from their data. For these theorists, 'disengagement' is a natural feature of good adjustment in older age. This contrasts with the next theory to be discussed.

Activity theory

Activity theory was proposed after disengagement theory (Neugarten, 1977), and presents a contrasting picture. It is based on the hypothesis that active older people are more satisfied than those who are not active. Self-concept is validated by participation in valued roles, and there are many socially valued roles characteristic of middle life which should replace lost roles – productive roles in voluntary associations, and religious and leisure organisations.

According to this view, support services which are based on disengagement theory are likely to embody (and may be an excuse for) ageism. They should instead take the responsibility to support community structures which encourage and make possible the continuing of activities from middle age into older age. In terms of societal well-being, older people should replace lost roles with new ones to maintain their place in society.

Activity theory is criticised for treating the problems of ageing as individual problems and ignoring the realities of older people's bodies, energies and choices.

Ageing is characterised by a progressive loss of the ability to adapt to stress: 'With progressing age, this falls below the level required for daily living' (Pendergast et al., 1993). If this is true, older adults more often operate near the limits of their ability to adapt. Faced with this, a typical strategy is to adapt to choose activities that leave them within their limits. Boyd and Bee (2015) suggest the example of giving up mountain climbing but continuing to walk regularly.

Chapter 5

Activity theory is supported by the finding in several studies that active older adults show slightly higher levels of life satisfaction and morale than others (Boyd and Bee, 2015, referencing Adelman, 1994, George, 1990 and others). As Boyd and Bee point out, however, the idea that disengagement is unproblematic gains support from the findings mentioned in Chapter 5: that although older people have fewer social contacts than younger people, it is younger people who report more loneliness (Revenson, 1982).

Both approaches have to be supplemented by a third set of research findings, about continuity. There may be significant continuity between earlier patterns and disengagement/activity in later life. People who tend to be satisfied with their own company and personal enthusiasms earlier in life tend to be so in later life, while those who gain satisfaction from social roles and physical activity earlier will tend in later life to continue these or to replace earlier roles with equivalents. Stuart-Hamilton (2012) gives some detail about American studies that support this view, including that of Reichard and colleagues (1962), who interviewed eighty-seven men aged 55 to 84. In a very long-running project, Haan studied a core sample of 118 subjects over a period of fifty years. She reports on dimensions both of continuity and of variability (Haan et al., 1986). Neugarten (1977) reports on a sample of people in their seventies and found different personality types which would link with the different approaches of disengagement or 'activity'. He concludes that 'older people adjust their personalities but do not change them radically'.

This is put forward formally by theorists such as Atchley (1989), who argue that life satisfaction is determined by how consistent current activities or lifestyles are with one's lifetime experience. The model is generally seen as an elaboration of activity theory and in opposition to disengagement theory. 'Continuity' is analysed in a subtle, rather than a static way. External continuity is distinguished from internal continuity, which allows people to have a sense of 'who they are' even as they change (Sugarman, 2009). *Continuity theory* emphasises a constantly moving dynamic.

This is taken a stage further by narrative theorists who explore *how* this continuity is created. They say that memory is essential in the process, involving constantly re-interpreting the past so as to create a coherent story with the individual as its subject (Sugarman (2009) quotes Cohler (1982) and McAdams (1997) as key authors).

Feminist approaches

Feminist approaches to understanding development in older age emphasise that here, as in other aspects of life, gender must be a primary consideration. Feminist writers and researchers adopt different views on many issues, but some of their key beliefs are:

■ The experiences of women are often ignored in attempts to understand human life unless an explicitly feminist perspective is taken.
■ These experiences must be analysed critically, taking into account how they are structured by women's unequal access to power.
■ Experiences of women in old age can only be understood in the context of the inequality they experience in caregiving, health and poverty across the life course.

They emphasise that feminist researchers should be explicit about the framework of power and knowledge from which they undertake research; they are likely to be middle-class, financially privileged and carrying out research with the prior beliefs outlined above, with the aim of benefiting women and involving them in the research as active participants.

Other views adopted by some feminists are that women occupy an inferior status to men in older age because of the structures of capitalist patriarchal society. Arber and Ginn (1995: 71; see also 1991), for example, use this perspective to explain how the differential age of entitlement to state pension (at the time, 60 for women and 65 for men) is a manifestation of male patriarchal power.

Until recently, the women's movement has tended to focus its attention on the need for out-of-family childcare to allow women to take on more paid employment, as well as the perceived injustice of the amount of (unpaid) care for older people provided by women. This has been compounded by some earlier perspectives which envisaged 'the death of the family' (Simon et al., 1968). It has paid less attention to the necessity of finding arrangements for the care of ageing parents which allow women to take an active role; arrangements which accommodate this as a 'normative family stress' (Brody, 1985), without neglecting the wishes of the parents or weighing excessively on the lives of these women. Conceptualising the requirements in terms of victimhood or burden has not created solutions to the potentially crippling problems of financial stress, depression and physical damage arising from 'the 36-hour day' (Mace and Rabins, 2007).

Reflective thinking

Can you briefly summarise disengagement theory, activity theory and feminist theories of ageing? If you can, have a conversation with a retired person in which you explain these views and ask for their observations.

POLITICAL, SOCIAL AND HISTORICAL INFLUENCES

The later stages of life are profoundly affected by specific historical circumstances, political factors, culture and social policy.

The social picture of older people has changed dramatically in the last hundred years. In 2003, 33 per cent of the population in the UK were over 50, and in 2007, life expectancy was 79. In 1901, the percentage was less than half this (15 per cent) and life expectancy was 47. The percentage of the population over 50 is projected to rise by a third, to 41 per cent, by 2031. People over retirement age now outnumber people under 16 for the first time (ONS, 2007a, 2008b; Tomassini, 2005: 1).

The 'oldest old' at the present time experienced the economic depression and mass unemployment of the 1930s, followed by the Second World War. They had to create a totally different picture of 'old age' and 'welfare' from their parents, many of whom regarded 'welfare' as a destructive ghost, haunting them with the spectre of the workhouse and degradation. The 'young old' were born during that war and just afterwards – they are the 'baby boom generation' who were brought up to take the welfare state for granted, and saw massive changes in the position of women. The image of 'old age' presented to the older of these generations was that it was likely to last only a couple of years after retirement from work, and public pensions at a realistic level were a new idea.

History and culture are intimately linked. Cultures change over time, and these changes are sometimes the outcomes of specific historical events. Afshar and colleagues (2002), in their study in the 'Growing Older' programme of the UK Economic and Social Research Council, found that:

> There was a connection between life course events and quality of life in later years. The curtailment of education, reduced employment opportunities, war time experiences and for Polish and Caribbean women being unable to use their previous training were all mentioned as having an effect. The African Caribbean women told of the horrific racism they had experienced on arrival in Britain.
> ... There are ethnic differences in how the women perceived ageing, with some Pakistani and Bangladeshi women reporting feeling older at a much earlier age than other groups.
>
> (Afshar et al., 2002)

This study illustrates the different experiences of ageing which may arise in different cultural groups. White women who were financially better off and had relocated on retirement were building new social networks and forms of social support; minority ethnic women who had migrated into this country during the course of their life and poorer white women who had lived in the same vicinity all their lives tended to have families who lived nearby, and had a sense of purpose linked to kinship ties – 'agreed tasks, obligations and reciprocities which bind families together'. Childcare tasks and grandparenting roles were important in their daily lives. Some, particularly Indian and Polish participants, made a link between a sense of well-being and being respected and valued by others, especially in terms of the status afforded to older people in their cultural circle. Only the white non-migrant women raised the issue of feeling ignored or dismissed because of their perceived age. The researchers noted that disadvantaged white non-migrant women can easily be excluded from consultation processes about social policy. Some minority ethnic groups felt over-researched (and saw few tangible results from the information they provided – Afshar et al., 2002: 4).

As has already been pointed out, people above pensionable age form only a small proportion of people in poverty in the UK. According to Age UK, the number of pensioners in poverty has fallen from 2.7 million to 1.6 million since the beginning of the century (Age UK, 2018). Those in the lowest income group were significantly more likely to suffer poor health, but the risk varied with age. Overall, about a third of people over 50 reported a limiting long-term illness, but this varied from 45 per cent of the poorest fifth to 19 per cent of those in the richest fifth. For those over 85, the risk is 70 per cent and is less dependent on income (Evandrou et al., 2002: 48).

Poverty after pension age for the oldest old and for single people – see Chaper 7.

Patterns of living vary substantially even between the countries of the European Union, among different subcultures in the UK and across different decades. In Italy, only just over a third (36 per cent) of older women live alone, whereas in the UK just under a half (46 per cent) do. In Sweden, the proportion is 51 per cent, just over a half. This represents a general pattern of greater family living in the Mediterranean countries which lessens progressively to the north. In each country the numbers had increased significantly over the last thirty years. Older Asian people in the UK (admittedly from a very small relevant population of 13,000) are much more likely than indigenous white people to live in a household including other generations. Tomassini points out that, assuming families provide care, these patterns have implications for the provision of care by the state (all these statistics are from Tomassini, 2005).

The national statistics analysed by Soule et al. (2005) show that compared with the general population in any age group there was a much greater proportion of single, widowed and divorced people living in communal establishments in 2003. They take this to indicate the extent to which spouses normally provide support for independent living. When care is provided by a partner, men are as likely to provide it as women. When provided by a younger generation, more women than men provide it – daughters-in-law as well as daughters. This group is sometimes called 'the sandwich generation' – 'women in the middle' – caring for their adolescent children or their children's children at the same time as providing care for their own parents (for more detail about multiple roles in mid-life, see Evandrou et al., 2002, and Brody and Saperstein, 2006).

Research has constantly found that the availability of social support plays a large role in enabling continuing development in older age. Further enquiries to understand the processes involved found that often, when it is effective, this 'social support' means enabling the older person to continue *offering* social support themselves (Boyd and Bee, 2015, citing Guse and Masesar, 1999). A satisfactory life means being of use to others – in family, friendship network or community. To provide a service which maintains a person in a position of dependency or as a passive recipient is not necessarily experienced as developmentally positive. This can present a particular challenge for the management of 'communal living' (often, residential establishments), where the support offered may emphasise that the older person is the recipient of support, not an active contributor to social life.

Family relationships are complex, and effective social support for older people has to fit in with family and cultural processes. Many adult children, for example, in some communities more than others, may feel not just a caring 'responsibility' towards their parents' generation but a sense of duty and obligation, which is a stronger dynamic. This may entail the feeling that to 'leave' a parent in a 'home' is a cause for shame. It could be a creative solution for the public services to support a residential facility which is culturally and psychologically 'owned' by the community. This might avoid the sense of 'abandonment' on the one hand and shame on the other.

As was mentioned earlier, the period after the age of 60 is as likely to be a time of providing care as of receiving it and the majority of social care is provided by family members. One in eight people (around 6.5 million people) are carers. About a quarter of carers are providing more than fifty hours each week. Of the younger old, more women provide care, but over 75, the proportion of men providing care is twice that of women. The proportion of people who provide care decreases with age, but of these, the proportion providing fifty hours each week increases. These are significant issues for any social care system to take into account. Social workers and other care workers have to understand the experiences of both the person who needs care and the person who provides it.

Whether the carer is young or old, this provision will have its own individual dynamics, containing a varied mixture of satisfaction, hatred, obligation and duty, love and self-sacrifice. Many women find it impossible to continue in paid employment and carry out necessary caring roles. The punishing physical responsibilities that may be involved, the isolation caused by constant attendance, or the depression brought about by the situation may damage the carer and their well-being (Brody and Saperstein, 2006). The job of the social worker and other providers is to work sensitively with each family or community network to offer as helpful a service as possible. This may involve tasks additional to the simple assessment of an individual's care needs, and is a subtle, sensitive process of fitting in with carers' development.

Do you know someone who has the role of carer in relation to an older person? Ask them if they would mind discussing with you some good things about this role and some areas which are negative or problematic.

Social exchange theory

Social exchange theory views social life as structured by what each participant exchanges with the other. Interactions continue as long as each feels they are profiting, and that there is some reciprocity. Writers such as Hendricks (2004), Dowd (1980) and Nelson (2000) apply this to ageing. They view withdrawal and social isolation not as a result of individual choice or functional system requirements, but as brought about by inequalities in the exchange available to older people. Younger adults can exchange work roles for financial income; partners exchange emotional goods; older people give up their place in the workforce and in exchange they receive a pension, increased leisure time and are relieved of the responsibility to work.

Dowd suggested that most old people do not see this as a fair exchange but feel they are unable to do anything about it. Their exchange goods become 'compliance' and 'dependence'. Nelson's research analyses this in relation to residential care, highlighting the non-symmetrical exchanges that exist. He finds that residents tend to adopt submissive influence strategies, whereas staff members tend to neglect, exploit, or abuse difficult or resistant residents. He argues that patient-directed advocates could rebalance power and eliminate inequities. Hendricks (2004) uses the framework to integrate the personal experiences of older people with broader factors: 'economics, [political social policy], and entitlements make a difference in how life is compiled ... [They] affect so fundamental a component of selfhood as sense of identity. The goal of this discussion is to provide a more inclusive template linking sense of self, identity, and public policies as meaning-making parameters affecting older actors.' This illustrates the way in which the different levels of Bronfenbrenner's analysis interact – the psychological is not independent of social structures.

Reflective thinking

Chapter 7 commented on identity – how it is created by social context and is also a personal 'sense of self'. This activity reflects on this subject in relation to ageing.

First, think about yourself. What aspects of your identity are common to others in your generation (perhaps, specific to your generation)? What aspects are formed by social expectations of 'someone in your position'? What aspects of your identity do you regard as specific to your personal qualities and experience?

Thinking of an older person whom you know, what aspects of their 'identity' do you think are common to others of the same generation (perhaps, distinctive to that generation)? Which are generated by social expectations of 'someone in their position'? Which aspects of their identity are specific to their personal qualities and experience?

The political economy of ageing

The **political economy of ageing** uses accounts previously applied to class, gender and race and applies them to the specific situation of older people. Marxist models of society had understood all social structure and function to flow from underlying economic factors. Those who own the means of production exploit those who don't. Politics, culture and social structures all rest on ownership and profit. In capitalist society workers have to sell their labour at less than its real value, the difference being taken as profit by the owners of the business. In capitalist society, argued Phillipson (1982), older people have no economic value, so few social resources are allocated to them. Older age is a period of structured dependency which is socially constructed, not biologically determined. Estes and colleagues (2003) further suggested that a service industry of agencies, providers and planners grows up that maintains the 'outsider' status of older people, but brings their situation into the profit-making economy to the benefit of planners, business people and service workers.

THE MATURE IMAGINATION

Simon Biggs (1999) uses the phrase 'the mature imagination' to introduce his account of the dynamic and varied sense of self in later life.

At each stage of growing older, people develop a fresh perspective on the matters which are the subject of this book and of your studies. All the issues listed so far in this chapter, and many others – the different situation of each older person – influence the understanding they bring to this appraisal. Someone who has had a life-threatening health experience may look in a different way on the whole significance of living and the pleasures (or satisfactions) that matter. Constant physical pain or low-level bodily discomfort may well prompt different explorations of the role of the body and the mind in the experience of pain – possibly a new sense of the ambiguity about the part played by biological and attitudinal factors.

Studies of relationship quality over time have to take account of changing partnership patterns, cultural effects and demographic effects. Nevertheless, most studies find that older married couples are happier than younger married adults, and report fewer negative interactions (Akiyama et al., 2003; Stuart-Hamilton, 2012).

A woman whose marriage has lasted sixty years will have insights and reflections about the meaning and management of a close relationship which are not available to others; a widow, in contrast, may have a unique sense of the contribution to personal identity made by being on one's own or in a couple. A same-sex couple who have stayed together through decades of differing public and legal attitudes will have their own conclusions about public morality. A woman born during the First World War who did not marry and worked until her seventies (or gave up work in her late forties to care for her mother) will have a specific view about social and emotional life. A person in the early stages of Alzheimer's disease will be able to describe the effects of losing memory, thinking power and ordered emotion (as well as articulating the way care should be managed) in a way that is not available to others. A daughter or partner caring for her experiences the loss of freedom, perhaps the loss of a work role, which only she is in a position to articulate. The most important lessons in social work come not from courses but from the people with whom you work.

Many may have insights to communicate about spiritual matters. They may consider that it is all-pervasive, even in secular life, and gives a fundamental meaning to what is done – or may now believe that, despite all the sacrifices they made for religion and the way they allowed it to structure their lives, it is in fact a social construct and cannot have the transcendence they once attributed to it.

As in so many matters, they may be able to comment in a way not available to younger people on the combination of decline and vitality they experience.

Erikson's analysis of the later stages of life is that it is a time when the older person reviews life. The two possible outcomes of the characteristic crisis of older age (see 'Essential background', section 6) are integration or despair. The positive outcome achieves a sense of integration of the experiences of life, valuing achievements and accepting realistically goals of middle life which turn out to be unattainable. Although this chapter has suggested that this is bound to oversimplify the long decades and diversity of the years grouped together as 'older age', it is worth noting that Erikson himself (1902–1994) published his last work, *Vital Involvement in Old Age*, at the age of 87. Feil (1989) suggested that a more realistic scheme would be to add a final stage to Erikson's, a stage in which the possible outcomes are to sink into a vegetative state or to integrate the experiences of life.

Chapter EB6

This chapter has looked at a number of the dimensions to this mature experience of self, the 'mature imagination'. The self is forming and re-forming in the context of a changing experience of the capabilities of body and mind, for many a changed experience of pain or discomfort. The chapter referred to the gap which can open up between the sense of self and restrictive, dependency-creating social structures. The research about social support indicated the importance of an individual feeling that he or she is still of use in society. As a study undertaken by older people themselves put it, the purpose of social support is to ensure 'you feel as though you are still someone' (CSAC and Age Concern Cumbria, 2006). Atchley's work emphasises the importance of being able to create 'continuity' in selfhood through the changes of life. Afshar's research indicated the difference between people in different life settings, white indigenous women who had not moved from their locality being the most likely in their study to feel ignored, marginalised and disregarded. Erikson's view that the developmental pathways arising in this particular life crisis can lead either to ego integration or to despair is a useful caution against romanticising the mature experience of self. (Boyd and Bee (2015) report studies which found that 'wisdom' is higher in young people than older people.) Statistics indicate the degree to which older people at different ages are themselves carers for others, with all that this entails in terms of health, experience, relationships, and self-identity. This active self-formation is structured by economic realities – of poverty or comfort, good or poor accommodation, physical neglect or care.

Chapter 9 takes our thoughts to death – the approach of death; the brute fact of death itself, at whatever age it arrives; the circumstances of death; and the impact on those bereaved.

SUMMARY

'Older age' refers to a very wide age span and widely varying experiences. One of the most striking features of any research into ageing is the extent of difference and diversity. A common scheme is to distinguish 'young old' (about 60 to 75), old old (about 75–85) and the oldest old (85 and older). The older people are, the longer they can expect to live. A 65-year-old man can expect to live until he is 83 whilst an 85-year-old can expect to live until he is 91 years old.

Loss of function in later life is related to social and psychological factors interacting with physical changes. The menopause is an example of changes that take place in the sexual system; arthritis is an example in joints and movement; strokes in the cerebrovascular system; dementia (through Alzheimer's disease or other causes) in cognitive functioning.

Disengagement theory views progressive social disengagement as a positive dynamic, for both the individual and society. Activity theory by contrast views participation in valued social roles as an important part of healthy ageing, and holds that active people are more satisfied than those who are not. Feminist perspectives emphasise that development in older age can only be understood if gender is taken into account. Exchange theory suggests that social life is structured by what people can offer to each other, and that dependency is characteristic in older people because it is all they have available to 'exchange'. The political economy of ageing regards older age as a period of enforced dependency caused by the lack of economic productivity.

Culture, social policy and history shape the ageing process. Social care should be flexible, designed to promote independence and choice. It is crucial for the social worker to be able to respect, appreciate and enter into the 'mature imagination' of each person.

FURTHER READING

Johnson, M. L., Bengtson, V. L., Coleman, P. G. and Kirkwook B. L. (eds) (2005) *The Cambridge Handbook of Age and Ageing.* Cambridge: Cambridge University Press. Standard resource on all aspects of ageing.

Bond, J., Peace, S., Dittmann-Kohli, F. and Westerhof, G. (eds) (2007) *Ageing in Society.* London: Sage. Thorough account of social aspects of ageing.

Brody, E. (2004) *Women in the Middle.* New York: Springer Publishing. This is a powerful account of the multiple competing demands on the time and energy of women who are the caregivers to ageing parents. The central focus is on the caregiving story from the perspective of women; its joys, demands and problems. It analyses the social background and subjective experiences of parent care, never losing sight of the experience of the older generation being cared for. The policy background is American, but that does not affect the universality of the studies in this remarkable book.

Stewart, S. and Vaitilingam, R. (eds) (2004) *Seven Ages of Man and Woman.* London: ESRC. Chapters 6 and 7, pp. 28–35, set older age in the context of the rest of life.

Statistics about older people – population profile, life expectancy, income, work, caring, gender, ethnicity and much more – are available from the Office for National Statistics, which holds a treasure house of information: www.ons.gov.uk.

For a comprehensive and readable account of ageing, with detail about many topics relating to older age, an (American) source is: Boyd, D. R. and Bee, H. L. (2015) *Lifespan Development.* Seventh edition. Boston: Pearson/Allyn and Bacon.

For topics related to social care and social policy, the Joseph Rowntree Foundation commissions and publishes much relevant research. Most of their research is accompanied by two- or three-page online summaries, found by using their search facility on www.jrf.org.uk/.

RESOURCES FOR SERVICE USERS

Resources for older people and their carers:

Age UK: www.ageuk.org.uk. Policies, campaigning and services about social care, inclusion, travel, safety, health, consumer issues and more.

The NHS Choices (patient resources): www.nhs.uk/pages/home.aspx. Information about all health matters relating to later life, including: healthy living, Alzheimer's disease, arthritis, Parkinson's disease, and many other topics.

Based on the text:

1. Write an essay titled: 'Anti-oppressive practice in social work with older people'.

    In suggesting this question, we make the assumption that you already have some knowledge of the meaning of 'anti-oppressive practice'.

    Note that the essay will not focus only on prejudice and discrimination about age, but will discuss how ageing can be negatively structured because of other factors like gender and ethnicity.

2. Are the following statements true or false?

    (i)   Social disengagement theory is critical of modern social structures for causing older people to be disengaged from society.
    (ii)   Activity theory states that older people who remain active are likely to be better adjusted.
    (iii) Continuity theory is particularly important at the present time because it emphasises the need for continuity, collaboration and person-centred care between social services and healthcare.
    (iv)   As you grow older, your life expectancy increases.

Prepare a poster or brief report on one of the following:

■ The presentation of older people in the newspapers, television and other media
■ Ageism
■ Assessing the social care needs of older people
■ Elder abuse

CHAPTER 9

Dying, grief and mourning

In this chapter you will find:

- **Death and dying**
- **Humanistic, psychodynamic and attachment approaches**
- **Kübler-Ross, Stroebe and Schut, and Worden**
- **Young people and death**
- **Context and meaning**
- **Understanding self**

INTRODUCTION

> Nicola's mother Ann is talking to the social worker. 'It just seems so hard at the moment. I was told about a death in the family at midnight last night. It's the godmother of my sister's children. So she's only our age. It's terrible news. It was quite quick, not expected, though she's been ill.
>
> 'And then there's my mother. She's been looking out for her neighbour Doris, who's got dementia as well as cancer. But now Doris has died. Mum's . . . quite getting on, you know, she's quite old now, so it's a kind of relief. But it's just so much.'

Freud described the experience of bereavement as 'living psychologically beyond our means' – that is, trying to do something we do not have the resources to do. Whatever one's personal history, one may be apprehensive about exploring this experience.

Every bereavement, and its effect, is different. For one person, the death of a mother after a long illness may be sad, an event which causes some simplification of day-to-day life, an event which brings home their own mortality. It may be an occasion which brings together family members, which brings the comfort of shared grief and the unusual experience of acceptable shedding of tears in public. Then and afterwards it allows the person's father,

brothers and sisters to talk about her, her admirable and her difficult qualities, to reflect in a new way about the totality of her life. They may feel able
to relate to her now in a less conflicted way, with affection released from
the day-to-day difficulties she presented. But in other circumstances, the
emotional experience may be intense, and the social worker who is involved
may be faced with emotional challenges.

> The doctors sought the consent of Robina and her husband to switch
> off Yasmin's life support machine. Yasmin was 10, and the hospital social
> worker had known the family for several years now. Yasmin had appar-
> ently been progressing well, and had been living at home for periods of
> up to six months. But when she came into hospital six weeks ago, there
> were unexpected complications, and it was evident that things were seri-
> ously wrong. In the last week, the doctors reported that her brain was not
> responding; on Tuesday, after discussions with the clinical team (includ-
> ing the social worker), the doctors held a meeting with the parents about
> switching off the equipment that was keeping Yasmin's body functioning.
> The social worker had met with different combinations of parents, aunts,
> children, and cousins four times during the week. 'Would you stay with
> me when they switch off the machine?' Robina had asked. In collabora-
> tion with the nurses, the social worker had asked whether the parents
> wanted some music played during Yasmin's last moments; whether they
> wanted incense burning; who they wished to be in the room; what time
> of day the final moments should take place; whether they wanted any
> photographs taken. Despite the comparative suddenness of the deterio-
> ration, the parents had reached a resignation, and there was a moving
> solemnity and calm about the final (technology-assisted) breaths taken
> by their daughter.

By contrast, Beryl's experience of the medical treatment and death of her
child forty years ago, followed by her attempts to establish her life afterwards,
is remembered as a nightmare. In recollection, the events are disjointed and
fragmentary. They cause a darkness to descend on her experience and
responses, a darkness she can neither describe nor manage. Now aged 60,
she leads a tightly organised life. In a way that she herself can hardly put her
finger on, she thinks of her child 'most days' or 'most weeks'. When there is
a 'new arrival' among acquaintances, she makes what she considers to be
appropriate social noises and finds her attention quickly turns to other matters. She and her husband separated nine months after the death of their
child, and she has not had the energy to invest in another close relationship
since. When the television news announced an inquiry into child deaths at
the hospital, they posted a phone number. She debated for days with herself
and then on an impulse rang the number. The social worker who took her
phone call invited her to see her. At the subsequent interview, it was explained
that there were no indications of any links between the news story and her
child, but that sometimes people appreciated the time to talk about what
had happened. In her meeting with the social worker, she talked for the first

time about the events that seemed burned into her memory. The day after the birth, she was allowed to see her baby for two periods of thirty minutes each. On the morning of the next day she was informed that her baby had died during the night, and she didn't see her body. 'They tried to shield me', she said. 'As if she was something ugly. But they didn't understand. To me she was beautiful. She was *mine*. And I never even gave her a name. I just call her "my angel". I blame them. I wish I had given her a name. They just sent me home. No one spoke to me.' On the whole, she kept her composure during this meeting. But the social worker sometimes felt her own eyes filling up, and felt unsure whether this was acceptable. Occasionally there were long pauses, too, and the social worker didn't know if she should say something. In truth, she didn't know what to say. At the end, she asked, 'Shall we fix another meeting?' There was no uncertainty in Beryl's response as she nodded agreement and took a small diary from her handbag.

DEATH AND DYING

Fears around death and dying loom large in many people's minds. Davidson and Gentry (2013) cite a recent opinion poll about people's fears and found that the top four out of seven fears people admitted to were around death:

- Dying in pain (83%)
- Dying alone (67%)
- Being told they are dying (62%)
- Dying in hospital (59%)
- Going bankrupt (41%)
- Divorce/end of a long-term relationship (39%)
- Losing their job (38%)

About 550,000 of the population (eight in every 1,000 people) die each year in the UK. This includes about four per 1,000 children at birth. Life expectancy at birth in the UK in 2016 was 83 for women and 79 for men. Mortality statistics can sometimes surprise people – a person has to be several years over 100 before the chances are that half of the people in their age group will have died within the year (all statistics from the Office for National Statistics – ONS, 2017c).

Over three-quarters of all deaths (79 per cent) take place in a hospital or other institution away from home (Marie Curie, 2017). The Department of Health (2005: 40, table 64) quotes research that shows a large discrepancy between the wishes of the public and current practice concerning where people die. Whilst there may be staff from other professions paying attention to this, it is clearly an area of core social work responsibility, involving psychosocial needs and practicalities. Munday and colleagues (2007) discuss the issues involved in paying greater respect to the wishes of people in these last stages of their development – which include funding issues, service availability, policy direction, and the competence and confidence of staff to hold (and sometimes initiate) the appropriate conversation with older people.

Having choice and control over where death occurs is one of the requirements for a 'good death' as identified by Meier et al. (2016), who conducted a literature review of thirty-two studies and identified eleven core themes of good death:

■ Preferences for the dying process – including the death scene (how, who, where and when), dying during sleep, preparation for death (advance directives, funeral arrangements).
■ Pain-free status.
■ Emotional well-being – receiving emotional and psychological support, opportunity to discuss the meaning of death.
■ Family – having family support, family preparation and acceptance of death, not to be a burden.
■ Dignity – being respected as an individual, having independence.
■ Life completion – an opportunity to say goodbye, a sense of a life well lived and acceptance of death.
■ Religiosity/spirituality – religious/spiritual comfort, faith, and opportunity to meet with clergy.
■ Treatment preferences – not prolonging life, belief that all available treatments were used, control over treatments, euthanasia/doctor-assisted suicide.
■ Quality of life – living as usual, sense that life is worth living, maintaining hope, pleasure and gratitude.
■ Relationship with the healthcare provider – trust, support and comfort from health professionals, professionals who are comfortable with death and dying, able to discuss spiritual beliefs/fears with professionals.
■ Other considerations – recognition of culture, physical touch, being with pets, healthcare costs.

If you consider the features listed above, it can be seen that some are purely medical, such as pain relief and treatment options. Most, however, are psychosocial and are therefore matters a social worker may have the responsibility to identify and implement. There is not the space here to discuss each in detail, but it is worth spending a few minutes to consider the information people need. This will come up in the form of questions, but sometimes the social worker must create a conversational opening for these to be asked. The social worker may or may not be the person to give the answers, but should always be alert to the psychosocial issues involved.

Questions about death

People who are dying and those close to them will have many questions about death. Lack of knowledge breeds unnecessary fears and disturbing fantasies. As Monroe (2004: 1109) points out in her description of social work responsibilities in end-of-life care, they will need knowledge about what happens at the moment of death; information about what normally happens and what their options are. They may wish for information such as how long after death, if the body is buried, will the digestive enzymes and bacteria in their stomach start to feed on their own flesh. If a relative has been buried (particularly, perhaps, in the case of children), they may wonder about the state of the body at different stages, weeks or months after death, and will want to be able to ask about these things without being thought peculiar or morbid. Social workers are unlikely to have the answers to these questions – their role is often to understand that they may legitimately be asked. Social workers are, however, particularly likely to be involved where there are family issues around the care of children as a parent faces death. In this situation they may need knowledge about the relevant issues and sometimes be involved in practical steps to tackle them. Either the surviving or the dying parent may want to know what to expect of their children after the bereavement, and how much to involve them in the death. The social worker needs to understand, as Monroe puts it, that helping to provide this information is as much a question of listening as of telling. What is certain is that asking these questions and assimilating the resulting information is a part of development around the time of death.

The social worker felt tears in her eyes as she listened to Beryl.

- Is this under the social worker's control?
- Is it wrong?
- What are some of the possible impacts on the person she is listening to?
- Is it something to be discussed in supervision?
- What are the requirements of supervision for this discussion to be possible?

Reflective thinking

Particularly when there is access to hospice care, many people experience a 'good death'. However, for whatever reason, death may be fundamentally unwelcome, and the idea of 'a good death' should not be idealised. Social workers in all fields are likely to be involved with 'the person-in-the-situation' (with the dying or the bereaved individual) precisely where there are complications, when the situation is additionally disturbing.

Deaths may be particularly difficult for many reasons. Untimely deaths, where the child dies before the parent for example, will seem to upset the natural order of things. There are insoluble aspects to the situation where the person who is dying has a young child. There are similar complications when there is an adult son or daughter with learning disabilities who has cognitive difficulties in grasping what has happened, and for whom the bereavement has serious consequences for day-to-day living arrangements.

Deaths which occur suddenly are likely to cause additional emotional complications, as are those where the manner of death is particularly distressing, as with road traffic accidents, murder or suicide. And in every age there are people who suffer 'disenfranchised grief' – grief in a relationship which is ignored, disapproved of or misunderstood by wider society. This may occur when the relationship is illicit (with a person married to someone else, for example, or with a teacher or pastor), or is an unacknowledged same-sex relationship, or when the person who experienced the loss is convicted of having caused it by murder or neglect.

In learning disability services, mental health, family support or work with older people, the social worker is often involved with the dying person and their family before, during and after the death. Where there is continuing psychological support required, the social worker will often (but not necessarily) be the provider of choice for the bereaved, because of the relationship and understanding already established. As in other aspects of social work, they may provide both practical and emotional support, or may focus almost entirely on the interpersonal support to be offered.

THE CONTRIBUTION OF HUMANISTIC, PSYCHODYNAMIC AND ATTACHMENT THEORIES

There can scarcely be any situation presented to social workers which does not involve loss. Given the great diversity of circumstances and personal responses, it is an enormous challenge to extract general descriptions without doing violence to diversity.

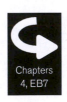

Some social workers, counsellors and psychologists would hold fast to that view, insisting that meaning can only be found in individual experience and individual response to others' experience. Such an approach may be broadly described as '**existentialist**', a term which has been briefly mentioned before as underpinning the humanistic model of psychology (Chapter 4 and 'Essential background', section 7). In practice (without the intellectual label), this mindset is one which characterises much sensitive social work. There is also a body of social work literature relevant to this view which examines how social workers use theory, emphasising that, in contrast to some disciplines, theory in social work often arises from the individual practitioner's experience, not from outside in the form of researched knowledge (Wilson et al., 2011).

Chapters 4, EB7

But there are others who attempt the difficult task of identifying common patterns in this area of human development. Becoming familiar with their work may sometimes give you words and ideas which will be found helpful by those with whom you work. It will give you appropriate concepts to consider in your writing, and enable you to build your understanding on the outcome of sensitive and persistent research into the subject.

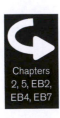

This part of the chapter first looks at the application of models introduced earlier in the book – the humanistic model (Chapter 5 and 'Essential background', section 7), psychodynamic theories (Chapter 2 and 'Essential

Chapters 2, 5, EB2, EB4, EB7

background', section 4), and attachment theory (Chapter 2 and 'Essential background', section 2). Following sections then analyse the issues around death and grief using three models: Kübler-Ross's model, which refers to stages of dealing with death; the work of Stroebe and Schut, who emphasised how people have two perspectives in their life after bereavement – one looking forward and the other looking back; and the approach of William Worden, who presents a description of the tasks which face bereaved people.

> The first paragraph of this section stated, 'There can scarcely be any situation presented to social workers which does not involve loss.'
>
> Choose one example, perhaps from your own experience or that of one of your fellow students. Write a paragraph which contains a sentence or two describing the loss (for example, 'Every time a child in care moves placement, he or she has to get used to a new bedroom, new carers, new people to share the house'), a brief reference to the ways in which social workers and other welfare staff can be helpful or unhelpful, and an explanation of why supportive supervision for these staff members is necessary. The 'loss' may not be in the present – social workers repeatedly provide service for people who have multiple or poorly handled losses in the past.

Reflective thinking

The humanistic model

In the humanistic model ('Essential background', section 7), the core feature which enables positive development after bereavement, or in the face of one's own death, is *unconditional acceptance*. Making links to relationships whose purpose is to facilitate or bring about development, what are the issues around '*empathy*' or '*congruence*' which arise in this area? The questions for reflection are about what is meant by 'self-actualising' (Maslow) or 'the fully functioning person' (Rogers), and what is meant by a motive to 'self-actualise' when a person is facing their own death or dealing with a severe loss. The following example, fictionalised so as to link with the lives of Tia and her mother, provides some prompts for your thinking about this. It should focus your thoughts on what kind of development a social worker might be fostering in the very last days of someone's life.

Chapter EB7

Bob

Bob has been in the hospice for three weeks now. It is increasingly difficult for him to retain any food, and the doctors are clear that he is unlikely to live another fortnight. His granddaughter Tia is unaware of anything about him, let alone that he is dying. Bella has not seen her father for twenty-five years, and has never spoken to her daughter about him. The final rift came when Bella, aged 19, came home at half past midnight. Bob let loose a tirade of vitriolic criticism and would not listen to Bella's explanations. As she tried to explain what had happened – 'Don't talk back to me, young lady', he said, as he pushed her against the wall. 'If you live in my house, you do as I say.' He blamed the lateness on her boyfriend, David, of whom he violently disapproved. Bob was repeating out loud arguments he had been rehearsing in his mind for weeks, and venting his fury at feeling he was not in control of the situation. Using tactics that had kept him in line in the army, he was expressing the views which had been rigidly instilled in him in his upbringing.

For Bella, this was the last thing she was prepared to tolerate. When she stormed out this time, she went back to David, and she did not return. The only message which reached her from her father was for her to stay away until she knew better, and she took him at his word.

The hospice nurses were quite fond of the old-fashioned 75-year-old with his tales of the army and his feisty spirit. Picking up his distress about his estrangement from his daughter (but knowing nothing of the details), they had put him in touch with the social worker.

As usual, the social worker was under pressure from a great volume of work. But she put lots of energy into tracing Bob's daughter, and after a number of frustrating attempts, made a telephone call on Wednesday evening arranging to meet Bella at her home, forty miles from the hospice, on Friday morning. At the end, Bella thanked her for taking the trouble to find her and give her the news of her father, saying she would think about it over the weekend and ring her on Monday.

On Monday Bella rang the social worker to explain that it had been painful for her to sort out what had happened in her childhood. Having found a way to deal with how her father had treated her, she could not face reopening the matter now. She had her own way of coping with what had happened; she had no feelings for her father, and did not want to meet him.

The social worker put the phone down and sat there. All the extra pressure she had put herself under last week – the stress she had created for herself, the evening phone calls – had come to this. She swore out loud, a single expletive. It crossed her mind that if she said nothing, Bob would not know it had been resolved so quickly and, given his condition, time would resolve the situation without her having to deliver this final message of rejection.

That afternoon, she sat beside Bob's bed. His drip had just been changed, and the dressings that covered him from his neck to his abdomen were more bulky than before. 'You've spoken to Bella.' His words were a statement, not a question. His eyes focused on hers and after a moment or two she put her hand over his, which was lying on top of the sheet . . .

During the conversation which followed, Bob said that he had always felt guilty about how he had treated Bella. There was little talk in this 'conversation' and long pauses. 'We were brought up you . . . had to do what you were told', he said. 'I didn't know what to do with her . . . It wasn't right, though. In the end, it didn't matter.'

He meant that, in the end, there were more important things than whether a person in authority could force another person to bend to their will. Relationships and care, human connectedness, were more important.

'You aren't responsible for how you're brought up', said the social worker.

'I didn't know any better', said Bob. 'No one told me.' There was a pause. 'No one . . . told me.'

The social worker had met Tia's mother (Bob's daughter) and knew how destructive his behaviour had been. Perhaps she thought of the cruelty and rejection he had displayed, but accepted that it came from his view of the world at that time. Her '**congruence**', in Rogers' terms ('Essential background', section 7), was to respond accurately to his experience. The interview was potentially very difficult. She had been frustrated because she had wasted time and effort; she had failed to deliver what he wanted (a meeting with his daughter), and did not know how this additional upset would affect his precarious physical condition. If she had analysed it later in supervision, she could have recognised the value and meaning in the simple fact of human contact, the value of comfort which came from the physical contact of her hand on his; and the recognition that, whilst only he could know the regret and guilt which belonged to his actions, he was entitled not to blame himself for how he was brought up, for not knowing things about relationships which he did not know. Specifically (see Chapter 3) we could analyse this as lessening punitive self-criticism. As we shall discuss in Chapter 10, the social worker would not have known in advance that this was what was needed, and is unlikely to have 'theorised' while she was with him (although being able to put it into words after one occasion may well strengthen her for the other ambiguous situations she would encounter in her work).

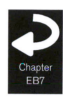

Chapter EB7

Chapters 3, 10

Does this have anything to do with human development which culminates in the high-sounding humanistic phrases 'self-actualisation' or 'fully functioning person'? Well, the social worker had failed in the practical task Bob had requested, but had given him some time of value – in which he had said out loud, to someone who understood, what really mattered to him, and spoken of his profound regret at his part in the destruction of a relationship which was part of the true meaning of life. Perhaps in a day or two she would phone Bella back and ask if she wanted to hear about her father's last days and have a word about what had happened with her dad.

Psychodynamic approaches

There is little in the previous paragraphs (about humanistic approaches) which would seem out of place in a psychodynamic perspective. However, there would be some characteristic additions. Earlier states of mind (Chapter 2 and 'Essential background', section 4) may be presented in the here and

Chapters 2, EB4

now. It is not infantilising to understand that the comfort offered to a man may be essentially the same as that offered to an infant (or whatever age-appropriate state of mind a client such as Bob may bring to the encounter). In dealing with the last stages of life or bereavement, the themes present to a psychoanalytic perspective are not new. Themes of death may be unconscious in earlier states of mind — present in the mind, but shut off from consciousness. The young person's pursuit of thrills in driving recklessly, group violence, or extreme sports may be a denial, an avoidance, of the reality of death in favour of a fantasy of immortality; and, indeed, one criticism of humanistic psychology is that its resounding affirmation of life and growth is a denial of death, decay and destructiveness, a firm shutting out of this reality. From the beginning of life, and in all its stages, the developing self has to deal with the fear (and sometimes the realistic proximity) of its own destruction. The approach of an individual's own death is linked to the way in which they have previously dealt with the death or other loss of those close to them.

According to this approach, the loss of a loved object has been experienced since infancy, when the baby cried for someone to come when it woke up alone at night. Relevant incidents thread through life, inevitable, but different for each individual — the first day at school, the first weeks of a student alone at college, the experience of being 'dumped' in a relationship. The external reality and degree of finality is different, but the individual's psyche has nevertheless been finding ways to deal with the absence of someone who seems essential for survival.

In relation to the action of the social worker in placing her hand over her client's — or in physically comforting a bereaved relative by holding their hand or putting an arm around their shoulder — note that different psychoanalytic practitioners take different views. Some (particularly, but not only, social workers) find the physical demonstration of care in this situation straightforward, the cue to its presence or avoidance being in the state of the client. Other psychoanalytic thinkers would see such contact as inappropriate, an unrealistic attempt by the worker to take away inevitable pain. They might argue that it arises at some level from the worker's own needs, and is not an appropriate part of the relationship between professional and service user.

The standard psychoanalytic understanding is that in grief, the person who has lost the object of their love must undertake the task of detaching the energy invested in that person. This frees them to attach it elsewhere. Many psychoanalytic commentators would expect that avoiding the expression of grief may prolong its effects and lead to complicated or pathological patterns later. It is true that this can sometimes happen — a social worker may need to listen and be with someone who says, 'I just wish I hadn't been so busy and unable to grieve at the time — I feel it's just made it worse later; it's unfinished, not sorted out.' And the person may gain relief from expressing the feelings they would have liked to have presented at the time of the loss. But there are many experienced practitioners who believe it is profoundly misleading to think that the avoidance of grief expressions at the time of a significant loss necessarily causes problems later on. Evidence supporting this view is cited by Boyd and Bee (2015).

Attachment theory and bereavement

Chapters 3, EB2

Attachment theory grew out of psychoanalytic theory, often paying much more attention to realistic observation (see Chapter 3 and 'Essential background', section 2). From an attachment perspective, bereavement is a disruption of an attachment relationship. Hazan and Zeifman quote the results of research showing that many of the responses of bereaved adults are similar to the responses of children separated from their primary caregivers (Hazan and Zeifman, 1999; Zeifman and Hazan, 2016). The experiences − of yearning, of protest and anger, of seeking so intently for the lost person that the brain thinks it has caught a glimpse of them when there is a likely figure in a crowd, of anxiety, of disorganisation and despair − can be understood as the activation of attachment systems after the breaking of affectional bonds.

In keeping with the psychodynamic background to attachment theory, Colin Murray Parkes and colleagues (1991) examined whether there was a link between the nature of the help requested by bereaved people and their descriptions of their earlier attachments (particularly with parents). In his sample of patient records reviewed retrospectively, he found that there was such a link − patients who described what might be expected to be secure attachments tended to be represented predominantly in relation to situations of 'traumatic' bereavements such as violent or obviously untimely deaths, and to use only a few sessions; whereas people who described problematic early attachment relationships tended to be equally present in relation to all kinds of bereavement.

In attachment theory, grief is understood as a process, not an event, and the process follows the response of the attachment system to the loss of an attachment figure.

Loss is a simple fact − the deprivation of something or the failure to get something.

Grief is a set of responses to loss − feelings and the expression of those feelings, a process people go through.

Does all loss result in grief? What are some of the components of grief, feelings that may be experienced or expressed?

Reflective thinking

THREE THEORIES ABOUT DEATH AND GRIEF

The work of Elisabeth Kübler-Ross

One way of making sense of responses to approaching death is to look for patterns. The psychiatrist Elisabeth Kübler-Ross (1989) was a strong advocate of listening to people's experiences during life-shortening illnesses. She describes her conversations with doctors (and others) in which she helped them to listen to their patients and not act out of their own discomfort or guilt or technical priorities. From her work with cancer patients (adults and children) and their relatives, she sets out a series of phases that people typically go through in the period between receiving a diagnosis and death.

Reflective thinking

'She helped them to listen to their patients and not act out of their own discomfort or guilt or technical priorities' (see paragraph above).

Thinking of the characteristics of a good death identified earlier in the chapter by Meier et al. (2016), in what way might social workers or medical staff act out of their own discomfort or guilt or technical priorities, instead of attending to the needs of someone who is going to die?

Obviously, there are many possible answers to this. You could point out:

- A social worker may be unsure of how to talk about death with a person whose needs they are assessing for discharge from hospital – so they don't enquire where the person wishes to die.
- Nurses may concentrate on their clinical tasks of medication and hygiene instead of taking the time to listen.
- Doctors may treat the person as a medical challenge and keep them alive without asking what the person wants.
- Social workers may keep rigidly to an assessment schedule about accommodation, activities of daily living, finance and independence, and not take the time to listen to the person's view of their situation.
- The topic may be avoided because the staff member is embarrassed, or the worker may think it is helpful to 'cheer the patient up' because it is too painful to stay with the real feelings.

Chapter 4

Kübler-Ross found that it is common for people to react initially with shock (you will recall from Chapter 4 that Hopson also identified this as the first reaction to life transitions in general – see Adams et al., 1976). In this phase they may find it hard to take the information in, may think there has been a mistake (perhaps the medical records have been mixed up), may find their ability to concentrate impaired, and have difficulty making decisions or managing their affairs.

This is followed by a phase of anger – perhaps directed at the people who conveyed the diagnosis, at people whom the individual blames for causing the illness, at friends and acquaintances, at 'God' or 'fate' for being so harsh.

Chapter EB9

The phases Kübler-Ross identifies are set out in 'Essential background', section 9. If full progress is made, the final phase is one of acceptance, in which the person is at ease with the reality of life, and can deal appropriately with tasks and relationships. This includes making appropriate financial arrangements, particularly as regards any dependants. It also means having a realistic sense of how to end close relationships – to say goodbye, exchange mementoes, to make space for things which need to be said but were not said earlier in life. It involves appreciating the needs of the other party in the relationship, who must face the loss. This too has echoes in Hopson's final phase of transitions, where he describes people coming to an understanding of their life and its meaning.

Kübler-Ross also applied her model to the experience of loss and bereavement. The bereaved person also goes through phases of shock, disbelief, guilt, sadness and so on – and if conditions are right, will finally reach acceptance.

This view highlights the varied support needed by a social worker working with people who are dying (or bereaved). If someone is in shock, and failing to cope appropriately with some of their affairs, it can be difficult to decide how much to do for them (or encourage friends or relatives to do), or whether it is more respectful of their independence to leave them to manage (that is, not manage) their own business. If someone disbelieves reality, the worker must decide how much to confront them, and implicitly dispute with them, about the situation; whereas when the person is accepting, it may be the worker's denial which is the challenge ('Don't give up hope', or, 'Don't say that', she may want to say when the individual says they don't need to get a card for their daughter's birthday or no longer need their pension book). Each phase presents different challenges for staff.

Having the words of Kübler-Ross available can help staff to respond appropriately. If incompetence (due to shock) or disbelief or unreasonable anger is understood as part of an expected stage, then responses may be more realistic. Otherwise the behaviour may be experienced as a personality trait of the individual; as undesirable behaviour to be managed. It is important to recognise that the dying person may come to an 'acceptance' which is beyond the social worker's own capacity; it may make them less likely to respond with 'cheering up' or 'denial'.

A rigid scheme?

Kübler-Ross emphasised that she did not regard the phases as part of a fixed scheme. She said people may move through them in a different order, or may move backwards and forwards, revisiting experiences they thought had gone away. One advantage of this framework is that it helps others not to overreact or pathologise the experiences of the bereaved and those facing the end of their life. They can be reassured that depression or guilt, disbelief in the reality of what is happening, or anger at people behaving in a genuinely helpful way, are natural responses. The model encourages staff not to confront and psychologically struggle with the individual, but to stay with them through a difficult and sometimes confusing journey. The difficulty for social workers is often that they are responsible for different people whose needs and timescales conflict.

Twenty-eight years ago Bella was 17. Her mother, Gracie, was 43, and had just returned to hospital two days before. The doctors were disappointed to find that her cancer had metastasised and was spreading rapidly. They estimated that she would die soon. Gracie, however, insisted (incorrectly) that the nurse had told her the most recent treatments had been successful, and that she had come in for checks to be made on her progress.

If anyone attempted to discuss her prognosis with her, she would say, 'I'm very tired just now', and bury herself beneath the bedclothes. Bella was a rebellious teenager who resented and feared her father's attitude. She took it out on her mum, blaming her for doing so little around the house now that she claimed to be getting better, and for being emotionally unavailable. Believing the words her mother told her, she came to the conclusion that her mum was just being weak and lazy.

This would be a typical situation referred to a social worker because of 'family issues', although then, as now, the pressure on the social worker would have been to give priority to discharge to make the bed available to other patients. The social worker would want to allow the teenager and mother to have a conversation in which Bella could be told the facts, and mother and daughter could say some of the things they needed to say. But Gracie would not even speak about the end of her life – she was in a phase of denial.

A scenario in which the problems are even more acute is one in which the mother is a lone parent and the children are only 11 or 12. As well as the emotional needs of mother and children, there may be practical arrangements to make about care for the children after the mother has died.

There are a number of difficulties with this 'stage' scheme. Chaban (2000) alleges that Kübler-Ross worked with patients only for a short time, and spent little time with them – directing her energies instead towards her career as a writer and publicist of her work. Subsequent academic empirical research has failed to validate the stages she identifies (Shneidman, 1995). It places much more emphasis on individual variation, the effect of particular circumstances and the impact of social context.

Kübler-Ross's work achieved great prominence, and has been taught widely on courses for nurses and counsellors. Despite her view that the stages should not be regarded as 'fixed', bereaved people have described how, if they didn't go through the stages described, they were made to feel that there was something wrong with them, that they hadn't 'grieved properly'. It is said that staff who receive a briefing about the model in their training tend to regard it as a blueprint for what people 'ought' to experience and try to fit people to the model. People who are deemed to be staying too long in one of the phases or not 'progressing' may be described as experiencing 'pathological grieving'.

Stage models are probably not the best way of understanding bereavement. In their work, Stroebe and Schut (1999) describe the process by looking at the varying focus of the bereaved person's emotional energy

– their 'orientation'. William Worden (2009) presented an influential account which describes the person as having to accomplish certain tasks.

Stroebe and Schut – looking backwards and looking forwards

Stroebe and Schut (1999; see also Stroebe, 2008) considered that in the process of coming to terms with a loss, people find they alternate between two contrasting orientations. One looks backwards to what they have lost, and the other looks ahead to dealing with life without the person who has gone. In one orientation they may feel the sadness, bewilderment and meaninglessness at the ending of a relationship, aware of the way in which their life is bound up with the person who has gone. In the other orientation, they may be considering a new intimate relationship. In one orientation they may feel disabled and disorganised without their partner. In the other, they may be making practical arrangements about new life choices, selling the house and moving to smaller accommodation. Stroebe and Schut describe this as a repetitive process in which the person experiences alternating orientations (see Figure 9.1).

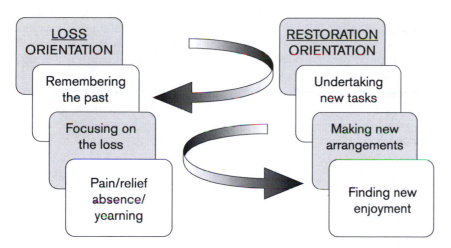

Figure 9.1 Dual process model of response to bereavement

Tasks to be accomplished – the work of William Worden

The function of grief is not easy to describe in ways that make sense to everyone. Where some theorists understandably see grieving as detaching the emotion which has been invested in a person who is now gone (or the internal representation of that person, its meaning to the bereaved individual), others find it makes more sense to speak of 'relocating' the person, 'to find a new place for the dead in their emotional lives' (Worden, 2009). We shall return to this in the final section of the chapter, about the process of creating meaning.

Worden analyses four tasks that face bereaved people. They have to come to terms with the reality of the loss, which is a cognitive component of the task. They have to work through the pain of grief, which involves a willingness to experience it – and not, for example, to avoid it by constantly being occupied instead by 'business' or by psychological denial so that it exists at some level but is always shut away, out of awareness and feeling; that would limit the richness of emotional life. This task also involves a willingness to face the additional pain that will be met during the other tasks of grief. The third task Worden identifies is the ongoing work of adjusting to an environment without the dead person, and the fourth task is to withdraw emotional energy from the loved one and invest in another relationship. Life can become meaningful once again when the cognitive and emotional aspects of grief have been experienced.

YOUNG PEOPLE AND DEATH

This section gives a brief introduction to young people's experience of death and bereavement, and looks also at the impact of the death of a child.

A questionnaire study by Harrison and Harrington (2001) of 1,746 adolescents concluded that as many as 92 per cent of young people in the UK are likely to experience a 'significant' bereavement before the age of 16. Between 4 per cent and 7 per cent will lose a parent – this is a figure in the region of half a million. The literature review by Ribbens McCarthy and Jessop (2005), noting that most studies were unlike Harrison's and used only samples known to professional staff, urged that more sociological studies of this sort were needed. They point out that mortality rates vary with class and locality and that therefore young people's experiences will vary similarly. Current literature tends to focus on the death of parents and siblings; the death of peers is the area to which research has paid the least formal attention.

Bereavement, then, appears to be a pervasive part of growing up and for some it is not notably problematic. The lasting pain or damage caused for others may only be truly evident several years later, and the cross-cutting features of gender, social class, personal and family characteristics which are relevant have not really been analysed adequately. Young people who experience multiple bereavements or bereavements alongside other difficulties are most at risk of negative outcomes – in such areas as education, depression, and risk-taking behaviour (Ribbens McCarthy and Jessop, 2005).

Some studies suggest that many bereaved young people never talk to anyone about their experiences. Friends and family can be either key sources of support or can contribute to additional subsequent problems. There are a number of adults who may be in a position to pay appropriate attention, but social workers may by virtue of their profession have specific day-to-day therapeutic relationship responsibilities with many of the most vulnerable; they have ethical responsibilities and a professional obligation to assess and provide for the continuing personal and social needs of the individual. Adults in a routine and non-stigmatising role such as club leaders and teachers also have a particularly important role to play. Some occupations involve only a specific and time-limited role (health staff whose contact with the family ends with the death of a child, or a year-tutor in school). They may not have a professional framework to take account of all the individuals in a social situation, or may be providing the support as 'befriending', additional to their core role and socially recognised expertise. This does not diminish the support received by the young person (indeed that may be enhanced), but it can create a vulnerability or lack of confidence for the adult, and indicates the importance of consultation and support for the professionals involved in these other roles about the important emotional services they offer young people.

Chapters 3, EB5

Many researchers from Piaget onwards (see Chapter 3 and 'Essential background', section 5) have studied the child's concept of death. Orbach and colleagues (1986) concluded that different aspects of 'death' (finality, causation and so on) are understood at different stages, and that intelligence and anxiety as well as age are relevant factors. Current research suggests children develop a concept of death about the age of 5, at the same time as they begin to construct a biological model of how the human body functions to maintain 'life' (Slaughter, 2005). One drawback of the Piagetian approach is that it tends to assess children's cognitions as imperfect and immature versions of adult thinking. The ideological stance of children's rights advocates is much more that children's views must be accepted as valid in their own right. This has particular relevance to children facing their own death or developing wisdom and maturity through their experience of the death of others. Valuing and listening to the voices of children can convey a humbling wisdom and knowledge about the world and its values. This is not appreciated if the adult is too aware of the 'imperfections' of childhood cognitions about death. That said, those working with children must understand their cognitive framework in order to respond appropriately and helpfully to their experience of death. This is equally true of work with adults who were bereaved as children. What lodges in their mind may be their understanding at the age of bereavement, which no one has thought to update in line with their age-developing powers of understanding.

> 'My father died when I was 5', Anna told me. 'I knew he was dead, but the last I saw him was when he went to hospital, and somehow in my mind I thought he was still there. It was only when I was 9 – I remember it vividly – that I realised he was dead; he was not in the hospital, he had been buried at the funeral, and he could not come back.'

It may be the task of the social worker in the course of their conversations with the adult to allow them to move on from their (now outdated) cognitions of the original event.

The death of a child

As Schwab (1998) puts it: 'Adjusting to the death of a child is among life's most challenging tasks. Parental grief is extremely intense and takes many years to resolve. Resolution of grief does not mean that parents put their loss behind them; it means that they come to accommodate the reality of their child's death into the way they live their lives, moving forward even though they grieve the death of their child as long as they live.' In a large-scale study in Denmark, Li and colleagues (2003) used population records to identify all children who died under the age of 18 and their family members over a sixteen-year period from 1980 to 1996. They compared the recorded sickness and deaths of the 21,062 parents identified with nearly 240,000 parents in the general population. They found statistically significant differences between the parents whose child had died and the comparison group. Among their many findings (looking at different causes of death in children and in parents, for example) they found that mothers had a statistically significant increased death rate from unnatural causes (accidents and suicides) throughout the eighteen-year follow-up period, and from natural causes between ten and eighteen years. Fathers had a statistically significant increased risk of death from unnatural causes in the first three years.

Many people – parents themselves, social workers, counsellors, nurses and researchers – have commented on the additional strain that the death of a child puts on the parental relationship. This has sometimes been extended by implication to say that the bereavement causes an increased risk of parental break-up. However, both Schwab (1998) and Murphy and colleagues (2003) found that empirical study did not bear this out, the risk of divorce being no greater than in the general population. The literature about bereavement increasingly identifies gender differences in patterns of grieving, and it is thought that this is one component of increasing tension in the parental relationship. One parent, for example, may respond to a death by looking for intimate physical comforting where the other may feel this is inappropriate selfishness and a distraction from their grief. There is some evidence using Stroebe and Schut's scheme that women tend to focus on the loss orientation and men on the restoration orientation, and this difference may lead one partner to feel that the other does not really feel the loss or does not understand their grief.

WIDER ISSUES

Culture and context

Death, grief and their management are woven into a cultural fabric. One function of culture is that it gives structure and meaning to the present. Rituals (whether at birth, adolescence, marriage or death) can be understood as part of the mutual human resourcefulness to support the creation and maintenance of meaning. Marris, an important researcher about death and bereavement, argued that death, bereavement and loss are central to culture – in its structure and function, culture has to take account of the constant passing away of the old, and has to be able to deal with the disruption when the 'imagined future' is suddenly torn away by bereavement (Marris, 1974). This links with Seale's view that 'social and cultural life can in the last analysis be understood as a social construction in the face of death' (Seale, 1998: 211, as quoted by Beckett and Taylor, 2010). The converse is also true – Eisenbruch (1984a, 1984b) identified the *cultural bereavement* of refugees as taking away the framework which gave meaning to their lives and death.

Death and grieving, therefore, as part of human growth and development, cannot be understood separately from their social and cultural context – dying is a social event.[1] Biological death occurs when the body dies; theorists distinguish this from social death, the point at which the person is treated like a corpse and is recognised to have no living social presence (Boyd and Bee, 2015).

Social work has tended to operate within a secular paradigm. Practitioners, perhaps applying 'pragmatic atheism' (Whiting, 2008), can feel anxious about exploring service users' religious beliefs, which can compromise cultural competence. Working with cultural difference and religious beliefs and practices requires reflection on one's own feelings, thoughts and attitudes (Briggs and Whittaker, 2018). It is important for practitioners to acknowledge that their own views about religion are likely to influence their practice (Horwarth and Lees, 2010). The culturally competent social worker must have the sensitivity to tune in to the meaning of death for both the individual and the social network that surrounds them.

Cultural ways of death are varied. Dominant Western practice regards the self as no longer present in a corpse, but expects respect to be shown, even in private. It is satisfied that this can be accomplished by strangers, and allows hospital and funeral staff to prepare the body. In some Islamic cultures, by contrast, dressing the body after death is a family duty and privilege, and it would be a strange abandonment for staff to be paid to do this. Contemporary Western culture takes the view expressed in this book that people – whether the relatives or the person with a short time to live – may wish to talk about their experiences, whereas a major Chinese cultural tradition regards doing so as impolite and an invitation to bad fortune.

One part of understanding the cultural place of death is to understand the **ontology** of the culture or religion – what is deemed to exist. In all the different Christian communions, each person has an immortal soul, so that the death of the body does not mean the end of the person – indeed for Catholics death may be seen as the end of a sojourn in 'this vale of tears'. For Hindus, the person will continue on their journey, to be manifested ('reincarnated') as a higher human or a lower animal, partly depending on the manner in which the person is dealt with around the time of death. Many bereaved people report seeing the dead person (Frankenburg, 1996: 3) and this has a different meaning for a culture in which this is taken to be a real sighting of a person whose spirit (or self) lives on, compared with a secular context in which it is treated as a hallucination or a psychological creation.

Only limited understanding, however, can be gleaned by reading about, or being told about, another culture, important though this general education is. In the first place, there is frequently no easy literal translation of meanings between two cultures – every word and practice ('relative', 'aunt', 'mourning') has meanings which can only be understood in relation to the lived practice of a host of other words. Also, cultural and religious practices change over time and between different local communities. The practices and expectations of an English Pakistani community, whose originators came in the 1970s, may by 2018 be different from the practices current in their Pakistani village of origin. They may be more conservative, Muslims and Hindus in the village being more intermarried than the expatriate community would allow. They may be subtly different from related families who went to live in South Wales, or Scotland. An Anglo-Indian community in the Punjab may have practices which are both influenced by Punjabi life and more like the cultural habits of 1950s England.

Finally, it is important to realise that the individual's experience and beliefs in facing death or bereavement may differ from those of their religion or culture. A lifelong Catholic may find that their experiences leading up to death destroy their belief in God and the afterlife; a man who has been brought up to keep a 'stiff upper lip' and not to show emotion may feel at a sombre and quiet funeral that he wants nothing so much as to give vent to his grief publicly and noisily. Conversely, a West Indian woman at the death of her close friend may wish everyone would go away, stop all the noisy celebrating and leave her in peace and privacy, to keep her emotions to herself. General cultural statements and patterns, cultural expectations placed upon people, do not tell us about the individual.

Life and its meaning

Attempts to research death and its consequences repeatedly return to the significance of mortality in shaking (and shaping) assumptions about the world which often lie otherwise hidden and unquestioned. The present is given meaning by the past. This is carried into the future by a picture (not necessarily conscious) of continuities about who will be there and what relationships will form the context and satisfactions of life.

To explore this as a social worker, and to understand the journey of those in close proximity to death, involves listening to clients, reflection, reading, thinking and discussion. The approach of the individual's own death, or the loss of a relationship with a significant figure, can undermine the assumptions which allow meaning to be created. Conversely, grief work can be understood as the route through which meaning is re-established. As Worden (2009) put it, 'Life can be meaningful once the cognitive and emotional aspects of grief and love have been experienced.'

The young person may take someone's life and vitality for granted. When this is taken away, the profound pain and disturbance caused in the young person by the loss may well force them to think about what they really value in life. The focus is on what really mattered in the person whose life is gone.

When my [great-grandfather] died I think it made me realise that I can't waste time and seeing the years were going by so quickly ... cause of that it made me realise that I don't have much time to waste.

(Shirleen, quoted in Ribbens McCarthy and Jessop, 2005)

The effect, as Ribbens McCarthy and Jessop observe (2005: 3), can be either that young people create high ideals for themselves, or that they become overwhelmed and demotivated. The effects, however, may have significance over long periods of time and reinforce the need for continuing attentiveness on the part of adults.

In the sixteenth century, Michel de Montaigne wrote a series of essays after the death of his father. Perhaps it is fitting to end with words which have a very different sense depending on whether they are uttered by a young, vigorous person speaking to an elder or an older person imparting words of wisdom: 'Make way for others,' advises Montaigne, 'as others did for you. Imagine how much more painful would be a life which lasts for ever' (de Montaigne: Bk 1, essay 20, 1580/1993).

UNDERSTANDING SELF

The subject of this chapter may be highly sensitive, for an experienced worker as much as for a student. Its emotional impact is specific to the person, their sensitivities and their previous experience. The subject matter may be particularly delicate because of current life events. As part of its review of the subject matter of the whole book, the next chapter reflects on the need for staff (and students) to receive competent and compassionate care for their feelings, and the need for them to understand their own responses.

SUMMARY

Experiences of death and grief are very diverse.

About eight in every 1,000 people die in the UK each year. Infant mortality varies between different social groups, including between ethnic groups; this is related to relative inequality in wealth as well as absolute levels.

There is a large difference between the expressed wishes of the public concerning where they would like to die and the reality of where the majority of deaths take place.

A review of research studies about a 'good death' found a range of themes, including preferences for the dying process, being pain-free and having support for emotional well-being.

Humanistic models emphasise the importance of unconditional acceptance, empathy and congruence. Psychodynamic models emphasise that 'states of mind' have been dealing with loss and deprivation since birth, and originally conceptualised 'grief work' as detaching emotion invested in the loved person. Attachment theory understands bereavement as a form of interruption to an attachment relationship.

Kübler-Ross developed a stage model of the processes experienced by dying people, and also applied it to grieving. It describes five stages, which include shock, anger, denial and finally acceptance. Kübler-Ross did not see these as a fixed sequence.

Stroebe and Schut do not describe stages – they analyse the person's fluctuating emotional orientation towards the past or towards the future. Worden identifies tasks which have to be accomplished – cognitive tasks such as accepting the reality of the death, and emotional tasks such as accepting the pain involved. When these tasks are accomplished, life can become meaningful again.

Harrison and Harrington concluded that most young people are likely to experience a 'significant' bereavement before they are 16. They point out that this experience will be different for different social groups, and that insufficient detail is known about it. For some it is not notably problematic, but for others it may still cause difficulties years later, and attention should be paid to the needs of young people. Factors such as intelligence and anxiety affect when the child develops an understanding of death, as well as the Piagetian idea of age-related cognition.

Dying and bereavement always have a cultural dimension to which social workers need to be sensitive, whilst realising that an individual's beliefs and experience will not necessarily follow cultural norms.

NOTE

1   The isolated death of a socially unknown individual does not seem to be an exception to this, as it has an important cultural meaning. The Beatles sang in 1964 of 'Eleanor Rigby, died all alone and was buried along with her name', and the city now has a bronze statue to her on one of its main streets; in 2008, the publicity about the death of Olive Archer, who had been unvisited for many years in a nursing home, drew a national response for fears that the funeral service would be attended only by the minister and the funeral director (*Salisbury Journal*, 14 January 2008).

FURTHER READING

About social work in palliative care:

Monroe, B. (2014) 'Social work in palliative medicine'. In G. Hanks, N. Cherny, N. Christakis, M. Fallon, S. Kassa and R. Portenoy (eds) *Oxford Textbook of Palliative Medicine*. Fourth edition. Oxford: Oxford University Press, pp. 1007–1017.

About cultural differences concerning death and bereavement:

Parkes, C. M., Laungani, P. and Young, B. (2015) *Death and Bereavement across Cultures*. Second edition. London: Routledge.

About social work, loss and grief:

Currer, C. (2007) *Loss and Social Work*. Exeter: Learning Matters.
Wilson, K., Ruch, G., Lymbery, M. and Cooper, A. (2011) *Social Work: An Introduction to Contemporary Practice*. Second edition. Harlow: Pearson.

RESOURCES FOR PEOPLE AFFECTED BY ISSUES DISCUSSED IN THIS CHAPTER

Resources for people facing their own death, and their families; for people affected by the death of someone close to them:

Turner, M. (2006) *Talking with Children about Death and Dying – A Workbook.* Second edition. London: Jessica Kingsley.

Macmillan Cancer Support provide a range of support resources for people with cancer and their families: www.macmillan.org.uk/information-and-support/index.html.

'Bereavement' – a leaflet from the mental health information site of the Royal College of Psychiatrists for 'anyone who has been bereaved, their family and friends, and anyone else who wants to learn more': www.rcpsych.ac.uk/mentalhealthinfoforall/problems/bereavement/bereavement.aspx.

Cruse Bereavement Care promotes the well-being of bereaved people. Leaflets include 'Advice for Older People' and 'Helping Children through Bereavement': www.cruse.org.uk.

SANDS is the Stillbirth and Neonatal Death Charity: www.sands.org.uk.

Questions

1. What are some of the words or phrases people use to avoid saying 'dead' or 'dying'? What are some of the reasons why they are used?
2. (i) Use Bronfenbrenner's model to describe briefly what you think may cause a large discrepancy between the wishes of the public and current practice concerning where people die.
   (ii) Expand briefly, in your own words, on what is meant by the following quotes from this chapter:

   a. 'People who are dying and those close to them will have many questions about death.'
   b. 'Stroebe and Schut considered that in the process of coming to terms with a loss, people find they alternate between two contrasting orientations.'
   c. 'Worden analyses four tasks that face bereaved people.'
   d. 'The need for staff (and students) to receive competent and compassionate care for their feelings, and the need for them to understand their own responses' (comment on why social workers working with people who are dying (and their relatives) should have someone to talk to about their emotions, and the sorts of matters that might be raised).

   Choose one of the topics in question 2(ii)a–d, and write a more extended discussion, using your own further reading and examples.

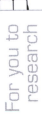

■ Helpful resources that people use when talking with a child about death
■ The core beliefs of Islam and the question of finding meaning in life after the death of someone close
■ Grief and loss

CHAPTER 10

Fitting the pieces together

In this chapter you will find:

- **Different kinds of knowledge about development**
- **Understanding your own growth and development**
- **The lifespan model of development**

INTRODUCTION

Human development is complex and often mysterious. We hope this book has helped you to create and refine your own picture of what happens in life. This chapter:

- reviews two different forms of knowledge and understanding involved;
- emphasises the importance of self-knowledge;
- concludes by outlining the 'lifespan approach' as a framework within which a number of other approaches can be located.

How do you learn about human development? Social workers should learn from the people to whom they provide service, through their own life experience, through reflective discussion and through professional study. At its best, a course in human development in your professional training will introduce you to the conversations, literature and concepts through which to tackle the subject effectively. A moment's reflection will indicate that these different methods can create different kinds of knowledge.

DIFFERENT KINDS OF KNOWLEDGE

Some knowledge about development is created so that it can be refined or disproved by other people. Other researchers can (at least in principle) repeat the observations and report whether they replicated the results. For the moment we can call this 'objective knowledge' – the discipline treats people and their development as outside objects of study. Understanding what goes into creating this 'objective' knowledge turns out not to be straightforward – it is the subject of the philosophy of science and also of social science research methods.

Other knowledge does not arise in this way. A mother may know accurately that her baby is troubled (or know what troubles it) when a developmental scientist does not. In the example used in Chapter 9, the social worker had no 'objective' knowledge that it was right for Bob's development at the end of his life for her to put her hand on his. Often, what we can call this 'subjective' knowledge is something like 'How would I feel if I were in the other person's situation? What would have led up to this, and what would be most helpful as a response?' It is unlikely that the worker would think explicitly like this in the interview, but it is an appropriate way to describe the thought processes. It may be one relevant part of a discussion in supervision afterwards.

Clearly, unlike objective knowledge, this subjective knowledge is not based on observations that can be reliably replicated by others. It arises from experiencing oneself and the other person as a 'subject'.

What we have here called 'objective' and 'subjective' knowledge arise from different methods of human enquiry, but we are not suggesting that the two are in totally separate categories. Research based on replicability and falsifiability may well be extended by further enquiries examining more subjective aspects of the topic. **Qualitative** research methods are explicitly designed as reliable ways to explore subjective matters. As a professional person, the social worker's 'subjective' judgement on a particular occasion may have been informed by supervision, discussions, seminars and research findings. The philosophical examination of knowledge, what it is and how it is validated, is known as **epistemology**.

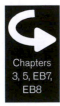

The theories discussed in this book have different epistemological frameworks. Behavioural and learning theory (Chapter 3 and 'Essential background', section 8) set out to be rigorously scientific. Researchers in that tradition excluded reports of thoughts and other mental events from the psychological study because they could not be independently verified. At the other extreme, humanistic psychology (Chapter 5 and 'Essential background', section 7) arose from existentialism, a philosophy which held that the most important feature of life is subjective human experience, and that the defining feature of this is that it cannot be 'objectified'. Psychoanalysis probably set out to be an empirical science of psychology (Freud was originally a neurologist and sought to establish a science of the mind); whilst some modern psychoanalysts would still hold that view, this is probably not the way it is usually regarded.

There are a number of well-established criteria for establishing objective validity, which you will examine in later study about research methods. Questions relevant to this appraisal are: 'What are the studies on which the theory is based, and have they been subsequently replicated?' There are detailed questions to ask about the studies, such as the method by which the study sample was chosen and whether it was biased towards a particular age group, social class, gender or geographical area. Key points are whether the method was appropriate to the research question, and whether the researcher's conclusion is justified by the findings. Different types of study – observation, experiment, cohort studies – all have different characteristics, with different critical questions to be asked. There are then related questions to ask of a theory or model which is claimed to be based on the studies. The evaluation of qualitative studies, which might explore how people make sense of some life experience, for example, is less clear-cut. There is a varied body of literature and much debate on what can be taken to constitute 'rigour' for these studies (Guba and Lincoln, 2005; Whittaker, 2012). When you consult reference books about the theories discussed in this book, any statements about their strengths and weaknesses are likely to place much emphasis on these ways of evaluating studies and theories. In using research findings in practice, the question is then, 'Is the finding or theory relevant to the service users I am considering?'

All this means that there are, in principle, readily understood ways of checking the analysis of 'objective knowledge'. The appropriate interpretation of what we have called 'subjective knowledge', on the other hand, raises many questions. One key implication relates to the importance of self-knowledge, and this is the subject of the next section.

UNDERSTANDING SELF

In using 'subjective' knowledge, one's own life experience is brought to bear on the life and development of someone else. This requires a combination of caution and confidence – confidence in one's perceptions and responses, but also caution that personal experience may be an unhelpful guide to the experience of someone else.

In the immediate interaction, a social worker's main focus of attention will be on the person with whom they are working. However, in many situations social workers will also have powerful feelings of their own, and it is much better that they should give free and accurate attention to these rather than allow them to be an unrecognised influence on how they behave. Mature workers, indeed, may develop the ability to hold an explicit awareness of themselves while they are paying attention to their client. Sometimes the worker's feelings may be important indicators of the emotional (as distinct from the verbal) interaction.

Self-awareness may not be straightforward. Some feelings may be kept out of awareness because they seem unacceptable. They may be suppressed as unsuitable for a man (or woman) or for a professional person; or they may be disowned, even to the self, because they conflict with the self-image. Disentangling the relative effects of self-generated stressors and external pressures can be confusing. It can sometimes be hard to know if particular experiences have a physical or psychological origin. Current experience may be strongly coloured by influences earlier in development – once again, present 'states of mind' have specific echoes from earlier times. Everyone is capable of self-deception.

There are, no doubt, many routes to self-knowledge. One of them is for the worker to make use of help for personal difficulties, especially for those which arise directly from work. In counselling and psychotherapy, it is taken for granted that the provision of this help is an essential component of training. Attitudes in social work are sometimes more mixed, even though social workers may have intimate and continuing involvement with the people and situations which are the most difficult in society. If this help is offered in a developmental way, the worker can learn much about themselves and the process of helping. It is important to be clear that using personal assistance for difficulties is not a sign of weakness or unsuitability. Mattinson (1975) explores how the very dilemmas faced by clients will often be precisely those which the worker experiences – and taking it a stage further, how they will in turn be the issues which confront the supervisor. The converse is also true, that when the supervisor effectively tackles the problem experienced by the worker, that may be the very support which enables the worker to be helpful with the person to whom they provide service.

Three examples

Like everyone else, social workers in their own development have needs:

- for care and support;
- for a helpful response to the anger they will sometimes feel;
- for assistance about feelings of self-reproach or depression.

Chapter 9

Here are three brief examples, referred to in the course of the book, which illustrate the link between careful support and self-knowledge. They expand in turn on the above bullet points.

Chapter 9 referred to the work of a social worker in a children's hospital. *Parents of a 10-year-old asked the social worker to be present when their daughter's life-support machine was switched off. The social worker helped with arranging the room, choice of time of day, whether they wanted incense burning, whether they wanted flowers or music, and so on.* During that day she may have been composed and supportive, but perhaps tears came to her eyes at the most emotional moments. She had known the child and her parents for several years. It was a day of intense emotion. It would not be surprising if afterwards, in supervision, she wept silently for a while as she described what had happened. If the supervisor is competent, there would be nothing inappropriate or out of place in this. The opportunity for expressing her feelings, along with the response by the supervisor and perhaps some reflective discussion afterwards, contribute to her sense of security about her emotions and their appropriateness. They are one part of what equips her not to shield herself from her emotional responses at work, to understand what is going on for herself in difficult situations, and indeed to allow her energies to be focused on the needs of her clients when she is with them.

In Chapter 4, we quoted the words of 'Emma', who at the age of 21 had kept in touch with Ann-Marie, her former foster carer – '*I speak to her on the phone I guess every couple of weeks.*' But when they had first met, Emma had been in the children's home where Ann-Marie worked – '*everyone was my enemy . . . me and Ann-Marie never used to get on, I used to hate Ann-Marie. I have threatened Ann-Marie with a knife, I've bitten her and everything because I didn't like her.*' What emotions might Ann-Marie have reported in supervision? Perhaps her dislike of the girl, her fury at Emma's lack of gratitude and the insolent way she behaved; how, for all her experience and training, she felt the urge to respond to the provocation, felt impulses of retaliation and aggression towards Emma. And then perhaps she would end by saying how much she enjoyed going shopping with Emma, how much fun she could be, reflecting that she just wished she could understand what troubled her. Perhaps this supervision would bring home in a vivid way that powerful feelings of one sort can conceal their opposites. And it was with Ann-Marie that Emma started talking about the abuse she had suffered when she lived with her father – abuse she said she had never talked about with anyone. Perhaps she needed to know that she was talking with someone who knew how to contain their own feelings of violence and hatred.

Chapter 4

Some troubles and needs are not about external relationships. As discussed at the end of Chapter 3, people doubt themselves, or are punitive towards themselves – they have a relationship with themselves as well as with other people. External reassurance will not remove that doubt – '*it doesn't matter what you say, I will still feel responsible*'. Social work has a particular tendency to trigger self-doubt in staff, and, once again, appropriate support not only tackles the immediate difficulty – if offered in a developmental way, it leaves staff with a greater understanding of the related issues faced by people they work with.

Chapter 3

A lack of self-awareness, on the other hand, can cause problems. The worker who is unclear about their own needs may be intrusive, or controlling, or too vulnerable to self-doubt. If their own development is unexamined, they may make clumsy and inaccurate assumptions about other people's lives. The influence of culture on development can be surprisingly invisible. To act in a culturally competent way, a worker has to be reflective and self-aware of these influences, and we are all required to recognise the extent to which the values and beliefs we hold may be culturally and gender specific.

Social workers are involved with intimate matters in people's lives, and they inescapably draw on 'subjective' knowledge. Whatever route they choose, they have a professional responsibility to pay as much attention to this knowledge as to 'objective' and research-based knowledge.

CONCLUSION – THE LIFESPAN MODEL

The first two parts of this chapter have referred to the place of 'objective' and 'subjective' knowledge. Checking the validity of these two forms of knowledge requires very different methods. Common to both is the appreciation that human development involves constant change, and also that our understanding of it is never static.

An essential starting point in many academic subjects is a definition of the terms used. In this book, we have taken a common-sense use of the word 'development' for granted. For further studies, however, a closer look at the terms used may become essential. 'Development' can refer to a field of study (the subject of this book) or it can refer to the progressive growth of an organism to maturity, a usage common in biology. Similarly, 'ageing' can refer to a subject of study or to a process of decline after peak maturity (again, the usage common in cell biology). There are a number of related concepts to be examined, and they overlap with questions such as whether development proceeds by stages, and what is implied by stage models.

'Lifespan' in itself refers to the period between conception and death. **'Lifespan development'** is the perspective developed in particular by Paul Baltes (1987) and now adopted in many reference books and textbooks, for example by Boyd and Bee (2015) and Sugarman (2009). It emphasises that development is a constant process of change and adaptation to new contexts through the whole of life. This has a number of implications:

1. Lifespan development focuses attention on the impact of different cultural and historical circumstances, highlighting the problems involved in searching for a 'universal' model of development.
2. Since it regards development as occurring throughout life, it contrasts with models which view development as a process leading to a static (or declining) 'maturity'.
3. It enlarges the range of academic disciplines which are concerned with 'human development'.

Reflective thinking

The activity in Chapter 1 suggested that you draw a lifeline and think about biological, psychological and sociological factors that are involved in development. Create your own lifeline again, and this time label it with specific topics you have covered in your course.

Here is the outline using some section headings from this book. The left-hand labels are specifically chronological, while the right-hand side picks out concepts, theories and themes.

Use one of the topics as a prompt, and reflect on its application to your life (this is a private exercise, and probably requires you to find a quiet, comfortable space and think reflectively, much more than it requires you to write). Perhaps you will repeat the exercise choosing a different theme.

A book such as this has to be selective, so many interesting themes and topics have been neglected. Thinking about your life and your development, list some important events or themes that, for you, are missing from the book. Ethnicity? Spirituality? Increasing knowledge and intellectual achievement through life? The impact of illness? Drugs and alcohol? Travel? Every person you work with has their own special themes and influences.

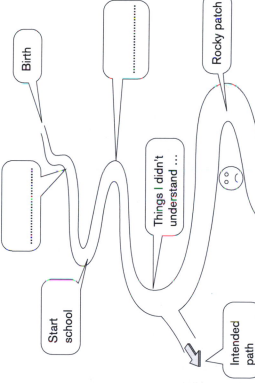

Chapter 1: Family circumstances about pregnancy and birth

Experience in the womb

Chapter 2: A secure base

Brain development in infancy – emotional factors

Infancy – before conscious memories

Birth of a sibling

Chapter 3: Early childhood

Piaget and other ideas of cognitive development, schooling

Chapter 4: Adolescence

Physical changes

Chapter 5: Living independently

Chapter 6: Adulthood

Chapter 7: Adulthood

Chapter 8: Adulthood

Chapter 9: Death, dying and bereavement

Attachment

- Infancy, childhood
- Separations in adolescence, in adult relationships; bereavements

Psychodynamic perspectives – earlier states of mind may be present in later experience; conscious and unconscious factors; internal conflict; self-attack

Erikson – psychosocial stages in life; identity formation

Living alone

Hopson's theory of transitions

Sex

Love

Children

Gender differences

Death of children

Mental health

Class and income affect lifetime development

Violence and aggression

Stigma

Disengagement and activity theories of ageing; continuity theory; feminist perspectives

Understanding self

Lifespan theory – the impact of economics and history on lifetime development

Birth

Start school

Things I didn't understand …

Rocky patch

Intended path

Baltes was particularly concerned with development in older age. 'Lifespan development' draws attention to the way changing life expectancy must change the discipline of 'human growth and development'. It makes subjects such as economics and anthropology (as well as biology, psychology and sociology) relevant. It examines historical differences in development, and explores the two-way influences in such topics as brain development, culture and environment. Lifespan researchers, therefore:

- emphasise that one unchanging feature of humanity is its changeability;
- for this very reason are also active in exploring the limits of plasticity – lifestyle, sex, ageing and child-rearing are variable across history and cultures, but not infinitely variable.

In whatever field social workers are engaged, they have constantly to develop their knowledge. They have to pay active attention both to new 'objective' knowledge developed by others, and to the constantly changing subjective knowledge which is theirs alone.

FURTHER READING

Research methods in the social sciences:

Bryman, A. (2015) *Social Research Methods*. Fifth edition. Oxford: Oxford University Press.
Whittaker, A. (2012) *Research Skills for Social Work*. Second edition. London: Sage.

Self-development and self-knowledge:

Howe, D. (2008) *The Emotionally Intelligent Social Worker*. Basingstoke: Palgrave Macmillan.
Wilson, K., Ruch, G., Lymbery, M. and Cooper, A. (2011) *Social Work: An Introduction to Contemporary Practice*. Second edition. Harlow: Pearson. This textbook empha- sises that relationship-based practice requires knowledge that comes through self-awareness as well as the knowledge that comes through 'objective' studies.
Casement, P. (2002) *Learning from Our Mistakes: Beyond Dogma in Psychoanalysis and Psychotherapy*. New York: Psychology Press. It is many years since Patrick Casement ended his work as a social worker and devoted his time to psy- choanalysis and psychotherapy. But his careful exploration of how it is that in professional conversations our mistakes and misperceptions lead us back to a greater understanding of what we actually need to understand is classic reading for all in professions concerned with human development.

1. Select a developmental theory or model. Outline its main features, and explain its strengths and weaknesses. Use an example to illustrate its application in a social work situation.

    Guidance: the theory or model may relate to the whole of life (such as Erikson's psychosocial theory, or attachment theory) or it may relate to one phase of life (such as William Worden's approach to bereavement).

2. 'Continuity, change and diversity': use this as an essay title to discuss an aspect of human development.

    Guidance: you may choose to discuss a model or theory, or to discuss a particular aspect or phase of life. If you decide on the first, you might choose attachment theory, and discuss what its adherents say about the continuity of attachment patterns over the life course, and about change and discontinuity; you could discuss diversity across different cultures and nationalities, including critiques of attachment theory. On the other hand, if you choose to apply the title to a phase in life, you might discuss adolescence, aspects of continuity in life before and afterwards, aspects of change, and areas of diversity – say between males and females, or across different cultures or historical periods. Or you could choose a concept such as 'identity' and look at areas of continuity, change and diversity.

3. 'When and where you were born predicts more about your life course than do your genes.' Discuss.

4. 'Self-awareness is the first necessity on the part of those who seek to help others' (Ferrard and Hunnybun, *The Caseworker's Use of Relationship*). Looking back to the example about the youth club in Chapter 6, or the meeting with Bob in Chapter 9, or choosing an example of your own, discuss why self-awareness is important and why it is not always straightforward.

5. Explicitly or implicitly, social workers are constantly assessing 'human development' (past, present and potential future). Discuss how their assessment is influenced by:

    (i)   both conscious and unconscious factors in themselves;
    (ii) both affective and cognitive factors in themselves;
    (iii) their own social and cultural background.

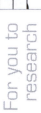

Prepare a seminar or poster presentation about:

■ The academic disciplines relevant to a lifespan approach to human development (explain what is covered by disciplines such as biology, psychology, sociology, social history, psychiatry, politics, philosophy, anthropology, economics and others, and why they are relevant to a study of human development)
■ Qualitative methods in social research

Essential background

1 The principles of heredity

Genes

Hereditary details are contained in the genes located in every cell of the body. There are about 20,000 genes comprising the 'instruction set' in each human cell, and they are arranged on twenty-three pairs of chromosomes, a chemical structure which has a single DNA molecule running its whole length.

Size

If all of the DNA molecules in your body were uncoiled and laid end to end, it has been estimated that they would reach to the moon and back 1,500 times.

There are more than 37 trillion cells in your body — if all the oceans in the world were divided into cups of water, there are more cells in one body than cups of water in the oceans. The scale of the units we are discussing is extremely small.

Babies combine 'instructions' from mother and father. Except for male sperm and female eggs, the cells in the body always contain two of each of the twenty-three chromosomes making up the 'instruction set'. The sperm and egg contain only one set each, and when they combine to form the beginnings of a new baby, this combined cell then has its double set — one from each parent. From then on, as this cell divides and multiplies, the cells it produces all have chromosomes in pairs. The DNA in chromosomes is self-copying, so one of the chromosome pair contains the mother's information and one contains the father's.

What happens when the instructions from the mother and father are different? The instructions from the mother may be for brown eyes, but from the father for blue. What happens then? Well, simplifying the situation, one version of the gene (signalling the creation of brown eyes) is 'dominant', whilst another (for blue) is called 'recessive'. If there are conflicting instructions, a dominant gene always 'wins'. There will therefore be blue eyes only if the instructions from both mother and father are for blue. In any other case, the brown-eyed signal will be put into effect. Another dominant gene is for normal colour vision versus colour blindness, and another is for Huntington's chorea (a distressing neurological condition leading to early dementia and death). An example of a recessive gene is for cystic fibrosis, which occurs in about one in 1,000 births.

Many genes display various types of 'incomplete' dominance and co-dominance. In these cases, one form of the gene fails to mask all the effects of the other. If the instructions are additive, the final characteristics are half-way between the two parental instructions – a white and red carnation producing pink offspring, for example. Another option is that the instructions 'multiply' each other, greatly intensifying the result of either signal on its own.

Most characteristics, particularly the psychosocial features at work in relationships, emotion and behaviour, involve the operation of numerous genes in complex interactions with each other.

Human variation

It is random which of the pair of chromosomes (one from the mother, one from the father) is chosen to be present on its own in the sperm or egg. With twenty-three pairs, this implies 2^{23} or over 8 million different combinations – each fertile person is capable of producing this number of different eggs/sperm. Theoretically, therefore, there are 65 trillion different possible fertilised eggs combining one of these from a father and one from a mother. In fact, because this is a simplified account, the number of possibilities is even larger, and this is why each person has a unique genetic inheritance. The one exception is when an existing fertilised egg splits identically into two. These form identical twins, a feature of approximately one in 270 pregnancies.

Other sources of genetic variation

An additional source of variation occurs because genetic information is occasionally not passed accurately through the generations. There may be copying errors, or environmental factors such as radiation may cause the DNA to mutate before it replicates.

Some 90 per cent of our genes have no function in producing a human – they are 'junk DNA' accumulated through the course of 1,000 million years of evolution. Most of the mutations occur in this junk DNA and therefore have no effects on the next generation. A small proportion produce a change which turns out later to be either harmful or helpful. The British royal family suffers from haemophilia – a dangerous condition in which blood does not clot, caused by a particular variation in a single gene. By tracing the family history of this disease, geneticists have been able to identify the individual (Queen Victoria) in whom the damaging gene mutation must have occurred. On the other hand, it is thought that a mutation long ago in a mosquito-infected area gave rise to a variation that is resistant to malaria. The offspring were better at surviving than people with the non-variant, and so the gene is quite prevalent in the population of these areas. Unfortunately, while having a single copy of this variant of the gene gives protection, having two copies causes the individual to suffer from sickle-cell anaemia. People whose ancestors came from these areas (particularly Africa, Italy and parts of Asia) are therefore at particular risk. So gene variations are 'blind' – they can have good effects in one situation and bad effects in different circumstances. As long as on balance they improve survival rates for the bodies which contain them, they will persist. This is the principle of 'natural selection', and it will operate to favour genetic variants even if they cause damage after childbearing age.

Sex

Twenty-two of the chromosomal pairs are similar for males and females. Chromosome 23 is an exception, and it controls sex. It comes in two forms, labelled X or Y because of their shape. If the fertilised egg has the combination XX, the individual is female; if it has the pair XY, the individual is male. The form of the embryo is initially female for all offspring. If the Y chromosome is present, it initiates the production of testosterone in the womb, and this heavy dose of testosterone causes the development thereafter of male characteristics.

Some diseases are linked specifically to the X or Y chromosome.

The nature/nurture debate

Much research has been devoted to understanding the relative influence of genes and environment in shaping us. Eye colour is determined by genes; which language we speak is totally determined by experience; a human's ability to use language is determined by genes. What about depression, or a woman's age when she has her first child?

There are a number of research designs which attempt to examine the relative contributions of genes and environment. *Twin studies* examine whether identical twins, who have identical genes, are more alike than non-identical twins or siblings in the quality under investigation. Studies of *identical twins who live apart* examine the degree to which they are similar or different – since they share all their genes, the degree to which they differ is an indicator of the influence of environment. *Adoption studies* examine whether adopted children are more similar to their birth parents (indicating the influence of heredity) or their adoptive parents (indicating the influence of upbringing). Some *communities* have been studied as they undergo massive changes in environmental variables, and measures then of such changes as illness patterns or intelligence indicate the influence of environment. *Home environment studies* measure relevant features of home environments and examine whether there is a correlation with children's characteristics. *Family studies* track the patterns of characteristics through family trees – the studies are most illuminating where there is a single-gene cause, which then produces a distinctive pattern of family transmission through the generations; most psychosocial traits, however, are not single-gene effects. *Population genetics*, using the techniques of molecular biology, compare the genetic makeup of 'populations' (samples of people) with and without a particular characteristic, and have generally been most effective in medical genetics rather than behavioural genetics.

For each characteristic which is studied – left-handedness, intelligence, mental illness, death from heart disease, and so on – there are different methodological problems, critiques and debates. As an undergraduate student, whenever you read of a 'headline' result about an experiment or observation indicating genetic or environmental influence in a psychosocial field, particularly if the issue is contentious, you should take for granted that there are probably complexities in the research design, results and conclusion that require careful exploration. That said, 'whilst opinions may reasonably differ on the strength of genetic influences in psychosocial behaviour, there can be no doubt that they are important' (Rutter, 2006: 6).

Genetics are referred to in: Chapter 1, where the final section is a discussion of the mode of interaction of genes and environment; Chapter 7, in relation to mental health; Chapter 8, in relation to ageing.

2 Attachment theory

Core features of attachment theory

- Infants are pre-programmed to seek proximity to an attachment figure, usually a parent or significant adult, who supplies comfort and protection from danger in times of distress, illness and fatigue.
- In the absence of threat this attachment figure offers a secure base – from which the infant begins to explore the (physical and emotional) environment.
- The hormone levels of the baby and its attachment figure co-regulate each other. Regulation of infant **affect** (emotion) occurs through the attachment relationship(s).
- When parted from the attachment figure the infant responds with separation protest – expressions of distress and aggression.
- The reciprocal relationship of the individual and the attachment figure is stored psychologically in the form of an **internal working model**. This guides the child's future assumptions about the responsiveness, reliability, proximity and intimacy of those to whom the child feels close.
- The attachment dynamic does not end in infancy but continues throughout life in a latent form and is particularly activated in adults at times of distress.

Attachment behaviours

Attachment behaviours are inborn behaviours that serve a function in establishing the attachment relationship. They include smiling, crying, clinging and following, which act to keep adults within a protective range. The 'kewpie doll' appearance – large forehead, chubby, protruding cheeks and so on – also causes highly favourable reactions and makes the infant appear cute or lovable. Adult responses which are evoked and then reinforce these behaviours include touching, holding and soothing.

After the attachment relationship has developed, separation from the attachment figure arouses the child's attachment system. Attachment behaviours then activated include loud protest, searching and refusal to be comforted (consider the response of a child in a busy shopping centre, when it realises it has inadvertently become separated from its parent).

Attachment relationships

An attachment relationship is defined by Bowlby as an emotional link, an 'affectional bond', between two people which serves certain functions (Bowlby, 1979). Infant/caregiver attachments serve to protect the young from prolonged discomfort and from predators. An attachment *relationship* for the child only develops through experience with an appropriate adult, whereas the child is born with the propensity to display attachment *behaviours.*

Howe and colleagues (1999: 19–21) draw on the work of Bowlby, Ainsworth and Schaffer to describe four phases in the development of a child's attachment, from early prosocial behaviour in newborns to goal-corrected partnerships over the age of 3 years. In this later stage, different attachment figures may serve different functions, and child and caregiver each consciously shape the nature of the other's attachment relationship (Ainsworth et al., 1978; Bowlby, 1979; Schaffer, 1996).

Co-regulation and physiology

The attachment system is described by Schore (1994), Fonagy (2016) and others as a 'biosocial co-regulatory system'. We are not born with the ability to regulate our emotions, and attachment combines biological and social features to enable regulation to be achieved. As described in Chapter 2, the mechanism is 'co-regulation' because child and caregiver are found to regulate each other's hormones and behaviour.

Internal working models

Attachment theorists consider that attachment behaviours and relationships are stored in the mind as an internal 'working model'. This 'working model' is a representation of what tends to happen in attachment relationships. It can be understood as a picture of three elements – the individual, the attachment figure and the relationship. In relation to the child, it contains beliefs about whether they are lovable, whether strong emotions usually get resolved, whether they remain safe after disturbance, and so on. Regarding the relationship between child and attachment figure, it contains beliefs about whether its security can be taken for granted or is dependent on placating, pleasing, avoidance or arbitrary external factors. On the basis of the developing internal working model, the growing child can organise its attachment behaviour to recover equilibrium when aroused by fear, pain or excitement. Internal working models tend to show consistency over the years, but change and develop according to experience.

Classification of attachment styles

Most developmental psychologists (and all who use attachment theory to describe development) regard children's attachments as falling into one of four 'attachment styles'. The 'attachment style' is primarily shown in a standard 'strange situation'. This is a specified sequence of eight events intended both to provoke the child's motivation to explore and to arouse a degree of security-seeking. The sequence begins with the child settled with its mother in an unfamiliar room. It includes a stranger entering the room, the mother leaving and her return after a short absence.

There is broad agreement about the categories into which children's responses fall, but the detail and boundaries vary between researchers. A common current scheme describes:

- **Secure attachment** – these children show a balance between exploration and play; they notice their caregiver leaving and their play activity is disrupted. Once reunited, they go to the caregiver for comfort and can be settled; they then return to play.
- **Insecure avoidant attachment** – these children display little visible distress on the caregiver's leaving or return, even though they may feel anxious; they may show greater emotional distance after separation, and they show little emotional display when playing.
- **Insecure ambivalent or resistant attachment** – these children are 'clingy' to start with and affected by the caregiver's leaving; their behaviour is again disrupted by the caregiver's return, but they don't settle. They constantly seek proximity, but are not settled by it. Howe (2005) describes this as the state in which the attachment system is constantly aroused, but cannot be brought back to equilibrium.
- **Disorganised attachment** – the child shows a variety of confused and contradictory behaviours, such as crying unexpectedly after having settled, or displaying a cold, frozen posture. The child wants to go to the caregiver, but finds them frightening. There is a strong link with child maltreatment.

Attachment through the life course

Attachment theory is one framework that has been extensively used to understand adult responses to bereavement (Parkes et al., 1991). The protest and searching behaviours often experienced by bereaved people have been analysed as the activation of attachment behaviours in response to the loss of an attachment figure.

A procedure commonly used to identify internal working models in adolescence and adulthood is the Adult Attachment Interview, developed by Mary Main and colleagues (1985). Researchers find that even though there is some continuity, the internal working model is modified by actual experience in attachment relationships.

Attachment behaviours tend to be activated particularly at times of illness or stress in adult life.

Response to separations

In examining the responses of children separated from their ordinary, 'good-enough' parents and not allowed to have contact with them (for example, in some hospital regimes), and in examining the responses of children in general to institutionalisation, Bowlby and his social work colleagues (see Bowlby and Robertson, 1953) claimed to observe three phases.

First there is a phase of protest, which is healthy, but of course can be problematic for staff. There is a phase of depression, when staff may mistakenly feel the child has 'settled down' and may prefer parents to stay away 'because he's only more upset when you come' – this is actually a sign that attachment systems are still functioning, even though the child is deprived of the attachment figure he needs. And if the child's attachment distress is not attended to, there is a phase of detachment/despair, when the attachment systems become deactivated. If this final stage is reached, the child may again be more compliant with adults, but the child has learnt to manage relationships both in the present and in the future without attachments. This is much harder to reverse.

Relation to other models of human development

Attachment theory evolved out of psychoanalytic theory, but with the intention of being based more firmly on observation. In his early formulation Bowlby saw his work as different from psychoanalysis because he postulated that the baby has intrinsic drives to form attachments. He saw this as contrasting with a psychoanalytic view that emotional attachments arose as the baby learned that there were gratifications (food, care and attention) from a particular person, the primary needs being biological. There is a similar contrast with behavioural and learning theories. These conceptualise behaviour as the result of rewards and punishments. Attachment theory, on the other hand, regards attachment behaviours as inbuilt, not learned. Attachment relationships develop as particular adults respond to these attachment behaviours. Bronfenbrenner ('Essential background', section 3, and Chapter 5) regarded his ecological theory as contrasting with theories such as attachment, which he saw as too individually based, placing too much emphasis on parent–child bonds and too little emphasis on ecological systems. Most attachment theorists, however, would have little difficulty in regarding the ecological model as a realistic way to describe the multitude of influences on development, of which attachment bonds form a part.

Chapters 5, EB3

Multiple attachments

One area of current interest is the exploration of children's use of multiple attachments. For example, it appears that in situations of shared caregiving, children form a hierarchy of attachments – looking when distressed first for their chosen attachment figure and then working through the list of possible attachments they have. Again, it appears that there may be patterns in the expectations and use children have for different attachment figures (for example, mother, father and grandmother).

Criticisms

Attachment theory is widely used to make sense of development, some researchers using it more systematically than others. Some psychologists have argued that it uses a single term to conflate a range of social influences and systems on development (see Thompson, 2005). For example, attunement is a measure of the degree to which a caregiver is openly responsive to the child's changing mindset and emotions, its inner world. Many attachment researchers refer to it as one component of the attachment relationship. On the other hand, in her research, Meins (2005; Meins et al., 2003) found attunement to be an effective predictive factor in its own right, and separate from other variables grouped into the concept 'attachment'.

There have been critics of attachment theory who argue that it is Eurocentric, or that it is sexist (see, for example, Burman, 2016). Feminists have argued that it is based on a particular orthodox ideology about the role of children and women. There have been concerns that it is an instrument for 'policing motherhood', specifically in the context of contemporary child protection activities.

From a different standpoint, Barth and colleagues (2005) argue that modern childcare social work (particularly in relation to support of adoptive parents) is over-reliant on attachment thinking to the detriment of other, more empirically based interventions. The prevalence of attributing the difficulties which some adults face with children to postulated 'attachment disorder' has been a significant concern among developmental psychologists. O'Connor and Nilson (2005), for example, argue that the consequent interventions described as 'attachment therapy' are based on a loose metaphor rather than a proper understanding of attachments.

Attachment theory is referred to in: Chapter 1, implicitly on pages 9–14, about Matthew and about Bella; Chapter 2, page 33, pages 40–44, describing brain development and describing the development of 'mind-mindedness'; Chapter 2, pages 50–61 – examining a variety of aspects of attachment theory in more detail; and Chapter 9, referring to the way in which attachment theory has been used to shed light on human bereavement and loss.

3 Bronfenbrenner's ecological model

Uri Bronfenbrenner argued that development can only be understood by considering the developing person and their surroundings together. A developmental relationship involving two people is a dyad, and both members of the dyad influence each other – for example, a mother changes at the same time as she has a baby and as her child grows. The change in her then affects the way her baby develops. Bronfenbrenner contrasts this *systems* view with one in which the development of the individual is considered on its own, as if it were independent of its environment. He considered that much research about the development of children either does not specify the changing environment in which the research took place, or takes place in a setting where the environment is in fact the psychologist's laboratory.

Theoretical ideas

Bronfenbrenner specified what should be counted as 'development' as distinct from 'behaviour currently shown'. He describes his model in terms of 'systems'. A 'system' is a collection of elements with relationships which describe how one element affects the others. A system has a boundary, and its behaviour may affect the behaviour of other systems through its outputs. It is in the nature of systems that changing one element (in a system, or one subsystem of a larger system) may cause changes in other elements or in the larger system as a whole. Understanding how systems behave is the subject matter of the academic discipline called 'systems theory', which has been applied to subjects from plant growth to economics and politics.

The ecological model of development

Bronfenbrenner's view of the systems which affect a person is illustrated in Figure E3.1.

He regards the developing individual (say, a child) as part of various systems. For example, the child may be a baby in a family comprised of two parents and an older brother. This same individual will be part of other systems (for example, the class at school comprising a teacher, a teaching assistant and thirty children). These are sometimes subsystems of a larger system – the sibling system of a younger sister and older brother is a sub-system of the family; the class is a subsystem of the school. All the systems mentioned in this paragraph are described by Bronfenbrenner as *microsystems* – the individual is a part of these systems and is directly influenced by them.

Microsystems are themselves elements in broader systems, and Bronfenbrenner analyses the *relationships between* different microsystems as the next level of influence on the child. The child is affected not just by the family and by the school, but also by how these microsystems relate to each other. For one child, the school may understand the values and beliefs of the family and reinforce them, while the family is in close contact with the school and works in tandem with the teachers. It is a very different situation if the school and family are hostile to each other and hold different beliefs and expectations. The system of relationships between the different microsystems is called by Bronfenbrenner the *mesosystem.*

Next there are various systems of which the child is not even a part, but which nevertheless affect the child's development. An example would be a father or mother's employment. Pressure or stress at work, unemployment or promotion and expected hours of work will all affect the child. Bronfenbrenner

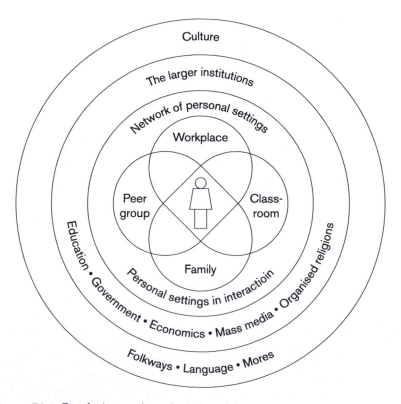

Figure E3.1 Bronfenbrenner's ecological model

describes this system as the *exosystem*. How children's services are organised is an exosystem for the child looked after by the local authority. Systems of parental support or religious community are other examples of exosystems.

Finally, Bronfenbrenner's ecological system draws attention to the *macrosystem* of society as a whole, in which attitudes, events and interactions at the large-scale level eventually affect the individual. The macrosystem includes cultural attitudes and the economy – how society views gender roles will have an effect on the expectations, self-image and behaviour of girls and boys; a negative panic about Islam may end up affecting the experience of a particular Muslim girl; national economic prosperity or crisis will affect the individual child. Bronfenbrenner was responsible for a major national project to support families with difficulties and regarded many attitudes and features of society as destructive for parents and their children (Bronfenbrenner, 1990; US Department of Health and Human Services, 2007).

These systems change over time, and the nature of that change has a significant effect on the individual. Bronfenbrenner incorporated this attention to change over time by adding to his model the idea of the *chronosystem*. When a family moves from Pakistan to Britain, there may be major changes that have an important effect on the development of the child and, of course, the parent. The chronosystem is the system of change over time.

Strengths of Bronfenbrenner's ecological model

The ecological model pays equal attention to the range of influences on a child's development, including those in which the child has no part. In this respect it is closely in tune with the classic concerns of social work – a concern with the individual-in-their-situation; not just the individual, not just the environment. In comparison with attachment theory or behavioural models it is explicitly concerned with social as well as individual interactions. It is concerned about the individual but does not consider individuals in isolation. It recognises the two-way influences at work in development – the child influences its parents as well as vice versa, and this influence is crucial in what happens next. It is a 'real world' model, in which the complexity of the real world is the starting point, as opposed to the laboratory or special situation.

Applications of the ecological model

Belsky (1980) applied an ecological perspective to child abuse – considering all the different features which increase the risk of abuse, from personal characteristics of the parents to the macro attitudes such as a societal acceptance of corporal punishment and attitudes towards children. The Framework for the Assessment of Children in Need (Department of Health, 2000) uses an ecological model as the underlying framework recommended to social workers in assessing the needs of children. Yu and Stiffman (2007) illustrate the use of an ecological model in relation to alcohol problems.

Evidence, theory and application

Bronfenbrenner proposes a theoretical framework for how theory needs to be understood. He uses a range of empirical studies (for example, Klaus and Kennel's observations of mothers' behaviour with newborn babies), and his model is deeply concerned with improving the care of children and support for families.

Limitations of the model

It can be argued that, whilst Bronfenbrenner's model is self-evidently accurate, it has produced no new information or insights about children's development – for that it is necessary to turn again to specific biological, psychological, or sociological research. Although it outlines a grand schema, it has not told us anything about the comparative strength of micro- versus meso-influences, of parental influence versus peer influence, and so on.

Practitioners and researchers using many different approaches have no difficulty using the model – it often summarises their own views of how to locate their work in a wider context. Bronfenbrenner himself, however, considered he was putting forward a new way of looking at development, which was a challenge to other perspectives. He attempted to set out a whole new framework for developmental research and practice. His work is not generally viewed in this way, and the elaborate detail of his conceptual framework is rarely used.

Bronfenbrenner's model could be used to summarise the underlying ideas of many parts of this book – Chapter 1 in explaining the developmental differences for Nicola, Tia and Naoko; Chapters 2 to 4 in setting out influences on the child and adolescent; Chapter 6 in the account of sexual development as involving biological, psychological and social influences; Chapter 7 in relation to mental health and to 'spoiled identity', both of which are presented as involving individual characteristics, face-to-face interactions, and societal influences; the different theories of ageing in Chapter 8 place differential emphases on aspects of the systems identified by Bronfenbrenner; and the experiences of dying and bereavement are similarly affected by the different systems, from the micro- to the macro- and the chronosystem. It is introduced explicitly in Chapter 5, at the end of which a more detailed example is given of how it might be interpreted.

4 Psychoanalytic theories

Variety

There is no agreed definition of the terms 'psychodynamic' or 'psychoanalytic'. Proponents argue about different theories and how they should be described. The ideas have a 'family resemblance' to each other, but no single set of core concepts is agreed by all. Many of the strands are named after the person who was influential in putting forward the ideas – Freudian ideas after Sigmund Freud, Kleinian theory after Melanie Klein, and so on. There are sometimes major disagreements in which one set of thinkers regard another as fundamentally mistaken, even though both may appropriately be described as 'psychodynamic'.

To use the terms appropriately requires reading the literature and working alongside psychoanalytic or psychodynamic practitioners. Until you are confident and authoritative, make it clear in your writing whose terms you are using.

Unconscious motivations

All psychodynamic and psychoanalytic thinkers regard actions and experiences as strongly influenced by forces which are not in conscious awareness. Some consider that these unconscious forces and conflicts can be brought into consciousness, with consequent improvements for self-awareness and emotional integration. Others regard 'the unconscious' as intrinsically and inevitably lying beyond consciousness – there will be forces whose effects can be seen, and whose content can be deduced but never directly brought into consciousness.

Unconscious forces can be dramatically contradictory – for example, at the unconscious level a person may want to be totally self-determined and independent, but also may want to be totally dependent and have someone else take all responsibility and make everything right. Unconscious motivations may be quite contrary to conscious behaviour and demeanour – for example, a person may behave and be aware of themselves as considerate and obliging, and yet their unconscious impulses may be ruthlessly self-seeking and ruthlessly antagonistic to anyone who thwarts them.

Conflicting motives

So it will be no surprise that psychodynamic thinkers take the presence of conflicting motives for granted. In this view, it is not out of the ordinary that a devoted mother should also potentially have murderous impulses towards her children (or that an abusive father experiences fierce devotion to his child). The conflicting impulses may be in consciousness, or may be between conscious and unconscious motivation, or may be entirely unconscious.

Orthodox psychoanalysts (and many other psychoanalytic thinkers) would find the root of many psychological symptoms and antisocial behaviour in problems caused by unconscious conflict. For example, constant opting-out of developmental opportunities in life may result from a feeling that approval of the father is essential, combined with a drive to rebel and attack the father; avoidance of commitment in relationships may come from a strong drive to be united with a parent, combined with a conviction that close love overwhelms and destroys the other person.

Three types of psychoanalytic theory

'Psychoanalytic theory' can refer to at least three different types of theory.

1. 'Psychoanalysis' began, and is still used, as a psychological therapy. This is widely used by people (who would not necessarily be identified by others as having 'psychological problems') as a means of self-exploration, a route to greater self-awareness and self-understanding. It involves consultations three to five times a week over a period of several (or many) years. The individual lies on a couch and cannot see the analyst, who sits behind their head. The only instruction given is to say whatever comes to mind. The analyst comments on what he or she sees emerging from these 'free associations'. From this point of view, psychoanalysis theorises what happens in the 'analytic relationship'. The ideas and theories derived from psychoanalysis may be used in briefer and less intensive services described as 'psychoanalytic therapy' or 'psychodynamic counselling'.
2. Psychoanalytic theory is also a theory about the structure and functioning of the mind. The reference above to *unconscious motivation* is an example. The concepts (explained below) of *psychological defences* and the *id, ego* and *superego* are others.
3. Psychoanalytic thinking provides theories about human development.

Psychoanalytic thinking has also been applied in other areas. For example, psychoanalytically based literary criticism might examine the plays of Shakespeare or the reasons for the popularity of the latest bestseller; the mass appeal of certain foreign policy or the media presentation of child abuse cases might be explored from a psychoanalytic point of view.

Id, ego, superego; other ideas about the structure of the mind

A characteristic of psychodynamic thinkers is that they regard the mind (or the self, or the personality) as comprised of different parts which interact with each other. Two of Freud's ideas about the structure of the mind are that it comprises a conscious and an unconscious part (see above), and that it comprises three areas called the *id*, *ego* and *superego*. In summary, the *id* comprises animal drives and totally self-seeking impulses, with no regard for others, morality or respect for the law; the *superego* develops as the part of the person which holds that they must be good, moral and law-abiding, regards punishment as a just response to wrongdoing and creates feelings of guilt if the individual does something 'bad'. These two parts, which may not be conscious, are at war with one another, and the part of the person which tries to find a balance, is primarily conscious, and tries to decide on everyday behaviour in a way that is rational, realistic and takes account both of legitimate need and of morality is the *ego*.

These two ideas about structure do not necessarily fit together logically. Freud, for example, developed the idea of conscious/unconscious and id/ego/superego at different times and there is no single view which explains how they fit together. Similarly there is no single account of exactly what is regarded as having this structure. In different contexts the ideas best refer to divisions of the 'mind', or of the 'self', or of the 'person', or indeed of what Freud called the 'ego'. These terms can be more or less similar in different contexts. 'Mind', for example, nearly always means something which is not the 'body'. The 'self' ('I', 'you' and so on) may or may not include bodily characteristics.

Woodmansey's concept (1966, 1989) of 'punitive superego' is that it is like another self, or another ego, which splits off from the original ego and develops with the aim of avoiding external punishment and keeping high self-esteem. It has the single (and, if necessary, self-attacking) purpose of controlling any natural impulses which tended to cause trouble when the person was young. It is like a conscience, but is not based on true morality but on what was approved or disapproved of during development.

Development – libido, stages of psychosexual development

Many orthodox psychoanalytic thinkers refer to the force which drives psychological development onwards from birth to death as *libido*. At the unconscious level, this pleasure-drive which contains the energy behind psychological life is attached in the early stages to the pleasure of feeding (oral stage), then to the pleasure experienced in defecating (anal stage), then for the boy to the pleasures discovered in the penis (phallic stage) and eventually for both sexes to full genital sexuality. Classic formulations of these ideas have been criticised for being wrong about feminine development and about gay experience, but there are nevertheless many examples of women theorists and gay thinkers who find psychodynamic ideas to be important.

Defence mechanisms

In most psychodynamic views, the developing self is sometimes faced with overwhelming anxiety, without the 'mature' resources to be able to cope. An example would be when the child wishes to destroy the very person it most loves and whom it totally depends on for survival and comfort. Psychoanalytic theory considers that the person copes by finding solutions which are not reality-based, but remove the overwhelming anxiety. For example, in Melanie Klein's view, the infant experiences the 'good mother' as a different person from the 'depriving mother'. It can love the one and hate the other without worry – this defence is described as 'splitting'. Other defence mechanisms include 'denial' – a physically abused child may be convinced its father loves it (better to believe that than that it is living with someone who wishes to harm and kill it); and 'identification with the aggressor' – a boy believes it is 'right' to become tough, bullying and domineering like his father, of whom he was originally afraid.

Defences may be essential for physical or psychological survival in one phase of life, but they are not realistic, and may be problematic later on. In a psychodynamic view, however, 'defences' had a reason for arising, and in the present they are a response to a situation which is experienced as the same as that which required the original response. There are also situations throughout life which require psychological defence reactions. For many psychoanalytic thinkers (beginning with Freud) important human achievements (Michelangelo's art, Gandhi's triumphant non-violence, for example) result from the *sublimation* of unconscious conflicts.

States of mind

Each 'state of mind' emerges seamlessly from those before it, and is not an isolated entity. Some psychoanalytic thinkers use this concept of 'states of mind' productively to describe how the present somehow often contains or reawakens experiences from the past (as when a scene in a film strikes an emotional chord with a viewer's past experience). Waddell (2002) describes how this way of thinking derives from the work of Melanie Klein (1975).

Transference and countertransference

In one sense, psychoanalysis is concerned with what happens when (in a very special, constant setting) one person's state of mind is in contact with another's. Psychoanalysts believe that when the individual is mentally (and emotionally) engaged with someone who is helping (or in authority), states of mind include elements relating to childhood experience. In effect, the individual experiences the helper/authority figure in part as if the latter were their parental figure; this phenomenon they call *transference*. The individual transfers onto the authority figure qualities and characteristics which actually belonged to their parent in the past. They relate with elements of openness, trust, fear, rebellion or anger which derive from the original experience with the parent.

Since the helper is human, they too bring experiences from the past, and attribute qualities to their client or service user which are not accurate. They may fear criticism, seek approval or anticipate anger in ways which are not reality-based. This is called *countertransference.*

When Freud first realised people transferred to him qualities which were not realistic, he saw it as a hindrance in his work. When he realised that actually in this transaction the client was presenting with great clarity (but not in words) the difficulties they experienced in relating, he stated that 'what had at first seemed the analyst's greatest enemy turned out to be his greatest ally'. As Paula Heimann put it later, 'On the stage of transference the original problem is brought up not just for re-enactment but for revision' (Heimann, 1959/1989).

The ideas about transference, developed originally in psychoanalysis, are applied by many people in situations such as social work. Because of their past experiences, service users may expect criticism, become angry before anything has been said, or be trusting because of earlier experiences. The worker brings their own attitudes to the encounter which are more or less realistic.

Like many psychoanalytic ideas, different writers have explored these concepts in different directions. What is described as transference and countertransference differs between different writers.

Critiques

Although psychoanalytic thought is widely used in many areas of study, it is equally widely criticised, ignored or ridiculed.

At a theoretical level, psychoanalytic ideas in general have traditionally been criticised for taking for granted (not questioning) a male-centred society as if universal truths about 'people' were being uncovered. There have been similar criticisms that it is based in very orthodox Western social and family arrangements at particular points in time and yet presents findings as if they were about 'all people'. There have also been numerous critiques and negative evaluations of the practice of psychoanalysis on which the ideas are based.

Each different psychoanalytic view has had its own response to these criticisms. In general, it is probably accurate to point out that psychoanalytic thought is based on an understanding of the common humanity of all people. It emphasises people as the *subject* of experiences, not the external *object* of study.

Many, but not by any means all, academic psychologists reject it in their discipline because they argue that it is not based on the scientific method and on empirical evidence, observation and testing (it tends to derive from individuals reflecting on their own life experience or their experience as therapists with other people). Some are of the view that where it has been subjected to testing, it has been found severely inaccurate. Some would see it more as 'storytelling' than science. Similar to this criticism is the problem (for example, about unconscious ideas) that the ideas may seem impossible to disprove – and one model of 'scientific truth' holds that scientific statements must always be expressed in such a way that they are capable of being disproved.

Psychoanalysis has had a reversal of fortunes more recently in relation to its evidence base for two reasons. First, developments in neuroscience technology have enabled key psychoanalytic concepts to be tested. For example, developments in functional magnetic resonance imaging (fMRI) that directly measures brain activity are providing growing evidence for the concepts of suppression and dissociation (Berlin and Koch, 2009; Berlin, 2011). Secondly, the psychoanalytic community has become more aware of the importance of research in establishing psychotherapy as a treatment. For example, there is now a more established evidence base that longer-term psychoanalytic psychotherapy is more effective than shorter forms of therapy for the treatment of complex mental disorders (Shedler, 2010). Similarly, individuals who undergo psychoanalytic psychotherapy appear to make considerable psychological gains after treatment has ended (Abbass et al., 2009; de Maat et al., 2009), whilst the benefits of other therapies tend to decay over time (de Maat et al., 2006).

The approach taken in all of the chapters, of encouraging your thought about 'states of mind' from within the person's frame of reference (the mother in Chapter 1, for example, or the infant and toddler in Chapter 2, or the dying person in Chapter 9) draws on the psychodynamic tradition. A central theme of the explanation about guilt and self-attack at the end of Chapter 3 is psychodynamic.

Further reading

Theoretical aspects:

Bower, M. (ed.) (2005) *Psychoanalytic Theory for Social Work Practice: Thinking under Fire*. London: Routledge.

Application to social work practice:

Ruch, G., Turney, D. and Ward, A. (eds) (2018) *Relationship-Based Social Work: Getting to the Heart of Practice*. Second edition. London: Jessica Kingsley.

Application to understanding social welfare systems:

Cooper, A. and Lousada, J. (2005) *Borderline Welfare: Feeling and Fear of Feeling in Modern Welfare*. London: Karnac Books.
Cooper, A. (2018) *Conjunctions: Social Work, Psychoanalysis, and Society*. London: Karnac Books.

5 Piaget's theory of cognitive development

In Piaget's view, the individual is always trying to construct reality out of their experiences. We are innately constructivists and we are innately scientists.

Table E5.1 Stages of cognitive development, after Piaget

	Cognitive stages	
Approximate age	Description	Cognitive stage – Piaget's descriptive term
Birth to 2 years	Mental processing consists of sensory perceptions and simple bodily responses.	Sensori-motor stage
2–6 years	Internal representation of the outside world gets more developed, begins to become more differentiated. However, many simple aspects of reality are misunderstood. The mental symbolisation still does not allow for the manipulation of thoughts and symbols.	Pre-operational stage
6–12 years	Child can reason about concrete objects, can perform mental 'operations' on them. They can mentally reverse procedures which they observe and develop the idea of generating general principles from their own experiences.	Concrete operational stage
12 years and beyond	Children develop the ability to reason about abstract ideas, understand the reason for distinguishing between valid and invalid conclusions. Can approach problems in a rational, thought-out manner using abstractions from reality.	Formal operational stage

How understanding grows

The term used in Piaget's theory for mental structures that represent, organise and interpret experiences is *schema*.

When new experiences are **assimilated** to existing ways of understanding the world, no new cognitive **schemas** are required. By contrast, when children create new models (schemas) to make sense of their experience, they **accommodate** to the external reality of the world. For example, the description of any four-legged animal as a dog occurs because a child assimilates their experience to an existing model; but to understand that some people are born ambiguously male or female, the process of accommodation requires modification of existing schemas about sex and gender.

> In the course of adaptation to the world, existing cognitive structures may be modified (assimilation) or the mind may have to create new cognitive structures for the new knowledge (accommodation).

Selected features of the stages identified by Piaget

Sensori-motor stage

Piaget identifies six substages:

- Primary use of reflexes (0–1 month). Primitive reflexes such as sucking adapt through small accommodations. No sense of persisting objects – just sense experiences.
- Primary circular reactions (1–4 months). Simple actions are repeated for their own sake. Beginnings of coordination of different senses – baby sucks on what it can reach/looks towards sound.
- Secondary circular reactions (4–8 months). Baby makes external events repeat by a kind of trial-and-error process. Imitation of actions already in the child's repertoire. Responds to visible objects, and will look over edge for dropped objects but acts as if objects out of sight don't exist.
- Coordination of secondary reactions (8–11 months). Child begins to solve problems – for example, by moving cushion to get toy. Is surprised by 'trick' behaviour of objects. Can imitate unfamiliar behaviour.
- Tertiary circular reactions (12–18 months). Child varies responses and tries out new ones. Active and purposeful experimentation. Most infants grasp the fact of the continuing existence of objects.
- Mental representation begins (from 18 months). Child able to solve some problems by thinking about them – there is a mental representation separate from the object.

Pre-operational stage

Four significant qualities of pre-operational thinking in children are:

- *The use of symbolism* – the child washes a doll as if she were a mother giving a baby a bath, for example.

- *Egocentrism* – the child interprets the world always from her own point of view (looking at a doll's house from the front, she is asked what the teddy bear in the back garden sees, and she picks out a picture which is of the front of the house, not the back).
- *Centration* – the child focuses on only one significant aspect of an object at a time (so animals walking on four legs are all dogs; a leaf that blows in the wind is alive).
- *Conservation* – during this period the child acquires the idea of conservation, that matter can change in shape or appearance without changing in quantity.

Concrete operational stage

This phase enables the child to think logically. Among the qualities of the child's thought: *decentration* allows the child to see the world from multiple points of view; *reversibility* allows the child to mentally undo a physical or mental transformation. The child is good at deriving general rules from observed concrete instances (inductive logic), but is not proficient at working from hypothetical general rules to the concrete consequences which would follow (deductive logic).

Formal operational stage

Problem solving by manipulation of abstract concepts becomes fully possible. Systematic problem solving is efficient because the underlying concepts are manipulated mentally, not the concrete examples. Logical deduction of outcomes from hypothetical premises is evident (in contrast to the preceding stage).

Later developments and alternative views

Piaget's work has been continued by many major research programmes. These have developed and refined his work, finding abilities in children a little earlier or a little later than he proposed and modifying substages, but generally working with the framework he identified.

There is debate about the degree to which Piaget studied 'actual performance' rather than 'competence'. A number of cross-cultural researchers find that abilities are much more linked to the tasks required in a particular culture (e.g. hunter-gatherer lifestyle versus modern Western) than Piaget allowed for. Some indigenous languages have number words only for 'one, two, three, many', but this may indicate difference in cognitive performance rather than cognitive competence.

Vygotsky's work places more emphasis on the role of culture and society in cognitive development. Whilst Piaget viewed children as 'little scientists',

Vygotsky viewed them as 'little apprentices' who learnt through others who were more skilled. He used the term 'zone of proximal development' to refer to the area in which learning will be possible, as long as adults (for example in school) provide the right 'scaffolding' to enable it to take place.

An alternative framework of 'information processing research' is more rigorously based in laboratory experiment and statistical/biological study. Regarding the brain as analogous to a computer, this approach analyses the different functional units and processes involved. It examines the development of each, providing a much more analytic picture than Piaget's more generalised approach. For example, this approach studies the development of 'working memory'. This is an area of memory which is used just in the performance of immediate tasks and is deleted after use – when you look up a phone number and hold the digits in mind while you concentrate on pressing the phone buttons, you use working memory. Researchers find that the number of items which can be stored in working memory grows as the brain develops. This is why children must be given only a number of instructions which fit in their short-term memory – a child may appear to be disobedient because 'close your books, stand up quietly, go to your desk and sit down' may contain too many items for their working memory.

 Piaget's work is discussed in Chapter 3.

6 Erikson's psychosocial theory of personality

Erikson developed his eight-stage model from the following origins:

- His basic psychoanalytic outlook – he accepted Freud's ideas of the conscious and unconscious and the functioning of the self at three levels – id, ego and superego (see 'Essential background', section 2).
- But he placed much more emphasis on conscious processes – emphasising the importance of the *ego*.
- And where Freud's developmental ideas explored childhood, Erikson's eight-stage framework describes the whole of life.
- Erikson paid systematic attention to social and cultural influences. He derived his model from an analysis of lives from a wide variety of cultural and ethnic backgrounds.
- He was particularly concerned with 'identity'. Many ideas in everyday use today about one's 'identity' use ideas developed by Erikson.

Chapter
EB2

Main features

Erikson (1950/1995) analyses the lifespan as involving eight stages. For each stage, there are positive or negative dimensions of outcome depending on experience, listed in Table E6.1. Each stage builds on the outcome of the previous stages. His work examines case studies to show how the individual's ego development is affected by the social environment. Each stage is characterised by a particular task, a problem in psychosocial development that is central to that life stage. Each therefore represents a particular turning point – in Erikson's terms, an unavoidable crisis arising from intrinsic physiological development combined with external social demand.

Table E6.1 Stages in Erikson's psychosocial model

Age	Stage	Potential positive outcome
Infancy	Basic trust vs basic mistrust	Basic security – underlying trust in the outside world
Early childhood	Autonomy vs shame and doubt	Sense of self-confidence and self-control – ability to manage one's own body
Play age	Initiative vs guilt	Experience of acting effectively on the outside world, ability to play
School age	Industry vs shame and doubt	Confidence that skills can be acquired and are effective
Adolescence	Identity vs identity confusion	Achievement of a coherent individual identity
Young adulthood	Intimacy vs isolation	Ability to love another
Adulthood	Generativity vs stagnation	Ability to show concern for another generation and for society in general
Old age	Integrity vs despair	Wisdom

Strengths of Erikson's theory

■ Erikson's model ranges over the whole of life, and is often used as a convenient summary description. This can then be used for more detailed analysis using a variety of other models and research methods (for example, in Hutchinson's social work textbooks about human development, 2003a and 2003b).

■ It is a psychosocial model that takes account of both psychological development and the influence of social and cultural factors.

■ All research needs a framework in which questions can be explored and hypotheses tested, and Erikson's model has provided this. For example, he describes the processes involved in identity formation in adolescence, and his concepts make a starting point for the research of Phinney and others into ethnic identity. They allow comparisons of identity development between males and females, and have informed research about young offenders.

Limitations

■ Erikson's model presents a highly abstracted presentation of a universal model. This contrasts with approaches such as the *life-course model*, which regards all development (even in theory) as inseparable from the specifics of culture, history, geography and individual circumstances. The question is whether Erikson's model takes full account of the different routes which can be taken through life.

- Even allowing for Erikson's view that the model must not be interpreted too rigidly, it is a stage theory, which thereby presents a linear picture. All elements in development are deemed to progress coherently to produce this single set of stages, each time with a 'crisis' which has a single summarising description.

- It has been criticised for reflecting a male perspective. Bingham and Stryker (1995) have presented models (sometimes a modification rather than an abandonment of Erikson's model) more reflective of women's experience in life (see Chapters 4 and 5).

Chapters 4 and 5

- Erikson's original scheme specified just one stage for 'old age'. This has been seen as inadequate for such a long and diverse period. Feil (1989) expanded his scheme to include a further stage after Erikson's eighth stage. Erikson himself (1985) expanded on the final stages of life in his book *The Life Cycle Completed*.

- Although Erikson based his work on his interest in people from different cultures (and quite possibly on his own experience of having more than one cultural heritage), his work nevertheless has the feel of being created from within a specific culture at a particular point in time.

Most of the chapters make at least a passing reference to Erikson's work: Chapter 2 where the ideas are introduced; Chapter 3 (Introduction); Chapter 4 in relation to adolescence; Chapter 7 in relation to models of the development of ethnic identity; Chapter 8 in relation to later life.

7 The humanistic models of Maslow and Rogers

Humanistic psychology

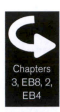

Chapters 3, EB8, 2, EB4

The humanistic movement in psychology reacted against two earlier ways of understanding people. Behaviourist psychology (Chapter 3 and 'Essential background', section 8) was regarded as too mechanistic to capture human psychology, and treated people as if their responses were essentially those seen in animals. Psychoanalytic theory (Chapter 2 and 'Essential background', section 4) was regarded as too 'expert'-based (ignoring the expertise people have about their own lives), and too concerned with destructive and self-centred motivations. Humanistic psychologists emphasised that all people set out with the capacity to become good people, to achieve their potential. If the conditions are right, this is what will happen; if the conditions are wrong, then the growth will go in other directions. This potential is highly individual, but distinctively human.

Both Maslow and Rogers regard people as having within them a 'self-actualising tendency'.

Humanistic theories – Abraham Maslow

Maslow considered that human beings have a **hierarchy of needs**. In different conditions, some needs are more prominent (**'salient'**) than others. So, in the very early stages of life, the needs to receive nourishment and to be kept safe are salient – without these, there is no survival. On top of these basic needs, there is built the need to be loved and respected. If this need is met, then the more complex and distinctively human need to respect oneself is salient – it is not enough to retain respect from others, one must have self-respect (see Figure E7.1). The highest motivations, reflecting the final set of needs, are those of 'self-actualisation' – a drive for self-fulfilment, to achieve one's potential, to contribute something to the world.

The first four levels were described by Maslow as 'deficit' needs, because they operate to reduce a felt sense of deficit or discomfort. They operate as 'tension reduction systems'. If one is hungry, one eats to reduce the tension and the motive to eat disappears. The final stage, in contrast, he described as a 'growth' need. Growth motives continue to act even when there are no

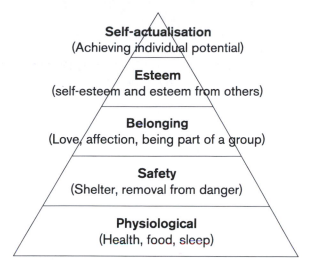

Maslow's hierarchy of needs

deficiencies. The parent, writer or artist continues to carry out their fulfilling activities even when there is no 'deficit' to be satisfied. The 'hierarchy' is not regarded as absolute – the earlier needs do not need to be fully satisfied before the higher ones become salient.

MASLOW – SOME CHARACTERISTICS OF SELF-ACTUALISING PEOPLE

- *Efficient perception of reality* – they perceive other people accurately and efficiently, see reality as it is rather than as they wish it to be, their perception is not distorted by expectations, anxieties, stereotypes, etc.
- *Acceptance of self and others* – they display a sense of respect and acceptance of self and others. Basic processses of life – sex, pregnancy, growing old – are graciously accepted without inhibition.
- *Spontaneity* – they are not afraid to express their independent judgements and express themselves honestly, but are not unconventional for its own sake.
- *Problem centring* – they are oriented to problems outside themselves, not egocentric or preoccupied with status.
- *Detachment* – they have a need for privacy, and are not dependent on friendship.
- *Autonomy* – they are able to be relatively independent of the general culture and social environment in which they live.

- *Social interest* – they show identification, sympathy and affection for mankind.
- *Democratic character* – they are free of prejudice.
- *Discrimination between ends and means* – they have strong moral standards.
- *Resistance to enculturation* – they get along in the culture but are detached from it.

Humanistic theories – Carl Rogers

In Rogers' view, there is fundamentally just one human motive, the *actualising tendency*:

> The inherent tendency of the organism to develop all its capacities in ways which serve to maintain or enhance the person.
>
> (Rogers, 1959: 196)

This is expressed through the *organismic valuing process*. Experiences that maintain the self and help it towards actualisation are valued. Rogers considered that in infancy this is straightforward – the infant experiences what is good or hurtful directly. The developing person, however, also has a need for *positive regard* – approval from others. As children grow, their self-concept becomes a combination of what is directly experienced as good and bad and what brings praise or rejection from others.

Unconditional positive regard enables the child to remain in touch with their organismic valuing process, so that they maintain, develop and enhance themselves according to their true potential. Unconditional positive regard does not stop the expression of parental emotion or displeasure, but the response is about the behaviour and not the person – the child remains secure that it is loved and accepted. Rogers regarded conditional positive regard ('I will love, accept and respect you only if you are the sort of person I want you to be') as damaging the child's potential to develop themselves to the full. It requires children to *disown* their feelings rather than inhibit their expression.

A simple example of the effects in later life might be a mother who has been taught that a good mother always feels loving towards her child. She has to have some process to deal with the fact of her 'organismic' experience of dislike, or of feeling angry or punitive. In Rogers' view, this process must be either denial of her true feelings (the defence mechanism of *denial*) or the distortion of reality – since a good mother would be angry with a child only if it deserves punishment, the child must be doing something which deserves punishment. In either case, the process has the negative effect of creating more distance between reality and how it is experienced.

Other typical examples of values which are introjected, but are not in accord with organismic valuing, are:

■ Sexuality (or sexual fantasies, or masturbation) is bad.
■ Unquestioning obedience to authority is good.

According to Rogers, the 'self' which is developed by each individual can be understood as having three components (see Figure E7.2): the area which is in awareness and is in accord with actual 'organismic' experience (area 1 in Figure E7.2); the area which is in awareness, but is a distortion of reality to fit in with what the person has been told about themselves or others (area 2) – for example, that when she was punished, it was for her own good, and because she had been bad; and the area of actual organismic experience that has had to be put out of awareness because it couldn't be accommodated (area 3) – for example, that her parents were wrong and hurtful to criticise and punish her.

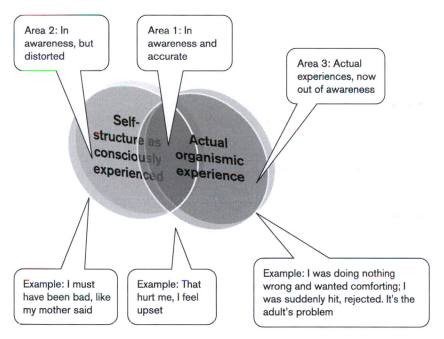

Figure E7.2 Rogers' self-structure

Applications

Many social workers find that humanistic models are a natural way to describe the developmental issues they face in their work with service users – children who have been neglected or abused, people with mental health problems, people in the last stages of their life, and so on.

Rogers was a psychologist and counsellor whose first unqualified job was in residential work with children. Aside from the fact that social work places a natural emphasis on practical as well as 'talking' help, and recognises the need people sometimes have for advice and guidance, the model of person-centred ('Rogerian') counselling he developed is very in tune with the principles of social work. Researchers working in the person-centred tradition found that the effectiveness of help depended not on the theories used by helpers, but on their personal qualities. These qualities are that the helper offers **unconditional acceptance** and **empathy**, and shows **congruence**. Unconditional acceptance is referred to above. Empathy is a continuing process whereby the counsellor lays aside her own way of experiencing and perceiving reality, preferring to sense and respond to the experiences and perceptions of her 'client', combined with the accurate communication of this perception. In brief, congruence is the ability to ensure that experience and awareness (the two circles in Figure E7.2) overlap as much as possible.

With modification over the years, the models developed by the humanistic psychologists have been widely adopted in other human services – education, conflict resolution, mental health and management.

Philosophical foundations and evidence

In general, the foundations of the humanistic models are not scientific, although Maslow was a workplace psychologist and was directly concerned about what actually mattered for people in their work. The models are based on a philosophy of what matters in human life. In particular, they place value on authentic human contact between people and authentic human experience. These ideas are based on existentialist philosophy, and would not necessarily be expected to support objective scientific investigation. However, as mentioned above, researchers in the humanistic tradition in the 1960s and 1970s (see, for example, Truax and Carkhuff, 1967) claimed to find that the significant factors in effective helping are those identified by the humanistic counsellors.

The account given in the previous section indicates how the values and approach of humanistic psychology can be widely applied in a general way. Nevertheless, the perspective originally arose in opposition to other traditions, and detailed adherents stress its incompatibility with many current approaches to helping. The emphasis on the developing self, on non-directedness, on the inner drive of the individual to find solutions for themselves, on the value of human encounter for its own sake, contrasts with didactic methods and targeted objectives decided by someone else in advance. The concept of the self in humanistic psychology, according to McLeod (2003: 142), stands in contrast to the 'problem management or coping model implicit in behaviourism', and 'identification of target problems or behavioural repertoires represent a distraction' from the aims of helping. 'Assessment procedures could well introduce into the therapeutic relationship an image of the therapist as expert and authority figure, which would run counter to the intentions of encouraging growth.' Seen in this way, the application of humanistic theory is very different from the didactic approaches of cognitive behavioural work. McLeod also emphasises that a rigorous humanistic theory of helping rejects the psychodynamic idea of transference because it is understood to diminish the significance of the human encounter in the here and now. More recently, Hill and Cooper (2016) argue that the person-centred approach in the twenty-first century consists of a range of approaches, from the classic non-directive client-centred approach to the more process-directive Emotion Focused Therapy, which combines an emphasis upon an empathic relationship with more task-focused elements.

Criticisms of the humanistic model

Despite this work about counselling and therapy based on humanistic psychology, the most fundamental criticism of the model is the difficulty of producing evidence which supports or disproves it. It is hard to see how the characteristics of 'self-actualising' people (Maslow) or the 'fully functioning person' (Rogers) can be put into objective measures, and the chances of relating these to a whole life history which identifies scientifically whether the person received 'unconditional positive regard' are even more remote. Chapter 10 explained that one criterion for a scientific theory is that it must be based on falsifiable statements, and it is argued that it is hard to see what would count to disprove these theories.

Chapter 10

It can also be argued that the theories are based on the idea of 'human nature' – and some have argued that this is a concept which is at best misleading and at worst non-existent.

The final section of Chapter 4 outlined the arguments put forward by a different criticism, one which applies to many general theories of human development. Some feminist thinkers have argued that, until recently, all descriptions of 'human' need were actually covert accounts of 'men', not including women (see, for example, Kagan and Tyndall, 2003). Society has oppressed women, it is argued, and all men benefited from the oppression; the meanings of all terms used in academic discourse have been necessarily implicated in this oppression. Attempts to describe the 'personal' independently of the 'political' were necessarily flawed. When Rogers, for example, states that he is explaining 'the most profound truth about man', the critics may say that, unwittingly, he is indeed thinking about only half the population.

Chapter 4

Humanistic theories are referred to in the last section of Chapter 4 (the discussion about general theories of 'human' development), and in Chapter 10.

Further reading

Many psychology textbooks summarise the humanistic approach to psychology – for example, Eysenck, M. W. (2000) *Psychology: A Student's Handbook*. Hove: Psychology Press, pp. 27, 713, 725.

Rogers, C. R. (1961/2004) *On Becoming a Person: A Therapist's View of Psychotherapy*. London: Constable; Boston: Houghton Mifflin.

For an account of the theory's application to contemporary practice, see Hill, A. and Cooper, M. (2016) 'Person centred therapy in the twenty-first century: growth and development'. In B. Douglas, R. Woolfe, S. Strawbridge, E. Kasket and V. Galbraith (eds) *The Handbook of Counselling Psychology*. London: Sage.

Gross, R. (2015) *Psychology: The Science of Mind and Behaviour*. Seventh edition. London: Hodder Arnold.

Rogers, C. R. (1959) 'A theory of therapy, personality and interpersonal relationships, as developed in the client-centered framework'. In S. Koch (ed.) *Psychology: A Study of Science*. New York: McGraw-Hill, pp. 184–256.

8 Learning and behavioural models

Behaviourism set out to be 'a purely objective, experimental branch of natural science' (Watson, 1913, quoted by Eysenck, 2000). Its goal was to explain, predict and control behaviour. Self-reports of feelings, moods and thoughts are not independently verifiable, so reference to these, and the use of introspection (thinking about oneself), was ruled out. Observations and experiments referred only to factors that are objectively and independently verifiable. Current approaches, however, include 'cognitive behavioural' methods, and the disciplines of experimental and biological psychology do take account of cognitions and emotions.

The main mechanisms of behavioural learning are classical conditioning, operant conditioning and social learning theory.

Classical conditioning

Dogs and cats salivate when they approach food. If a bell is sounded every time food is put down for them, they begin to salivate at the sound of the bell, even without the presence of food. This is classical conditioning. An *unconditioned response* (salivating in the presence of food) has changed into a *conditioned response* (salivating in the presence of a stimulus that has constantly been associated with the food). Chapter 3 gave the example of an abused boy who has an anxiety response as soon as he hears the door slam when his father returns home.

Chapter 3

The target behaviour is affected by what precedes or accompanies it.

Operant conditioning

Behaviour which is consistently rewarded is likely to persist. When a baby gets a round of applause, smiles and laughter for his first few steps, he is encouraged to try again, and looks round for a similar response. A girl who is praised for looking pretty pays attention to clothes, hair and make-up. The responses which make the behaviour more likely are described as 'reinforcements'.

In operant conditioning the behaviour is shaped by rewards or punishments which follow.

Social learning theory

Behaviour which is typical of gender, culture or class, as well as the particular forms taken by aggressive behaviour, is learnt by observation of others as much as by direct reinforcement. For observational learning to be effective, Bandura (1977) found that the models should appear to the observer to have *high prestige*; they should appear to *get rewards* for the action; the observer should *focus attention* on the behaviour; they should be *capable of reproducing it* (a golfer can learn observationally from an expert golfer, but will not learn brain surgery by watching a surgeon).

Behavioural interventions

Behavioural models have had extensive applications to control or influence behaviour. Some phobias, for example, arise through classical conditioning, a neutral stimulus such as a dog becoming associated with a response such as panic. The therapy might consist in reversing this association by systematically associating dogs with relaxation. Operant conditioning has been used to systematically modify the behaviour of children (or autistic people, or people with learning difficulties, or youth offenders) using rewards and punishments.

Cognitive behavioural therapy

Cognitive behavioural therapy (often referred to as CBT) is the most common modern approach. It applies principles of learning to personal difficulties, including emotional problems. Unlike the original formulations of behavioural learning, the theoretical framework incorporates the importance of cognitions – for example, what is understood to be a reinforcer (such as verbal praise or a star on a star chart) depends on cognition. It recognises the role of information processing as well as conditioning in affecting behaviour. In this respect, it has links with Bandura's social learning theory (see above) which had shown a *perceived* reinforcer was as potent as an actual reinforcer.

As the name implies, the approach combines cognitive therapy with behavioural learning principles. Faulty thought patterns ('cognitions') are seen to underlie many problems of behaviour and emotion, including depression and anxiety. Therapy is directed at identifying and changing these faulty cognitions, using the principles of learning – systematic reinforcement and stimulus-response. In experimental studies, cognitive behavioural therapy has been found to show the most promising results for many problems of mental health.

It is a didactic model of intervention, in which a number of different aspects of coaching and teaching may be combined. The person directing the modification is the expert, always in the method and sometimes in the behaviour that should be achieved. Often, the therapist works initially with the client to identify the thought patterns which are causing the problem, and then works out a schedule which will lead to reinforcement of accurate thought patterns. For example, the faulty cognitions may relate to a conviction that the person always has to please others. The therapist may identify this as a problem, and enable the person to see theoretically for themselves that they are just as socially effective when they don't act on this belief. They may then work out a schedule which enables the person to internalise the new convictions, to gain reinforcement from the resulting behaviour and emotions, and to achieve social satisfaction by being less dependent on others' good regard.

Chapter 3, about cognitive development in children and about learning; Chapter 7, about mental health difficulties.

Further reading

Corcoran, J. (2014) *Collaborative Cognitive-Behavioral Intervention in Social Work Practice*. Oxford: Oxford University Press.

Theoretical background as well as practical applications:

Corr, P. J. (2006) *Understanding Biological Psychology*. Malden, MA: Blackwell Publishing.
Leahy, R. L. and Dowd, E. T. (2002) *Clinical Advances in Cognitive Psychotherapy: Theory and Application*. New York: Springer.

There are many accessible instructional manuals about CBT in relation to specific fields, of which the following are examples:

- Youth offending
- Alcohol and drug services
- Mental health problems
- Parental support
- Illness and chronic pain (Winterowd et al., 2003).

9 Models of ageing: social disengagement theory, activity theory, feminist perspectives and political economy theory

As with many areas of development, there are different lenses through which development in later life can be viewed. What follows is a quick guide to social disengagement theory, activity theory, feminist perspectives and political economy theory. A reference is also made to Simon Biggs's term 'the mature imagination'. This is not usually presented as a single coherent theory, but it is an attempt to capture and explore the developing sense of self and the creation of a mature identity in adulthood.

Social disengagement theory

Using data from a study of 279 men and women between the ages of 50 and 90, Cumming and Henry (1961) concluded that progressive disengagement from social roles benefited both the individual older person and wider society. The older person is relieved of more onerous work and family responsibilities, and the new generation is given space to take over active and creative responsibilities. This disengagement is therefore seen as positive, 'normal' and healthy. Elaine Cumming (1975) suggests that with increasing age comes: decreasing life space – fewer interactions with others; an active choice of disengagement; and a change in style of interaction, towards a less socially controlled style.

Chapter 8

As Chapter 8 above points out, the theory has been criticised for not looking sufficiently at the details of different cultures and social settings; at the degree to which some societies establish useful roles for older people and some exclude them. Hochschild (1975) criticised the research for not distinguishing 'maturational' effects of ageing from 'cohort' effects ('cohort' effects are those which arise simply because people are born into a particular society in a particular decade). Bengtson and Achenbaum (1994) summarise in addition that it fails to explain or allow for individual choice and individual differences – for example, many people may resent or dislike 'disengagement' or may be financially disadvantaged by it.

Cumming herself (1975: 187) considers that the dispute over activity is 'an unenlightening controversy' which is not relevant to the theory, but many others have seen a contrast between disengagement theory and activity theory.

Activity theory

Activity theory (Neugarten, 1977) maintains that the healthiest approach to older age is to be active and socially engaged. Roles from middle life which are no longer appropriate should be replaced by relevant alternatives. Services which build on an implicit model of disengagement theory are likely in this view to be overtly or covertly ageist. The role of services should be to support and maintain community structures which allow for the continuing engagement and activity of older people.

The evidence for activity theory is that research generally finds (small) positive advantages for older people who are active and socially engaged. Politically oriented perspectives criticise it for being overly individual-oriented and ignoring structural inequality.

The mature imagination

Both of the above theories have to be supplemented (or supplanted) by recognition of the enormous individual variety among older people. Some wish to remain active whilst some create a new lifestyle which is much less socially engaged. Some undertake new activities which were not possible before. Some may move from full-time work to a different part-time occupation. For much of the population, there are many years of life ahead after 50. There is time, as in earlier decades, for the experience of self to show both continuity and change. Simon Biggs (1999) explores the way in which 'an identity is constructed in maturity which is serviceable and will take the bearer through to deep old age'. He tries to portray how a vigorous identity is constructed in the face of social pressures to see ageing as decline; the paradoxical finding for the individual that although the picture of decline is wrong, the body changes in negative ways and becomes less reliable. A new mature identity is constructed in a world which defines identity through consumption and change, which is often not the mode of identity expression for an older person.

Stuart-Hamilton (2012) quotes research showing that there is often, but not invariably, continuity between personality style in earlier and later ages in life – this may account for some of the controversy between activity theory and disengagement theory, as people are more or less active and more or less isolated than in their earlier lives. Atchley (1989) argues for *continuity theory*. He describes how people create both internal and external structures to their lives. The core of the theory is that people make efforts to support and maintain these structures as they progress through maturity. Circumstances may change, but they develop strategies and lifestyles in the new circumstances which provide continuity and links to the past as they perceive it. This approach arises particularly from a life-course perspective.

Like other theories referred to so far, continuity theory is criticised for paying insufficient attention to sociological and structural disadvantages that affect ageing. The final two theories summarised here, on the other hand, are based on a model of society that assumes continual conflict, with vested interests always oppressing and exploiting those with less power.

Feminist theories of ageing

Feminist perspectives are very diverse. However, major feminist theories of ageing have taken the view that women occupy an inferior position in older age because of exploitative patriarchal structures. Socialist feminist theories would add that this is exacerbated in a capitalist system because their productivity does not wrest economic advantage from men with capital resources. Arber and Ginn (1991, 1995) put the case strongly that gender, age and class interact to form a complex of unequal social categories – changes in any of the three change the relationship between the other two. More generally, feminist researchers argue that models of ageing have in the past taken men's experience as 'standard', ignoring the fact that women form the majority of older people and their experience in this phase of their life is heavily structured by the personal experience, economic situation, social position and social policy of earlier decades. Social structure, it is argued, enforces dependency and limited choices for women in old age.

Whether or not the arguments are seen as feminist, there is clearly an urgent need to identify policy and social structures that take full account of women's lifetime experience, which ensure security in older age and allow women in particular (but men as well) to combine caregiving and employment as they would wish, to the benefit of individuals and society.

The political economy of ageing

Marxist social theory regarded all power as arising from the control of economic resources. This analysis leads primarily to social structures based on class. Phillipson (1982) used the same analysis to examine the social position of older people. He argued that in a capitalist society the lack of economic productivity of older people left them with no social power. They are allocated few resources and are put into a position of enforced dependency. Estes et al. (2003) applied this analysis further to the 'industry' of care provision, arguing that a service industry of agencies, providers and planners grows up that maintains the 'outsider' status of older people, but brings their situation into the profit-making economy to the benefit of planners, business people and service workers.

10 Three approaches to loss and grief

This section summarises three models which have been put forward to describe the human response to bereavement. Kübler-Ross's work (1989) considers the path experienced by the bereaved person as a series of *stages*. Stroebe and Schut (1999) analyse the experience not as stages which may be followed, but as involving two mindsets which can alternate in the bereaved person. Worden (2009) sees the process as involving *tasks* which have to be accomplished by the bereaved person.

Elisabeth Kübler-Ross

Elisabeth Kübler-Ross identified stages people went through as they approached their death, but her work has been widely used also as a framework for understanding the experience of bereavement. The terms she uses are in the first column of Table E10.1 (the notes are ours). The stages do not have to be followed in strict order, and the person may move forward and back between them.

Table E10.1 Kübler-Ross's model: stages of grief

Stage	Notes
Denial	A typical reaction of people in relation to awareness of a terminal illness is to respond with the statement, 'No, not me. It cannot be true.' A similar response is often the first reaction to the news of the death of someone close. Denial is a defence mechanism that, in the short term, protects us from the trauma of the loss.
Anger	After the initial shock, a common reaction is 'Why me?' The bereaved person may be angry with the dead person for leaving them; with people, such as doctors, associated with the circumstances of death; or aware in general of a rage within themselves. It is as though someone must be blamed for this overwhelming disaster.
Bargaining	Examples are the wish in anticipatory grieving that they be taken instead of the person who is dying. Bargaining is also evident when a bereaved person copes by offering imaginary 'deals': if I do this, adopt such and such a strategy, the pain and the disruption will diminish, things should stabilise for me.

(continued)

Table E10.1 continued

Stage	Notes
Depression	People may experience feelings of guilt, a lack of purpose to life; a great sense of loss, as the person is aware of how much they have lost. This marks the beginning of acceptance.
Acceptance	This represents the end of the struggle. People experience the realisation that life can and does go on, coping positively with feelings. This can be accompanied by a lifting of the depression.

Stroebe and Schut

Stroebe and Schut recognised the weaknesses of a stage theory, and proposed that the experience is better conceptualised as alternation between two processes:

- A *loss orientation* focused on the gap and the pain caused by the loss of the person who has gone.
- A *restoration orientation* focused on building a future without the person.

There is no single path through 'stages' or any expected trajectory. Rather, they identify two kinds of work that bereaved people are engaged in, and they point out that there are individual differences in people's allocation of time and energy to the two types of task.

William Worden

William Worden emphasises that bereavement is a process rather than a state, and analyses the experiences of bereaved people as they work through their reactions. He understands them to be tackling four overlapping tasks:

- to face the reality;
- to work through the emotional pain of their loss;
- to adjust to the new reality – changes in their circumstances, roles, status and identity;
- to reinvest in the future.

He would understand the tasks to be complete when the bereaved person has integrated the loss into their life and let go of emotional attachments to the deceased.

These and other theories of bereavement are referred to in Chapter 9 (many writers about loss and grief have made use of psychoanalytic theory and attachment theory). Chapter 2, explaining 'states of mind', refers also to the experience of loss, as does Chapter 3 in the context of guilt; Chapter 4 about transitions; Chapter 5 about loneliness and aloneness; Chapter 6 about the loss of children; and Chapter 8 in relation to older people.

Glossary

accommodation the term in Piaget's theory of cognitive development to indicate that an individual's scheme of understanding has changed to accommodate a new experience in the world – the opposite of **assimilation**.

activity theory the theory of ageing which holds that older people who remain active will have better psychological well-being and be better adjusted than those who do not.

affect the experience of feeling or emotion (**affective**: relating to affect); affect may often be discussed in relation to cognition or thought processes – affect is partly in contrast to cognition and partly interlinked with it.

ambivalent holding opposite attitudes at the same time – as when a person both loves and hates another.

assimilation the term in Piaget's theory of cognitive development to indicate that a new experience from the outside world is made to fit (assimilated into) existing schemes of understanding – the opposite of **accommodation**.

attachment theory the theory of development which states that individuals are born with a drive to seek attachments. These are affectional bonds which provide comfort in times of threat and a secure base from which to explore; separation from the attachment figure activates attachment behaviours.

attunement in **attachment theory** the process demonstrated by an attachment figure when their responses are 'in tune with' the internal experiences of the individual (in contrast, for example, to self-centred responses based on the impact of behaviour on the caregiver).

avoidant children in attachment research show individual differences in attachment behaviour. If a child's attachment is categorised 'avoidant' in the 'strange situation' test, they tend to treat the stranger in the same way as the caregiver: on separation they are unlikely to be distressed; on reunion the child shows signs of ignoring. The infant is unlikely to show emotional 'sharing' with the caregiver, although they may turn to them for practical help and support.

bioregulation mechanisms by which the body brings itself back to equilibrium after disturbance. Physically – for example, sweating to reduce the effects of heat; emotionally – mechanisms to return to a steady state after panic or exhilaration.

Bronfenbrenner's ecological model model of human development in which development is always viewed as taking place in systems – for example, the **microsystem** of immediate face-to-face contexts, through to the **macrosystem** of society and its processes.

chromosomes structures (large molecules) which contain genetic information about the individual. Within the chromosome, this information is stored in units called **genes**. There are twenty-three pairs of chromosomes in each cell of the body.

chronosystem in Bronfenbrenner's ecological model of development, the influence on the person's development of changes (and continuities) over time in the environments in which the person is living.

classical conditioning learning process in which an unconditioned response (such as a dog salivating in the presence of food) becomes associated with a conditioning stimulus (such as the bell which is always rung when the food is presented). After conditioning, the response can be produced by the conditioned stimulus.

cognitive behavioural therapy therapy which combines behavioural learning (using ideas of stimulus and behavioural response) and cognitive therapy (emphasising the importance of thoughts).

congruence in humanistic psychology, the condition in which a person's self-awareness matches their actual experience; also used to mean that the therapist's attitude and awareness matches the client's experience.

controlled (or independent) variable in an experiment, the feature under the researcher's control, which can be varied in order to find the change caused in the **uncontrolled (or dependent) variable**.

co-regulation process by which **bioregulation** occurs not within the individual but between two people – the excited biological state of one person is brought back to equilibrium by the other.

corporate parent an organisation which has the responsibilities of a parent (used to describe a UK local authority when it has parental responsibilities towards a child by virtue of the Children Act).

cosmopolitanism the situation in which it is increasingly common for individuals living in one country to owe allegiance and identity to cultures in other countries, in contrast to strongly local or nationalistic societies. This is also associated with the idea that all peoples are part of a single moral community, and contrasts with Eurocentric, Afro-centric or radical Islamic philosophies.

countertransference in psychoanalytic theory, aspects of the analyst's experience of the analysand (the client). Different schools of thought limit the definition to different aspects of experience. See **transference**.

determinist theories in which clear rules or laws enable the present situation to have been exactly predicted from a state existing in the past.

didactic based on teaching by an expert.

disorganised attachment in attachment theory, children's attachment behaviour typically falls into one of a limited number of patterns (see also **secure**, **avoidant** and **ambivalent**). In the disorganised pattern, parents evoke contradictory behaviours in the child, of simultaneous avoidance and approach. In the 'strange situation' observation, children display disorganised and disrupted behaviour – such as wandering around whimpering, banging their head against a wall, or 'freezing'. **Co-regulation** is absent, and the child does not develop a coherent sense of self.

empathy the capacity to think and feel oneself into the inner life of another person; it also involves the ability to communicate with the other person so that they feel this sense of being understood.

epigenetics inherited changes which are not caused by changes in genes. Variations in the effects of **genes** which are not caused by changes in core genetic information.

epistemology the branch of philosophy dealing with knowledge – what it is, the different forms it can take, how it is acquired, how its truth is established or disproved.

Erikson's psychosocial model a model of development through the life course, it combines a psychoanalytic approach about inner psychological development with a formulation about the influence of social conditions and culture. It divides the life course into eight stages from infancy to old age.

eugenics ideology that if care is not taken, 'poor quality' breeding lines will be perpetuated into later generations (and conversely, that careful breeding can improve the human stock). Associated with racist ideologies and the sterilisation of people with learning disabilities.

existentialist a school of philosophy which placed emphasis on the importance of subjective experience; this could not form an 'object' of study (because that would again leave unexamined the subject who was doing the study).

exosystem in **Bronfenbrenner's ecological model** a system which affects the growing individual even though they themselves are not part of it. In particular, the exosystem involves other people in the individual's **microsystem**. The parent's workplace is an exosystem for the child.

expressive role a role in which the personal qualities of an individual are relevant (as in the role of lover or friend), in contrast to an **instrumental role**.

gender dysphoria or gender identity disorder a condition where a person experiences distress as a result of a mismatch between their biological sex and gender identity.

gender-variant a general term to describe young people whose gender identity differs from what is normative for their biological sex in a particular time and culture.

gene a tiny component of the body which contains information about the way the body should be built. Each of the more than 100 trillion cells in a human body contains a complete set of the 22,000 genes. They are arranged on twenty-three **chromosomes**.

genetics the science studying the transmission of information from one generation to the next through genes.

gerontology the study of ageing.

hereditable able to be passed from one generation to the next by heredity. In a group of people, some differences (such as eye colour) may be totally caused by heredity. These qualities are described as 100 per cent hereditable. Other qualities (which particular language is spoken) may be totally independent of heredity and are 0 per cent hereditable. Many qualities lie between these extremes, with some of the variation caused by heredity and some by environment.

hierarchy of needs in Maslow's theory, the arrangement of different kinds of needs, such that some are more prominent (**salient**) than others at different times in life (for example, food and shelter are salient in infancy, whereas the need for self-esteem becomes prominent after other more basic needs have already been met).

hormones chemicals released into the body that affect other aspects of functioning; hormones carry signals or messages between different systems in the body.

humanistic a loose grouping of psychological models which emphasised the distinctive nature of human experience to strive for personal and social improvement.

instrumentality in psychology, the degree to which individuals act as directive agents in their lives as distinct from having matters determined by someone else.

instrumental role in social psychology or sociology, a role in which the personal quality of the person is not relevant to performance (for example, street cleaner) – contrasts with **expressive role**.

internal working model in attachment theory, the individual's mental representation of attachment relationships. It contains a view of: (1) the individual themselves – whether they are basically likeable or not; (2) the attachment figure – whether they are well disposed and competent when needed; (3) the relationship – whether it is usually available and competent. The internal working model is particularly important in the regulation of negative emotions such as fear, panic and anger.

life course the course of life from conception to death.

lifespan development an approach which emphasises that development occurs throughout life and must be understood in the light of social and historical factors; its study therefore involves a range of academic disciplines.

lifespan theory theory which regards development as the system's adaptation to changing circumstances and environment. It therefore occurs throughout life, and valid research about it has to explore historical, economic, political and cultural dynamics as well as the biological and psychological. Lifespan theorists have paid particular attention to development in older age.

life structure a concept in Levinson's theory. It represents the character of an individual's life at a given time. In adulthood, this often focuses on family and work. In Levinson's view, there are characteristic periods of structure-building and structure-changing.

macrosystem in Bronfenbrenner's ecological theory of development, the broadest system of social and cultural influences.

mesosystem the system of relationships between microsystems.

microsystem in Bronfenbrenner's ecological theory of development, a system in which the developing individual is directly involved – for example, both the family and the school class are microsystems for the child.

modernist a term with different meanings in different academic fields. In relation to the social sciences, it is a fairly vague term referring to theories which seek to find general patterns of development thought to have universal applicability. The theories assume that it is possible to identify truths which are independent of the observer.

multifactorial arising from the combination of several causes – the cause of heart disease may be multifactorial, involving genetic predisposition, diet in childhood and current lifestyle.

neural to do with the nervous system, including the brain.

neuroses category of psychiatric diagnosis referring to mental imbalance or distress not primarily affecting the capacity for rational thought; modern psychiatric categories stay much closer to specific behavioural definitions of problems, and do not use the term.

ontology branch of philosophy dealing with existence; within a particular view (such as a religion) the beliefs about what exists.

operant conditioning in learning theory, the process by which actions become more (or less) frequent because of rewards or punishments. The target behaviour is affected by its consequences.

paradigm a set of assumptions, procedures and values which inform a particular approach to an academic discipline; the feminist paradigm, for example, assumes that if gender is not specifically referred to in social research, it is likely that differences between men and women are being overlooked.

phenotype an observable characteristic of an individual, which can include shape, appearance and behaviour.

play therapy work with troubled children which recognises that children normally communicate in play (not necessarily using words), and that they work on problems in their play. For example, a child who has been sexually abused and then lived with two different foster carers before being adopted may have many questions and conflicts. The therapist may work with the child in painting, in play with dolls, or in sand play.

political economy of ageing a model which views the ageing process as structured by the position of older people in a given political and economic system.

political economy theory referred to particularly in connection with ageing – emphasises the importance of social structure, power, hierarchy and distribution of resources, all of which can impact negatively on older people.

positivist research which insists that terms should be reducible (at least in principle) to verifiable observational statements, that effects have deterministic causes, that the goal of (social) science is to create hypotheses and laws which account for the observed diversity of the world. One of several possible **paradigms** for social science; positivism is limited in its ability to explore and value the subjective states of individuals.

postmodernist a vague term used in many different ways and deriving from the contrast with **modernist**. In social science, postmodern theorists tend to regard knowledge as always presented from particular points of view, and as having implicit connections with social power structures; often, the distinction between 'objective' and 'subjective' is doubted, and reality is regarded as constructed by society and language. This approach is sometimes criticised for further complicating ideas which are already complex.

primary healthcare normally the first point of contact for people entering the healthcare system. In the UK it is typically the family doctor, health centre or walk-in centre.

primary sex characteristics the sex organs of reproduction; in the female, the uterus, ovaries and vagina; in the male, the penis.

privilege term used to indicate how different people have unearned advantages (including basic human rights) over others in different social networks – typical examples may be males over females, welfare professionals over welfare applicants, white Europeans over others, women over children, able-bodied over disabled people – but there are many others depending on the attribution of power to specific characteristics in particular social arrangements.

psychiatry the medical speciality concerned with 'mental illness'.

psychoanalysis (psychoanalytic) a method of investigating the mind; a form of therapy; a theory developed from these practices. The method places particular emphasis on free association (the subject saying whatever comes into their mind), and self-exploration rather than expert direction; the theory includes attention to conscious and unconscious components of the mind.

psychodynamic theories and practices which draw on psychoanalytic ideas, and emphasise that different parts of the mind are in dynamic interaction with each other. 'Psychodynamic' is often a broader term including, but not limited to, 'psychoanalytic'. There is no authoritative distinction between the two terms.

psychosis (plural: **psychoses**) in traditional psychiatric classification, a mental impairment in which thought disorders are prominent. No longer used in the main official diagnostic manuals.

psychosocial paying attention both to external social factors and to internal psychological states. Social work is a psychosocial activity.

qualitative studies research investigations which pay attention to factors which are not necessarily countable – for example, to the way in which people make sense of their lives; there are many qualitative studies about reactions to a cancer diagnosis, or to the experience of belonging to a youth gang.

resilience factors which distinguish people who are not permanently negatively affected by adverse events from those who are.

salient prominent.

scaffolding term in Vygotsky's model of cognitive development. It indicates the support given by knowledgeable adults to enable the child to develop their cognitive skills; this support is gradually withdrawn as the child acquires the skill.

schema term in Piaget's description of cognitive development. Refers to the various types of mental routines. For example, an infant's schemas are largely bodily responses of the brain, nervous system and muscles to experience; the sucking response is one such 'schema'. But in the 'formal operation' stage, schemas may be complex mental operations based on abstractions – solving complex mathematical problems using advanced algebra, for example.

secondary sex characteristics features that distinguish the sexes but are not reproductive organs – for example, facial hair.

secure attachment in attachment theory, children's attachment behaviour typically falls into one of a limited number of patterns (see also **avoidant**, **ambivalent** and **disorganised**). Secure attachment is built up by sensitive and attuned responses by a caregiver to the child's attachment behaviour. Arousal states are **co-regulated**, and the attachment figure provides a 'secure base' – for exploration of the world, and for help in managing powerful emotions of fear, anxiety, pain or sadness.

serial monogamy monogamy is the practice of having only one sexual partner at a time. 'Serial monogamy' is pair bonding which does not last for life but is replaced by another.

social constructionism the idea that groups construct reality out of their discourse and culture; often used specifically to apply to concepts which are thought by others to be naturally arising and existing in nature. There are many different degrees of social constructionism – many accept that 'family' is a social construct; some would regard the existence of mountains as a social construct.

social disengagement theory in relation to ageing, the idea that the process of gradually withdrawing from social roles benefits both the individual and society.

social exchange theory a model which views social life as structured by what participants exchange with each other. Interactions continue as long as each feels they are profiting, and that there is some reciprocity.

social learning theory learning theory associated with Albert Bandura – that behaviour is shaped not just though stimuli and reinforcements, but also through social observation.

transference in psychodynamic thinking, the re-creation in the present of states of mind which originate in earlier (particularly parent–child) relationships.

transgender a term used to describe a person whose gender identity does not match their biological sex. Can also be used as an umbrella term to include people who do not have an exclusively male or female identity, e.g. non-binary or gender-fluid.

unconditional acceptance/unconditional positive regard acceptance of the value of a person without conditions being placed upon their behaviour. A concept of Rogers' humanistic model of psychology and (person-centred) helping.

uncontrolled (or dependent) variable in an experiment, the feature which changes because the experimenter manipulates the **controlled variable**.

References

Abbass, A., Kisely, S. and Kroenke, K. (2009) Short-term psychodynamic psycho-therapy for somatic disorders: systematic review and meta-analysis of clinical trials. *Psychotherapy and Psychosomatics*, 78: 265–274.

Abbott, P., Wallace, C. and Tyler, M. (2005) *An Introduction to Sociology: Feminist Perspectives*. London and New York: Routledge.

Abbott, R. and Burkitt, E. (2015) *Child Development and the Brain*. Bristol: Policy Press.

Adams, J. D., Hayes, J. and Hopson, B. (1976) *Transition: Understanding and Managing Personal Change*. Bath: Pitman Press.

Adelman, P. (1994) Multiple roles and psychological well-being in a national sample of older adults. *Journal of Gerontology*, 49: S277–S285.

Afshar, H., Maynard, M. and Franks, M. (2002) *Women, Ethnicity and Empowerment in Later Life*. Sheffield: ESRC Growing Older Programme.

Age UK (2018) How we can end pensioner poverty. Available at: www.ageuk.org.uk/Documents/EN-GB/Campaigns/end-pensioner-poverty/how_we_can_end_pensioner_poverty_campaign_report.pdf?dtrk=true. Accessed 2 January 2018.

Ainsworth, M., Waters, E., Blehar, M. and Wall, S. (1978) *Patterns of Attachment: A Psychological Study of the Strange Situation*. Hillsdale, NJ: Lawrence Erlbaum.

Akiyama, H., Antonucci, T. C., Takahashi, K. and Langfahl, E. S. (2003) Negative interactions in close relationships across the lifespan. *Journal of Gerontology: Psychological Sciences*, 58(2): 70–79.

Allott, P. (2004) What is mental health, illness, and recovery? In T. Ryan and J. Pritchard (eds) *Good Practice in Adult Mental Health*. London and Philadelphia: Jessica Kingsley.

American Psychiatric Association (2013) *Diagnostic and Statistical Manual of Mental Disorders: DSM-5*. Washington, DC: American Psychiatric Association.

Andrews, G. (2001) Should depression be managed as a chronic disease? *British Medical Journal*, 322: 419–421.

Appiah, K. A. (1997) Europe upside down: fallacies of the new Afrocentrism. In R. R. Grinker and C. Steiner (eds) *Perspectives on Africa* (pp. 728–731). London: Blackwell.

Arber, S. and Ginn, J. (1991) *Gender and Later Life: A Sociological Analysis of Resources and Constraints*. London: Sage.

Arber, S. and Ginn, J. (1995) *Connecting Gender and Ageing: A Sociological Approach*. Buckingham and Philadelphia: Open University Press.

Aries, P. (1996) *Centuries of Childhood*. London: Pimlico.

Association of Directors of Children's Services (ADCS) (2016) *Unaccompanied Asylum Seeking and Refugee Children* (November), 36. Available at: http://

adcs.org.uk/assets/documentation/ADCS_UASC_Report_Final_FOR_PUBLICATION.pdf. Accessed 20 October 2017.

Association of Reproductive Health Professionals (ARH) (2005) *Women's Sexual Health in Midlife and Beyond*. Washington, DC: Association of Reproductive Health Professionals.

Atchley, R. C. (1989) A continuity theory of normal aging. *The Gerontologist*, 29(2): 183–190.

Ayotte, W. (2000) *Separated Children Coming to Western Europe: Why They Travel and How They Arrive*. London: Save the Children.

Baillargeon, R. (1987) Object permanence in 3½- and 4½-month-old infants. *Developmental Psychology*, 23: 655–664.

Baillargeon, R. (2017) Infant cognition lab. Online: http://internal.psychology.illinois.edu/infantlab/index.html. Accessed 2 December 2017.

Bales, K. L. and Carter, S. (2009) Neurobiology and hormonal aspects of romantic relationships. In M. De Haan and M. R. Gunnar (eds) *Handbook of Developmental Social Neuroscience*. New York: Guilford Press.

Baltes, P. B. (1987) Theoretical propositions of life-span developmental psychology: on the dynamics between growth and decline. *Developmental Psychology*, 23(5): 611–626.

Bamber, C. (2004) From grassroots to statute: the mental health user movement in England. In T. Ryan and J. Pritchard (eds) *Good Practice in Adult Mental Health*. London and Philadelphia: Jessica Kingsley.

Bandura, A. (1977) *Social Learning Theory*. Englewood Cliffs, NJ: Prentice Hall.

Barn, R., Andrew, L. and Mantovani, N. (2005) *Life after Care: The Experiences of Young People from Different Ethnic Groups*. York: Joseph Rowntree Foundation. Available at: www.jrf.org.uk/report/experiences-young-care-leavers-different-ethnic-groups.

Barth, R. P., Crea, T. M., John, K., Thoburn, J. and Quinton, D. (2005) Beyond attachment theory and therapy: towards sensitive and evidence-based interventions with foster and adoptive families in distress. *Child and Family Social Work*, 10(4): 257–268.

Bartlik, B. and Goldstein, M. Z. (2000) Practical geriatrics: maintaining sexual health after menopause. *Psychiatric Services*, 51: 751–806.

Bartlik, B. and Goldstein, M. Z. (2001) Practical geriatrics: men's sexual health after midlife. *Psychiatric Services*, 52: 291–302.

Bass, S. (2006) Gerontological theory: the search for the Holy Grail. *Gerontologist*, 46: 139–144.

Basson, R. (2005) Women's sexual dysfunction: revised and expanded definitions. *Canadian Medical Association Journal*, 172(10): 1327–1333.

Bateson, P. (2001) Where does our behaviour come from? *Journal of Biosciences*, 26(5): 561–570.

BBC (2007) *Woman's Hour* message board, 22 April 2007. www.bbc.co.uk.

BBC (2017) *The Sex Lives of Us*. Radio 4, 13 September. Information available online at www.bbc.co.uk/radio4/arts/sexuality.shtml. Accessed 2 December 2017.

Beart, S. (2005) 'I won't think of meself as a learning disability. But I have': social identity and self-advocacy. *British Journal of Learning Disabilities*, 33(3): 128–131.

Beart, S., Hardy, G. and Buchan, L. (2004) Changing selves: a grounded theory account of belonging to a self-advocacy group for people with intellectual disabilities. *Journal of Applied Research in Intellectual Disabilities*, 17: 91–100.

Beck, A. T. and Weishaar, M. (2005) *Cognitive Therapy*. Belmont, CA: Thomson Brooks/Cole Publishing Co.

Beck, U. (2000) The cosmopolitan society and its enemies. *Theory, Culture and Society*, 19(2): 17–44.

Beckett, C. and Taylor, H. (2010) *Human Growth and Development*. Second edition. London: Sage.

Belsky, J. (1980) Child maltreatment: an ecological integration. *The American Psychologist*, 35(4): 320–335.

Belsky, J., Melhuish, E. and Barnes, J. (2007) *Evaluating Sure Start: Does Area-Based Early Intervention Work?* Bristol: Policy Press.

Bengtson, V. L. and Achenbaum, W. A. (1994) The changing contract across generations. *Gerontologist*, 34(4): 564.

Bennett, A. (2005) *Untold Stories*. London: Faber and Faber.

Bentovim, A. (2002) Preventing sexually abused young people from becoming abusers, and treating the victimization experiences of young people who offend sexually. *Child Abuse and Neglect*, 26(6–7): 661–678.

Beresford, P. and CPAG (1999) *Poverty First Hand: Poor People Speak for Themselves*. London: Child Poverty Action Group (CPAG).

Berlin, H. A. (2011). The neural basis of the dynamic unconscious. *Neuropsychoanalysis*, 13(1): 5–31.

Berlin, H. A. and Koch, C. (2009). Neuroscience meets psychoanalysis. *Scientific American Mind*, 20(2): 16–19.

Biddle, B. J. (1979) *Role Theory: Expectations, Identities, and Behaviors*. New York: Academic Press.

Biggs, S. (1999) *The Mature Imagination: Dynamics of Identity in Midlife and Beyond*. Buckingham: Open University Press.

Bilton, T. (2002) *Introductory Sociology*. Basingstoke: Palgrave.

Bingham, M. and Stryker, S. (1995) *Things Will Be Different for My Daughter: A Practical Guide to Building Her Self-Esteem and Self-Reliance*. New York: Penguin Books.

Blackwell, D. (1997) Psychotherapy, politics and trauma: working with survivors of torture and organized violence. *Journal of Social Work Practice*, 11(2): 81–90.

Blakemore, S.-J., Ouden, H., Choudhury, S. and Frith, C. (2007) Adolescent development of the neural circuitry for thinking about intentions. *Social Cognitive and Affective Neuroscience*, 2: 130–139

Blum, R. W., Resnick, M. D., Nelson, R. and St Germaine, A. (1991) Family and peer issues among adolescents with spina bifida and cerebral palsy. *Pediatrics*, 88(2): 280–285.

Bohannan, P. (1970) *Divorce and After: An Analysis of the Emotional and Social Problems of Divorce*. Garden City, NY: Anchor.

Botcherby, S. and Hurrell, K. (2004) *Ethnic Minority Women and Men*. Manchester: Equal Opportunities Commission.

Bowlby, J. (1951) *Maternal Care and Mental Health: A Report Prepared on Behalf of the World Health Organization as a Contribution to the United Nations Programme for the Welfare of Homeless Children*. Geneva: WHO.

Bowlby, J. (1979) *The Making and Breaking of Affectional Bonds*. London: Tavistock Publications.

Bowlby, J. and Robertson, J. (1953) A two-year-old goes to hospital. *Proceedings of the Royal Society of Medicine*, 46(6): 425–427.

Boyd, D. and Bee, H. (2014) *The Developing Child*. Thirteenth edition. Boston, New York and London: Pearson.

Boyd, D. R. and Bee, H. L. (2015) *Lifespan Development*. Seventh edition. Boston: Pearson/Allyn and Bacon.

Boyd, C. and Bromfield, L. (2006) *Young People Who Sexually Abuse: Key Issues*. Melbourne: Australian Institute of Family Studies. https://aifs.gov.au/publications/young-people-who-sexually-abuse.

Brennan, D. (2016) *Annual Report on Cases of Femicide in 2016*. Available at: www.femicidecensus.org.uk. Accessed 3 December 2017.

Briggs, S. (2008) *Working with Adolescents and Young Adults: A Contemporary Psychodynamic Approach*. Second edition. Basingstoke: Palgrave.

Briggs, S. and Whittaker, A. (2018) Protecting children from faith-based abuse through accusations of witchcraft and spirit possession: understanding contexts and informing practice. *British Journal of Social Work*. Available at: http://researchopen.lsbu.ac.uk/1725. Accessed 7 January 2018.

British Red Cross (2018) *Our Services for Refugees*. Online: www.redcross.org.uk/What-we-do/Refugee-support. Accessed 2 January 2018.

Brody, E. M. (1985) Parent care as a normative family stress. *Gerontologist*, 25(1): 19–29.

Brody, E. M. and Saperstein, A. R. (2006) *Women in the Middle: Their Parent Care Years*. New York: Springer.

Bronfenbrenner, U. (1979/2006) *The Ecology of Human Development: Experiments by Nature and Design*. Cambridge, MA: Harvard University Press.

Bronfenbrenner, U. (1990) Discovering what families do. In D. Blankenhorn, S. Bayme and J. B. Elshtain (eds) *Rebuilding the Nest: A New Commitment to the American Family*. Milwaukee, WI: Family Service America.

Brown, S. (2005) *Understanding Youth and Crime: Listening to Youth?* Second edition. Maidenhead and New York: Open University Press.

Burman, E. (2016) *Deconstructing Developmental Psychology*. Third edition. London and New York: Routledge.

Burton, J. M. and Marshall, L. A. (2005) Protective factors for youth considered at risk of criminal behaviour: does participation in extracurricular activities help? *Criminal Behaviour and Mental Health*, 15(1): 46–64.

Buss, D. M., Abbott, M., Angleitner, A., Asherian, A. et al. (1990) International preferences in selecting mates: a study of 37 cultures. *Journal of Cross-Cultural Psychology*, 21(1): 5–47.

Buss, C., Davis, E. P., Shahbaba, B., Pruessner, J. C., Head, K. and Sandman, C. A. (2012) Maternal cortisol over the course of pregnancy and subsequent child amygdala and hippocampus volumes and affective problems. *Proceedings of the National Academy of Sciences*, 109(20).

Butler, I. (2011) *Social Work with Children and Families: Getting into Practice*. Third edition. London and New York: Jessica Kingsley.

Butler, J. (1990) *Gender Trouble: Feminism and the Subversion of Identity*. New York: Routledge.

Butler, J. (1993) *Bodies That Matter: On the Discursive Limits of 'Sex'*. New York: Routledge.

Butler Sloss, E. (1988) *Report of the Inquiry into Child Abuse in Cleveland, 1987: Presented to Parliament by the Secretary of State for Social Services by Command of Her Majesty, July 1988*. London: HMSO.

Bynner, J., Elias, P., McKnight, A., Pan, H. and Pierre, G. (2002) *Young People's Changing Routes to Independence*. York: Joseph Rowntree Foundation/YPS. www.jrf.org.uk/report/young-peoples-changing-routes-independence.

Cafcass (Children and Family Court Advisory and Support Service) (2018) *Putting Your Children First: Divorce and Separation*. Available at: www.cafcass.gov.uk/leaflets-resources/leaflets-for-adults.aspx#%20Putting%20Your%20Children%20First. Accessed 4 January 2018.

Cann, J., Falshaw, L., Nugent, F. and Friendship, C. (2003) *Understanding What Works: Accredited Cognitive Skills Programmes for Adult Men and Young Offenders.* London: Home Office.

Casement, P. (2002) *Learning from Our Mistakes: Beyond Dogma in Psychoanalysis and Psychotherapy.* New York: Psychology Press.

Cass, V. C. (1984) Homosexual identity: a concept in need of definition. *Journal of Homosexuality*, 9(2–3): 105–126.

Cassidy, J. and Shaver, P. (eds) (1999) *Handbook of Attachment: Theory, Research and Clinical Applications.* New York and London: Guilford Press.

Cassidy, J. and Shaver, P. (eds) (2016) *Handbook of Attachment: Theory, Research and Clinical Applications.* Third edition. New York and London: Guilford Press.

Ceci, S. and Williams, W. (1999) *The Nature-Nurture Debate.* Oxford: Blackwell.

Centre for Social Justice (CSJ) (2015) Finding their feet; equipping care leavers to reach their potential. Available at: www.centreforsocialjustice.org.uk/UserStorage/pdf/Pdf reports/Finding.pdf. Accessed 21 November 2017.

Centrepoint (2018) Youth homelessness: the issues. Online: https://centrepoint.org.uk/youth-homelessness/the-issue/. Accessed 3 January 2018.

Chaban, M. (2000) *The Life Work of Dr. Elisabeth Kübler-Ross and Its Impact on the Death Awareness Movement.* New York: Mellen Press.

Chapman, M. G. T. and Woodmansey, A. C. (1985) Policy on child abuse. *British Journal of Clinical and Social Psychiatry*, 3 (supplement).

Charlton, L., Crank, M., Kansara, K. and Oliver, C. (1998) *Still Screaming: Birth Parents Compulsorily Separated from Their Children.* Manchester: After Adoption.

Chisholm, J., Quinlivan, J., Petersen, R. and Coall, D. (2005) Early stress predicts age at menarche and first birth, adult attachment and expected lifespan. *Human Nature*, 16(3): 233–265.

Chivers, M. L., Seto, M. C. and Blanchard, R. (2007) Gender and sexual orientation differences in sexual response to sexual activities versus gender of actors in sexual films. *Journal of Personality and Social Psychology*, 93(6): 1108–1121.

Chodorow, N. (1999) *The Reproduction of Mothering: Psychoanalysis and the Sociology of Gender. With a New Preface.* Berkeley: University of California Press.

Cicchetti, D. and Rogosch, F. A. (1997) The role of self-organization in the promotion of resilience in maltreated children. *Development and Psychopathology*, 9(4): 797–815.

Citizens as Trainers Group, Young Independent People Presenting Educational Entertainment (YIPPEE), Rimmer, A. and Harwood, K. (2004) Citizen participation in the education and training of social workers. *Social Work Education*, 23: 309–323.

Clarke, A., Burgess, G., Morris, S. and Udagawa, C. (2015) *Estimating the Scale of Youth Homelessness in the UK.* Cambridge: Cambridge Centre for Housing and Planning Research; DCLG Live Table 781.

CLS (2008) *National Child Development Study.* Online: www.cls.ioe.ac.uk. Accessed 3 December 2017.

Cobb, N. J. (1995) *Adolescence: Continuity, Change, and Diversity.* Mountain View, CA: Mayfield.

Cohler, B. (1982) Personal narrative and the life course. In P. B. Baltes and O. G. Brim (eds) *Life-Span Development and Behavior.* New York: Academic Press.

Colborn, T. and Clement, C. (1992) *Chemically-Induced Alterations in Sexual and Functional Development: The Wildlife/Human Connection.* Princeton, NJ: Princeton Scientific Publishing Co.

Cooley, C. H. (1902) *Human Nature and the Social Order*. New York, Chicago and Boston: Scribner.

Cooper, A. and Lousada, J. (2005) *Borderline Welfare: Feeling and Fear of Feeling in Modern Welfare*. London: Karnac.

Cooper, A. and Whittaker, A. (2014) History as tragedy, never as farce: tracing the long cultural narrative of child protection in England. *Journal of Social Work Practice*, 28(3): 251–266.

Cooper, C., Selwood, A. and Livingston, G. (2008) The prevalence of elder abuse and neglect: a systematic review. *Age and Ageing*, 37(2): 151–160.

Corr, P. J. (2006) *Understanding Biological Psychology*. Malden, MA: Blackwell Publishing.

Crawford, C., Dearden, L. and Meghir, C. (2007) *When You Are Born Matters: The Impact of Date of Birth on Child Cognitive Outcomes in England*. London: Institute for Fiscal Studies.

Crispin, T., Milliken, D. and Bews, K. (2005) *Armbands in Deep Water: A Summary of Research into Home Start's Home-Visiting Volunteers*. Leicester: Home Start. Online: www.home-start.org.uk/research-and-evaluation.

Crittenden, P. M. (2016) *Raising Parents: Attachment, Parenting and Child Safety*. Second edition. Abingdon: Routledge.

Crowley, A. and Vulliamy, C. (2007) *Listen Up! Children and Young People Talk: About Poverty*. London: Save the Children.

CSAC and Age Concern Cumbria (2006) *You Feel as Though You Are Still Someone*. Report presented at CSAC conference, Rheged, June 2006. Cumbria, UK: CSAC.

Cumming, E. (1975) Engagement with an old theory. *International Journal of Aging and Human Development*, 6(3): 187–191.

Cumming, E. and Henry, W. (1961) *Growing Old: The Process of Disengagement*. New York: Basic Books.

Damasio, A. R. (1997) Emotion in the perspective of an integrated nervous system. Paper presented at the Nobel Symposium: Towards an Understanding of Integrative Brain Functions – Analysis at Multiple Levels, Stockholm, Sweden, June 1997.

Davidson, S. and Gentry, T. (2013) *Age UK End of Life Evidence Review 2013*. Available at: www.ageuk.org.uk/Documents/EN-GB/For-professionals/Research/Age UK End of Life Evidence Review 2013.pdf?dtrk=true. Accessed 29 December 2017.

Davies, C. and Jenkins, R. (1997) She has different fits to me; how people with learning difficulties see themselves. *Disability and Society*, 12: 95–109.

Davoren, E. (1974) The role of the social worker. In R. E. Helfer and C. H. Kempe (eds) *The Battered Child*. Second edition (p. 262). Chicago and London: University of Chicago Press.

DCFS/DfES (2004) *Parental Separation: Children's Needs and Parents' Responsibilities*. London: The Stationery office. Online: www.standards.dfes.gov.uk/eyfs/resources/downloads/dfeschildrensneeds.pdf.

Dean, J. and Goodlad, R. (1998) *Supporting Community Participation? The Role and Impact of Befriending*. Brighton: Pavilion Publishing in association with the Joseph Rowntree Foundation. Research summary available online: www.jrf.org.uk/sites/files/jrf/scr038.pdf. Accessed 23 April 2009.

de Bernières, L. (1994) *Captain Corelli's Mandolin*. London: Secker & Warburg.

De Maat, S., Dekker, J., Schoevers, R. and De Jonghe, F. (2006) Relative efficacy of psychotherapy and pharmacotherapy in the treatment of depression: a meta-analysis. *Psychotherapy Research*, 16(5): 566–578.

De Maat, D., De Jonghe, F., Schoevers, R. et al. (2009) The effectiveness of long term psychoanalytic psychotherapy: a systemic review of empirical studies. *Harvard Review of Psychiatry*, 17: 1–23.

de Montaigne, M. (1580/1993) *The Essays* (M. A. Screech, trans.). London: Allen Lane.

Department for Education (DfE) (2015a) Outcomes for children looked after by local authorities as at 31st March 2014. London: DfE.

Department for Education (DfE) (2015b) Special Educational Needs in England (January 2015) National Tables. Available at: www.gov.uk/government/uploads/system/uploads/attachment_data/file/539158/SFR29_2016_Main_Text.pdf. Accessed 3 January 2018.

Department for Education (DfE) (2015c) Working together to safeguard children: a guide to inter-agency working to safeguard and promote the welfare of children. London: HM Government. Available at: www.gov.uk/government/uploads/system/uploads/attachment_data/file/592101/Working_Together_to_Safeguard_Children_20170213.pdf.

Department of Health (2000) *Framework for the Assessment of Children in Need and Their Families*. London: The Stationery Office.

Department of Health (2001) *Valuing People: A New Strategy for Learning Disability for the 21st Century*. London: The Stationery Office.

Department of Health (2005) *Tackling Cancer: Improving the Patient Journey*. London: The Stationery Office. Online: www.nao.org.uk/publications/NAO_reports/04-05/0405288.pdf.

Diamond, L. M. (2008) *Sexual Fluidity: Understanding Women's Love and Desire*. Cambridge, MA: Harvard University Press.

DiPietro, J., Novak, M., Costigan, K., Atella, L. and Reusing, S. (2006) Maternal psychological distress during pregnancy in relation to child development at age two. *Child Development*, 77(3): 573–587.

Dirie, W. and Miller, C. (2006) *Desert Flower: The Extraordinary Journey of a Desert Nomad*. London: Virago.

Dirie, W., Milborn, C. and Alabaster, S. (2005) *Desert Children*. London: Virago.

Dowd, J. J. (1980) *Stratification among the Aged*. Monterey, CA: Brooks/Cole Publishing Co.

Drobnic, S., Blossfeld, H.-P. and Rohwer, G. (1999) Dynamics of women's employment patterns over the family life course: a comparison of the United States and Germany. *Journal of Marriage and the Family*, 61(1): 133–146.

Dunk-West, P. and Hafford-Letchfield, T. (eds) (2016) *Sexual Identities and Sexuality in Social Work: Research and Reflections from Women in the Field*. Abingdon: Routledge.

Dunn, J. and Layard, P. R. G. (2009) *A Good Childhood: Searching for Values in a Competitive Age*. London: Penguin.

DWP (2017) *Households below Average Income: An Analysis of the UK Income Distribution 1994/95–2015/16*. London: Department for Work and Pensions. Online: www.gov.uk/government/uploads/system/uploads/attachment_data/file/600091/households-below-average-income-1994-1995-2015-2016.pdf.

Eapen, V., O'Neill, J., Gurling, H. M. and Robertson, M. M. (1997) Sex of parent transmission effect in Tourette's syndrome: evidence for earlier age at onset in maternally transmitted cases suggests a genomic imprinting effect. *Neurology*, 48(4): 934–937.

Eisenbruch, M. (1984a) Cross cultural aspects of bereavement 1: a conceptual framework for comparative analysis. *Culture, Medicine and Psychiatry*, 8(4): 283–309.

Eisenbruch, M. (1984b) Cross cultural aspects of bereavement 2. Ethnic and cultural variations in the development of bereavement practices. *Culture, Medicine and Psychiatry*, 8(4): 315–347.

Elliott, E. and Kiel, L. (2001) *Chaos Theory in the Social Sciences: Foundations and Applications*. Ann Arbor, MI: University of Michigan Press.

Emerson, E. and Hatton, C. (2008) *Research Report 2008(1): People with Learning Disabilities in England*. Lancaster: CEDR/Lancaster University.

Emerson, E., Azmi, S., Hatton, C., Caine, A., Parrott, R. and Wolstenholme, J. (1997) Is there an increased prevalence of severe learning disabilities among British Asians? *Ethnicity and Health*, 2(4): 317–321.

Emerson, E., Malam, S., Davies, I. and Spencer, K. (2005) *Adults with Learning Disabilities in England, 2003/4*. Leeds: NHS Health and Social Care Information Centre.

Erikson, E. H. (1950/1995) *Childhood and Society*. London: Vintage.

Erikson, E. H. (1985) *The Life Cycle Completed: A Review*. New York and London: Norton.

Estes, C. L., Biggs, S. and Phillipson, C. (2003) *Social Theory, Social Policy and Ageing*. Maidenhead: Open University Press.

Evandrou, M., Glaser, K. and Henz, U. (2002) Caregiving – multiple role occupancy in midlife: balancing work and family life in Britain. *The Gerontologist*, 42(6): 781.

Eyman, R. K. and Call, T. L. (1991) Life expectancy of persons with Down's syndrome. *American Journal of Mental Retardation*, 95(6): 603–612.

Eysenck, H. J. (1968) *The Scientific Study of Personality*. London: Routledge & Kegan Paul.

Eysenck, M. W. (2000) *Psychology: A Student's Handbook*. Hove: Psychology Press.

Feil, N. (1989) *Validation: The Feil Method: How to Help Disoriented Old-Old*. Cleveland, OH: Edward Feil Productions.

Ferri, E., Bynner, J. and Wadsworth, M. (2003) *Changing Britain, Changing Lives: Three Generations at the Turn of the Century*. London: Institute of Education, University of London.

Firth, M., Dwyer, M., Marsden, H., Savage, D. and Mohamad, H. (2004) Non-statutory mental health social work in primary care: a chance for renewal? *British Journal of Social Work*, 34: 145–163.

Fitzpatrick, S., Kemp, P. and Klinker, S. (2000) *Single Homelessness: An Overview of Research in Britain*. Bristol: Policy Press.

Flavell, J. H., Miller, P. H. and Miller, S. A. (2002) *Cognitive Development*. Upper Saddle River, NJ: Prentice Hall.

Fonagy, P. (2016) Reconciling psychoanalytic ideas with attachment theory. In J. Cassidy and P. Shaver (eds) *Handbook of Attachment Theory and Research* (pp. 780–804). New York: Guilford Press.

Forde, L. (1999) *Report of the Commission of Inquiry into Abuse of Children in Queensland Institutions*. Brisbane: Queensland Government.

Frampton, P. (2004) *The Golly in the Cupboard*. Manchester: Tamic.

Frankenberg, R. (1996) Cogito ergo doleo. *Mortality*, 1(2): 213–217.

Frankham, J., Edwards-Kerr, D., Humphrey, N. and Roberts, L. (2007) *School Exclusions: Learning Partnerships outside Mainstream Education*. York: Joseph Rowntree Foundation.

Freud, S. (1905/1991) *On Sexuality: Three Essays on the Theory of Sexuality and Other Works* (J. Strachey and A. Richards, trans.) London: Penguin.

Friendship, C., Blud, L. and Erikson, M. (2002) *An Evaluation of Cognitive Behavioural Treatment for Prisoners*. London: Home Office, Research, Development and Statistics Directorate.

Galinsky, E. (1982) *Between Generations: The Six Stages of Parenthood*. New York: Berkley Books. Online: www.dushkin.com/connectext/psy/ch03/parenthood. mhtml.

Garfield, S. (2005) *Our Hidden Lives: The Remarkable Diaries of Postwar Britain*. London: Ebury.

Gaskell, C. (2010) 'If the social worker had called at least it would show they cared': Young care leaver's perspectives on the importance of care. *Children & Society*, 24(2): 136–147.

GBHGIS (Great Britain Historical Geographical Information System) (2008) *General Report of the 1921 Census, with Appendices, 1927*. Online: www.visionofbritain. org.uk/census/report_page.jsp?rpt_id=EW1921GENand show=ALL. Accessed February 2009.

Gelles, R. (1998) The youngest victims: violence towards children. In R. K. Bergen (ed.) *Issues in Intimate Violence*. Thousand Oaks, CA: Sage.

George, L. K. (1990) Social structure, social processes, and social-psychological states. In R. H. Binstock and L. K. George (eds) *Handbook of Aging and the Social Sciences* (pp. 186–204). San Diego: Academic Press.

Gerhardt, S. (2015) *Why Love Matters: How Affection Shapes a Baby's Brain*. Second edition. London: Routledge.

Giarrusso, R., Feng, D. and Bengtson, V. L. (2005) The intergenerational-stake phenomenon over 20 years. In K.W. Shaie and M. Silverstein (eds) *Annual Review of Gerontology and Geriatrics; Focus on Intergenerational Relations across Time and Place*, 24: 55–76. New York: Springer.

Giddens, A. and Sutton, P. W. (2017) *Sociology*. Cambridge: Polity Press.

Gilligan, C. (1982/1993) *In a Different Voice: Psychological Theory and Women's Development*. Cambridge, MA: Harvard University Press.

Glasser, M., Kolvin, I., Campbell, D., Glasser, A., Leitch, I. and Farrelly, S. (2001) Cycle of child sexual abuse: links between being a victim and becoming a perpetrator. *British Journal of Psychiatry*, 179: 482–494.

Goffman, E. (1959/2008) *The Presentation of Self in Everyday Life*. New York: Anchor Books.

Goffman, E. (1963/1990) *Stigma: Notes on the Management of Spoiled Identity*. Harmondsworth: Penguin Books.

Gordon, D., Adelman, L., Ashworth, K., Bradshaw, J., Levitas, R., Middleton, S. et al. (2000) *Poverty and Social Exclusion in Britain*. York: Joseph Rowntree Foundation.

Goudarzi, S. (2008) Double-edged sword: education delays dementia, but memory declines faster once it hits. *Scientific American Mind*, 19(1).

Granqvist, P., Hesse, E., Fransson, M., Main, M., Hagekull, B. and Bohlin, G. (2016) Prior participation in the strange situation and overstress jointly facilitate disorganized behaviours: implications for theory, research and practice. *Attachment and Human Development*, 18(3): 235–249. http://dx.doi.org/10.1080/14616 734.2016.1151061.

Granqvist, P. L. Sroufe, A., Dozier, M., Hesse, E., Steele, M. et al. (2017) Disorganized attachment in infancy: a review of the phenomenon and its implications for clinicians and policy-makers. *Attachment and Human Development*, 19(6): 534–558. https://doi.org/10.1080/14616734.2017.1354040.

Green, G., Hayes, C., Dickinson, D., Whittaker, A. and Gilheany, B. (2003). A mental health service user's perspective to stigmatisation. *Journal of Mental Health*, 12(3): 223–234.

Guba, E. G. and Lincoln, Y. S. (2005) Paradigmatic controversies, contradictions, and emerging influences. In N. K. Denzin and Y. S. Lincoln (eds) *The Sage Handbook of Qualitative Research.* Third edition (pp. 191–215). London: Sage.

Guse, L. and Masesar, M. (1999) Quality of life and successful aging in long-term care. Perceptions of residents. *Issues in Mental Health Nursing*, 20: 527–539.

Haan, N., Millsap, R. and Hartka, E. (1986) As time goes by: change and stability in personality over fifty years. *Psychology and Aging*, 1(3): 220–232.

Hakamies-Blomqvist, L. (2006) Are there safe and unsafe drivers? *Transportation Research, Part F: Traffic Psychology and Behaviour*, 9(5): 347–352.

Halsey, A. H., Heath, A. F. and Ridge, J. M. (1980) *Origins and Destinations: Family, Class, and Education in Modern Britain.* Oxford and New York: Clarendon Press/ Oxford University Press.

Hanisch, C. (1968/2006) The personal is political. *Notes from the Second Year: Women's Liberation.* New York: Radical Feminism. Online: http://scholar.alexander street.com/download/attachments/2259/Personal+Is+Pol.pdf?version=1.

Hansard (2007) House of Commons Written Answers, 9 January 2007. Online: www. parliament.the-stationeryoffice.co.uk.

Harris, J. R. (2009) *The Nurture Assumption: Why Children Turn out the Way They Do.* New York: Free Press.

Harrison, L. and Harrington, R. (2001) Adolescents' bereavement experiences. Prevalence, association with depressive symptoms, and use of services. *Journal of Adolescence*, 24: 159–170.

Hausdorff, J. M., Levy, B. R. and Wei, J. Y. (1999) The power of ageism on physical function of older persons: reversibility of age-related gait changes. *Journal of the American Geriatrics Society*, 47(11): 1346–1349.

Hazan, C. and Zeifman, D. (1994) Sex and the psychological tether. In K. Bartholomew and D. Perlman (eds) *Advances in Personal Relationships.* Vol. 5. London: Jessica Kingsley.

Hazan, C. and Zeifman, D. (1999) Pair bonds as attachments: evaluating the evidence. In J. Cassidy and P. Shaver (eds) *Handbook of Attachment: Theory, Research and Clinical Applications.* New York and London: Guilford Press.

Healy, T. (1999) A struggle for language: patterns of self-disclosure in lesbian couples. In J. Laird (ed.) *Lesbians and Lesbian Families: Reflections on Theory and Practice.* New York: Columbia University Press.

Heath, A. and McMahon, D. (2001) Ethnic differences in the labour market: the role of education and social class origins. In H. Goulbourne (ed.) *Race and Ethnicity: Critical Concepts in Sociology* (pp. 35–59). London and New York: Routledge.

Hecht, D. T. and Baum, S. K. (1984) Loneliness and attachment patterns in young adults. *Journal of Clinical Psychology*, 40(1): 193–197.

Heimann, P. (1959/1989) Countertransference. In P. Heimann and M. Tonnesmann (eds) *About Children and Children-No-Longer: The Work of Paula Heimann* (pp. 151–160). London: Routledge.

Hendricks, J. (2004) Public policies and old age identity. *Journal of Aging Studies*, 18(3): 245–260.

Henry, J. D., MacLeod, M. S., Phillips, L. H. and Crawford, J. R. (2004) A meta-analytic review of prospective memory and aging. *Psychology and Aging*, 19(1): 27.

Hersch, J. and Stratton, L. (2002) Housework and wages. *Journal of Human Resources*, 37(1): 217–229.

Hesse, E. and Main, M. (1999) Second-generation effects of unresolved trauma in nonmaltreating parents: dissociated, frightened, and threatening parental behavior. *Psychoanalytic Inquiry*, 19(4): 481–540.

Hetherington, R., Cooper, A., Smith, P. and Wilford, G. (1997) *Protecting Children: Messages from Europe.* Lyme Regis: Russell House.

Hicks, S. (2000) 'Good lesbian, bad lesbian . . .': regulating heterosexuality in fostering and adoption assessments. *Child and Family Social Work*, 5(2): 157–168.

Higgins, J. and Hirsch, J. (2007) The pleasure deficit: revisiting the 'sexuality connection' in reproductive health. *International Family Planning Perspectives*, 33(3): 133–139.

Hill, A. and Cooper, M. (2016) Person centred therapy in the twenty-first century: growth and development. In B. Douglas, R. Woolfe, S. Strawbridge, E. Kasket and V. Galbraith (eds) *The Handbook of Counselling Psychology.* London: Sage.

Hirsch, D. (2007) *Experiences of Poverty and Educational Disadvantage.* York: Joseph Rowntree Foundation. Online: www.jrf.org.uk (use publication ref. no. 2123).

Hirst, J., Formby, E., Parr, S., Nixon, J., Hunter, C. and Flint, J. (2007) *An Evaluation of Two Initiatives to Reward Young People.* York: Joseph Rowntree Foundation.

Hirst, M. and Baldwin, S. (1994) *Unequal Opportunities: Growing up Disabled.* London: HMSO.

Hobbs, G., Hobbs, C. and Wynne, J. (1999) Abuse of children in foster and residential care. *Child Abuse and Neglect*, 23(12): 1239–1252.

Hobson, C., Cox, J. and Sagovsky, N. (2008) *Deserving Dignity: The Independent Asylum Commission's Third Report of Conclusions and Recommendations.* London: Independent Asylum Commission in association with the Citizen Organising Foundation.

Hobson, R. (1974) Loneliness. *Journal of Analytical Psychology*, 19(1): 71–89.

Hochschild, A. R. (1975) Disengagement theory: a critique and proposal. *American Sociological Review*, 40(5): 553–569.

Hokanson, J. E., Megargee, E. I., O'Hagan, S. E. and Perry, A. M. (1976) Behavioral, emotional, and autonomic reactions to stress among incarcerated, youthful offenders. *Criminal Justice and Behavior*, 3(3): 203–234.

Hollander, N. C. (2000) Exiles: paradoxes of loss and creativity. In U. McCluskey and C.-A. Hooper (eds) *Psychodynamic Perspectives on Abuse: The Cost of Fear.* London: Jessica Kingsley.

Holmes, J. (2000) Attachment theory and abuse: a developmental perspective. In U. McCluskey and C. A. Hooper (eds) *Psychodynamic Perspectives on Abuse: The Cost of Fear.* London: Jessica Kingsley.

Holmes, T. H. and Rahe, R. H. (1967) The social readjustment rating scale. *Journal of Psychosomatic Research*, 11(2): 213–218.

Holt, N., Bremner, A. J., Sutherland, E., Vliek, M. and Passer, M. (2015) *Psychology: The Science of Mind and Behaviour.* Third edition. New York: McGraw-Hill Education.

Home Office (2008) Domestic Violence Mini-Site. Online: www.crimereduction. homeoffice.gov.uk/dv/dv01.htm. Accessed 2 February 2009.

Home Office (2016) Domestic violence and abuse. Guidance originally issued 26 March 2013, updated 8 March 2016. Available at: www.gov.uk/guidance/domestic-violence-and-abuse#domestic-violence-and-abuse-new-definition. Accessed 17 December 2017.

Horrobin, D. F. (2002) *The Madness of Adam and Eve: How Schizophrenia Shaped Humanity.* London: Corgi.

Horwarth, J. and Lees, J. (2010) Assessing the influence of religious beliefs and practices on parenting capacity: the challenges for social work practitioners. *British Journal of Social Work*, 40(1): 82–99.

Howe, D. (2005) *Child Abuse and Neglect: Attachment, Development and Intervention.* Basingstoke: Palgrave Macmillan.

Howe, D. (2008) *The Emotionally Intelligent Social Worker*. Basingstoke: Palgrave Macmillan.

Howe, D., Sawbridge, P. and Hinings, D. (1992) *Half a Million Women: Mothers Who Lose Their Children by Adoption*. London: Penguin.

Howe, D., Brandon, M., Hinings, D. and Schofield, G. (1999) *Attachment Theory, Child Maltreatment and Family Support*. Basingstoke and New York: Palgrave.

Huber, D., Veinant, P. and Stoop, R. (2005) Vasopressin and oxytocin excite distinct neuronal populations in the central amygdala. *Science*, 308: 245–248.

Humm, M. (1992) *Feminisms: A Reader*. New York and London: Harvester Wheatsheaf.

Hutchison, E. D. (2003a) *Dimensions of Human Behaviour: The Changing Life Course*. Second edition. London: Sage.

Hutchison, E. D. (2003b) *Dimensions of Human Behaviour: Person and the Environment*. Second edition. London: Sage.

Iacovou, M. (2004a) *Life Chances: The Impact of Family Origins and Early Childhood Experiences on Adult Outcomes*. London: ESRC. Online: www.esrc.ac.uk. Accessed 1 July 2009.

Iacovou, M. (2004b) Life chances: the impact of family origins and early childhood experiences on adult outcomes. In S. Stewart and R. Vaitilingam (eds) *Seven Ages of Man and Woman* (pp. 12–15). London: ESRC. Online: www.esrc.ac.uk.

Jackson, S. and Scott, S. (2002) *Gender: A Sociological Reader*. London: Routledge.

Jahoda, M. (1982) *Employment and Unemployment: A Social-Psychological Analysis*. Cambridge: Cambridge University Press.

Jencks, C. and Phillips, M. (1998) The black-white test score gap: an introduction. In C. Jencks and M. Phillips (eds) *The Black-White Test Score Gap* (pp. 1–51). Washington, DC: Brookings Institution.

Johannesen, M. and Logiudice, D. (2013) Elder abuse: a systematic review of risk factors in community-dwelling elders, *Age and Ageing*, 42(3): 292–298.

Jordan, B. (1991) *Social Work in an Unjust Society*. Hemel Hempstead: Harvester Wheatsheaf.

Joseph Rowntree Foundation (JRF) (2016) UK poverty: causes, costs and solutions. Available at: www.jrf.org.uk/report/uk-poverty-causes-costs-and-solutions.

Joyce, A. (2005) The first six months. In E. Rayner, A. Joyce, J. Rose, M. Twyman and C. Clulow (eds) *Human Development: An Introduction to the Psychodynamics of Growth, Maturity and Ageing*. Fourth edition (pp. 47–70). London and New York: Routledge.

Kaati, G., Bygren, L. O. and Edvinsson, S. (2002) Cardiovascular and diabetes mortality determined by nutrition during parents' and grandparents' slow growth period. *European Journal of Human Genetics*, 10(11): 682–688.

Kagan, C. and Tindall, C. (2003) Feminist approaches to counselling. In R. Woolfe, W. Dryden and S. Strawbridge (eds) *Handbook of Counselling Psychology*. London and Thousand Oaks, CA: Sage.

Kaplan, H. S. (1979) *Disorders of Sexual Desire and Other New Concepts and Techniques in Sex Therapy*. New York: Simon and Schuster.

Kawaguchi, M. C., Welsh, D. P., Powers, S. I. and Rostosky, S. S. (1998) Mothers, fathers, sons, and daughters: temperament, gender, and adolescent-parent relationships. *Merrill-Palmer Quarterly*, 44(1): 77–96.

Keizer, P., Dykstra, A. and Jansen, M. (2008) Pathways into childlessness: evidence of gendered life course dynamics. *Journal of Biosocial Science*, 40: 863–878.

Kennedy, A. (2008) Eugenics, 'degenerate girls', and social workers during the progressive era. *Affilia*, 23(1): 22–37.

Kermode, F. (2007) The long life. *The London Review of Books*, 29(24): 17.

King, G. A., Shultz, I. Z., Steel, K., Gilpin, M. and Cathers, T. (1993) Self-evaluation and self-concept of adolescents with physical disabilities. *American Journal of Occupational Therapy*, 47(2): 132–140.

Kirkwood, T. B. L. (2001) *The End of Age*. London: Profile Books.

Klaus, M. H., Kennell, J. H., Plumb, N. and Zuehlke, S. (1970) Human maternal behavior at the first contact with her young. *Pediatrics*, 46(2): 187–192.

Klein, M. (1975) *Envy and Gratitude and Other Works*. London: Hogarth.

Klentrou, P. and Plyley, M. (2003) Onset of puberty, menstrual frequency, and body fat in elite rhythmic gymnasts compared with normal controls. *British Journal of Sports Medicine*, 37(6): 490–494.

Klusmann, D. (2002) Sexual motivation and the duration of partnership. *Archives of Sexual Behavior*, 31(3): 275–287.

Klusmann, D. (2006) Sperm competition and female procurement of male resources as explanations for a gender-specific time dependent course in the sexual motivation of couples. *Human Nature*, 17(3): 283–300.

Koenig, A. L., Cicchetti, D. and Rogosch, F. A. (2004) Moral development: the association between maltreatment and young children's prosocial behaviors and moral transgressions. *Social Development*, 13(1): 97–106.

Kohlberg, L., Levine, C. and Hewer, A. (1994) *Moral Stages: A Current Formulation and a Response to Critics: 3. Synopses of Criticisms and a Reply; 4. Summary and Conclusion*. New York: Garland Publishing.

Kohli, R. (2007) *Working with Unaccompanied Asylum Seeking Children: Issues for Policy and Practice*. Basingstoke and New York: Palgrave Macmillan.

Kristensen Whittaker, M., Brown, J., Beckett, R. and Gerhold, C. (2006) Sexual knowledge and empathy: a comparison of adolescent child molesters and non-offending adolescents. *Journal of Sexual Aggression*, 12(2): 143–154.

Kübler-Ross, E. (1989) *On Death and Dying*. London: Routledge.

Lamb, M. E. (2004) *The Role of the Father in Child Development*. Hoboken, NJ: Wiley. Online: www.abc.net.au/rn/talks/lm/stories/s1099987.htm.

Leahy, R. L. and Dowd, E. T. (2002) *Clinical Advances in Cognitive Psychotherapy: Theory and Application*. New York: Springer.

Levinson, D. J. (1978) *The Seasons of a Man's Life*. New York: Ballantyne.

Levinson, D. J. (1986) A conception of adult development. *American Psychologist*, 41: 3–13.

Levy, B. and Banaji, M. (2006) Implicit ageism. In T. Nelson (ed.) *Ageism: Stereotyping and Prejudice against Older Persons*. Cambridge, MA: MIT Press.

Lewin, K. (1935) *A Dynamic Theory of Personality*. New York: McGraw-Hill Custom Publishing.

Li, J., Precht, D. H., Mortensen, P. B. and Olsen, J. (2003) Mortality in parents after death of a child in Denmark: a nationwide follow-up study. *Lancet*, 361: 363–367.

Lunney, J. R., Lynn, J., Foley, D. J., Lipson, S. and Guralnik, J. M. (2003) Patterns of functional decline at the end of life. *Journal of the American Medical Association*, 289(18): 2387.

Mace, N. L. and Rabins, P. V. (2007) *The 36-Hour Day*. New York and London: Warner.

Main, M., Kaplan, N. and Cassidy, J. (1985) Security in infancy, childhood, and adulthood: a move to the level of representation. *Monographs of the Society for Research in Child Development*, 50(1–2): 66–104.

Malina, R. (1990) Physical growth and performance during the transition years. In R. Montemayor, G. R. Adams and T. Gullotta (eds) *From Childhood to Adolescence: A Transitional Period?* Newbury Park, CA: Sage.

Mallon, G. P. (1998) *We Don't Exactly Get the Welcome Wagon: The Experiences of Gay and Lesbian Adolescents in Child Welfare Systems*. New York: Columbia University Press.

Marie Curie (2017) *Can Giving Patients Choice Be Cost Effective for the NHS?* London: Marie Curie Cancer Care. Available at: www.mariecurie.org.uk/global assets/archive/www2/pdf/patient-choice-v-cost_graphics.pdf. Accessed 27 December 2017.

Marris, P. (1974) *Loss and Change*. New York: Pantheon Books.

Maslow, A. H. and Frager, R. (1954/2003) *Motivation and Personality*. New York: Longman.

Masters, W. H. and Johnson, V. E. (1966) *Human Sexual Response*. London: Churchill.

Mattinson, J. (1975) *The Reflection Process in Casework Supervision*. London: Institute of Marital Studies, Tavistock Institute of Human Relations.

Mayo Clinic (2018) *Male Menopause: Myth or Reality?* Minnesota: Mayo Foundation for Medical Education and Research. Online: www.mayoclinic.org/healthy-lifestyle/mens-health/in-depth/male-menopause/art-20048056. Accessed 5 January 2018.

McAdams, D. P. (1997) *The Stories We Live By: Personal Myths and the Making of the Self*. New York: Guilford Press.

McAuliffe, D. and Sudbery, J. (2005) 'Who do I tell?' Support and consultation in cases of ethical conflict. *Journal of Social Work*, 5(1): 21–43.

McCarron, M., Swinburne, J., Burke, E., McGlinchey, E., Mulryan, N., Andrews, V., Foran, S. and McCallion, P. (2011) Growing older with an intellectual disability in Ireland in 2011: first results from the Intellectual Disability Supplement of the Irish Longitudinal Study on Ageing. School of Nursing and Midwifery, Trinity College Dublin. Available at: https://nursing-midwifery.tcd.ie/assets/research/doc/ids_tilda_2011/ids_tilda_report_2011.pdf. Accessed 27 November 2017.

McCarthy, M. (1999) *Sexuality and Women with Learning Disabilities*. London and Philadelphia: Jessica Kingsley.

McCluskey, U. and Hooper, C.-A. (2000) *Psychodynamic Perspectives on Abuse: The Cost of Fear*. London and Philadelphia: Jessica Kingsley.

McGuire, J. (ed.) (1995) *What Works: Reducing Reoffending – Guidelines from Research and Practice*. Chichester: Wiley.

McKittrick, D. (2007) Life expectancy of Irish travellers still at 1940s levels despite economic boom. *Independent* (world edition), 28 June.

McLeod, J. (2003) The humanistic paradigm. In R. Woolfe and W. Dryden (eds) *Handbook of Counselling Psychology* (pp. 140–160). Thousand Oaks, CA: Sage.

McManus, S., Bebbington, P., Jenkins, R. and Brugha, T. (eds) (2016) *Mental Health and Wellbeing in England: Adult Psychiatric Morbidity Survey 2014*. Leeds: NHS Digital.

McMurray, I., Connolly, H., Preston-Shoot, M. and Wigley, V. (2008) Constructing resilience: social workers' understandings and practice. *Health and Social Care in the Community*, 16(3): 299–309.

Meier, E. A., Gallegos, J. V., Thomas, L. P. M., Depp, C. A., Irwin, S. A. and Jeste, D. V. (2016) Defining a good death (successful dying): literature review and a call for research and public dialogue. *The American Journal of Geriatric Psychiatry*, 24(4): 261–271.

Meins, E. (2005) *Developmental Outcomes of Joint Attention and Maternal Mind-Mindedness*. Swindon: ESRC.

Meins, E., Fernyhough, C., Wainwright, R., Clark-Carter, D., Gupta, M. D., Fradley, E. and Tuckey, M. (2003) Pathways to understanding mind: construct validity and predictive validity of maternal mind-mindedness. *Child Development*, 74(4): 1194–1211.

Mencap (2007) *Death by Indifference*. London: Mencap. Available at: www.mencap. org.uk/sites/default/files/2016-06/DBIreport.pdf. Accessed 20 November 2017.

Mencap (2018) Children and young people with a learning disability. Available at: www.mencap.org.uk/learning-disability-explained/research-and-statistics/.

Mental Health Foundation (2016) *Fundamental Facts about Mental Health 2016*. London: Mental Health Foundation.

Mental Health Foundation (undated) *My Daddy Wasn't Scared of Anything Except Feeling Sad*. London: Mental Health Foundation.

Michael, J. (2008) *Healthcare for All: Independent Inquiry into Access to Healthcare for People with Learning Disabilities*. London: Independent Inquiry into Access to Healthcare for People with Learning Disabilities. Available at: www.dh.gov.uk/ prod_consum_dh/groups/dh_digitalassets/@dh/@en/documents/digitalas- set/dh_106126.pdf. Accessed 1 November 2017.

Mickelson, K. D., Kessler, R. C. and Shaver, P. R. (1997) Adult attachment in a nation- ally representative sample. *Journal of Personality and Social Psychology*, 73(5): 1092–1106.

Minsky, R. (1996) *Psychoanalysis and Gender*. London: Routledge.

Mir, G., Nocon, A., Ahmad, W. and Jones, L. (2001) *Learning Difficulties and Ethnicity: Report to the Department of Health*. London: Department of Health.

Monroe, B. (2004) Social work in palliative medicine. In D. Doyle, G. Hanks, N. Cherny and K. Calman (eds) *Oxford Textbook of Palliative Medicine*. Third edition (pp. 1007–1017). Oxford: Oxford University Press.

Moore, K. A. and Glei, D. (1995) Taking the plunge: an examination of positive youth development. *Journal of Adolescent Research*, 10(1): 15–40.

Morgan, R. and Lindsay, M. (2006) *Young People's Views on Leaving Care. What Young People in, and Formerly in Residential and Foster Care Think about Leaving Care: A Children's Rights Director Report*. Great Britain: Commission for Social Care Inspection.

Morningstar, B. (1999) Lesbian parents: understanding developmental pathways. In J. Laird (ed.) *Lesbians and Lesbian Families: Reflections on Theory and Practice*. New York: Columbia University Press.

Morris, J. K. and Alberman, E. (2009) Trends in Down's syndrome live birth and antenatal diagnoses in England and Wales from 1989 to 2008: analysis of data from the National Down Syndrome Cytogenetic Register. *British Medical Journal*, 339: b3794. Available at: http://doi.org/10.1136/bmj.b3794.

Morrison, L. L. and L'Heureux, J. (2001) Suicide and gay/lesbian/bisexual youth: implications for clinicians. *Journal of Adolescence*, 24(1): 39–49.

Morrow, D. and Messinger, L. (2006) *Sexual Orientation and Gender Expression in Social Work Practice Working with Gay, Lesbian, Bisexual, and Transgender People*. New York: Columbia University Press.

Morrow, V. and Richards, M. (1996) *Transitions to Adulthood: A Family Matter?* York: York Publishing Services.

Munday, D., Dale, J. and Murray, S. (2007) Choice and place of death: individual pref- erences, uncertainty, and the availability of care. *Journal of the Royal Society of Medicine*, 100(5): 211–215.

Murphy, S. A., Johnson, L. C. and Lohan, J. (2003) Challenging the myths about par- ents' adjustment after the sudden, violent death of a child. *Journal of Nursing Scholarship*, 35(4): 359–364.

Myers, J. E., Madathil, J. and Tingle, L. R. (2005) Marriage satisfaction and wellness in India and the United States: a preliminary comparison of arranged marriages and marriages of choice. *Journal of Counseling and Development*, 83(2): 183–190.

Myerscough, G. (1981) *I'm Not a Bloody Label*. Southsea: Issness.

Myhill, A. (2015) Measuring coercive control: what can we learn from national population surveys? *Violence Against Women*, 21(3): 355–375.

NACRO (2000) *The Forgotten Majority: The Resettlement of Short Term Prisoners*. London: National Association for the Care and Resettlement of Offenders.

National Audit Office (2015) Care leavers' transition to adulthood. HC 269 Session 2015–16. Published 17 July 2015.

National Institutes of Health (2005) *Tourette Syndrome Fact Sheet*. Bethesda, MD: NINDS.

Nelson, H. W. (2000) Injustice and conflict in nursing homes: toward advocacy and exchange. *Journal of Aging Studies*, 14(1): 39–61.

Neugarten, B. (1977) Personality and ageing. In J. E. Birren and K. W. Schaie (eds) *Handbook of the Psychology of Aging*. New York: Van Nostrand Reinhold.

Newman, T. (2002) *Promoting Resilience: A Review of Effective Strategies for Child Care Services*. Exeter: Centre for Evidence-Based Social Services. Online: www.nursingacademy.com/uploads/6/4/8/8/6488931/promotingresilience newman.pdf. Accessed 5 November 2017.

Nirje, B. (1999) How I came to formulate the normalization principle. In R. J. Flynn and R. A. Lemay (eds) *A Quarter-Century of Normalization and Social Role Valorization: Evolution and Impact*. Ottawa: University of Ottawa Press.

O'Brien, J. (1989) *What's Worth Working For? Leadership for Better Quality Human Services*. Syracuse, NY: Center on Human Policy, Syracuse University.

O'Connor, T. G. and Nilson, W. (2005) Models versus metaphors in translating attachment theory to the clinic and community. In L. J. Berlin, Y. Ziv, L. Amaya-Jackons and M. T. Greenberg (eds) *Enhancing Early Attachments: Theory, Research, Intervention and Policy* (pp. 313–326). New York and London: Guilford Press.

Office for National Statistics (ONS) (2004) *Life Expectancy – More Aged 70 and 80 Than Ever Before*. London: ONS.

Office for National Statistics (2005) *Focus on Older People*. Online: www.statistics. gov.uk/focuson/olderpeople/.

Office for National Statistics (ONS) (2006) *Cancer Survival: England and Wales, 1991–2001*. Online: www.statistics.gov.uk/StatBase/Product. asp?vlnk=10821andMore=Y. Accessed 11 April 2009.

Office for National Statistics (ONS) (2007a) *Calculating Expectations of Life*. Online: www.statistics.gov.uk/cci/nugget.asp?id=1898. Accessed 11 April 2009.

Office for National Statistics (ONS) (2007b) *Mortality Statistics General Review of the Registrar General on Deaths in England and Wales, 2005*. London: ONS.

Office for National Statistics (ONS) (2008a) *Focus on Gender*. Newport: Office for National Statistics. Online: www.statistics.gov.uk.

Office for National Statistics (ONS) (2008b) *Ageing: More Pensioners Than Under-16's for First Time Ever*. Online: www.statistics.gov.uk/cci/nugget.asp?ID=949. Accessed February 2009.

Office for National Statistics (ONS) (2013) *Interim Life Tables*. Online: www.ons.gov. uk/peoplepopulationandcommunity/birthsdeathsandmarriages/lifeexpectancies/ bulletins/interimlifetables/englandandwales20102012. Accessed 2 January 2018.

Office for National Statistics (ONS) (2017a) *Suicides in Great Britain: 2016 Registrations*. Statistical bulletin, released 7 September 2017.

Office for National Statistics (ONS) (2017b) *Divorces in England and Wales (2016).* Statistical bulletin, released 18 October 2017. Available at: www.ons.gov.uk/peoplepopulationandcommunity/birthsdeathsandmarriages/divorce/bulletins/divorcesinenglandandwales/2016/pdf.

Office for National Statistics (ONS) (2017c) *National Life Tables, UK: 2014 to 2016,* released 18 October 2017. Available at: www.ons.gov.uk/peoplepopulationand-community/birthsdeathsandmarriages/lifeexpectancies/bulletins/nationallifetablesunitedkingdom/2014to2016. Accessed 3 November 2017.

Office for National Statistics (ONS) (2017d) *Domestic Abuse in England and Wales: Year Ending March 2017.* Statistical bulletin, released 23 November 2017. Available at: www.ons.gov.uk/peoplepopulationandcommunity/crimeandjustice/bulletins/domesticabuseinenglandandwales/yearendingmarch2017.

Office for National Statistics (ONS) (2017e) *Births by Parents' Characteristics in England and Wales: 2016.* Statistical bulletin, released 27 November 2017. Available at: www.ons.gov.uk/peoplepopulationandcommunity/birthsdeathsandmarriages/livebirths/bulletins/birthsbyparentscharacteristicsinenglandandwales/2016. Accessed 23 November 2017.

Office for National Statistics (ONS) (2017f) *Divorces in England and Wales: 2015.* Statistical bulletin, released 21 June 2017. Available at: www.ons.gov.uk/people-populationandcommunity/birthsdeathsandmarriages/divorce/bulletins/divorcesinenglandandwales/2015#how-long-do-marriages-of-opposite-sex-couples-last. Accessed 3 January 2018.

Office for National Statistics (ONS) (2017g) *Families and the Labour Market, England: 2017.* Statistical bulletin, released 26 September 2017. Available at: www.ons.gov.uk/employmentandlabourmarket/peopleinwork/employmentan-demployeetypes/articles/familiesandthelabourmarketengland/2017#mothers-with-a-youngest-child-aged-between-three-and-four-years-old-have-the-lowest-employment-rate-of-all-adults-with-or-without-children-and-are-the-most-likely-group-to-work-part-time. Accessed 3 December 2017.

Office for National Statistics (ONS) (2017h) *Annual Survey of Hours and Earnings.* Statistical bulletin, released 26 October 2017. Available at: www.ons.gov.uk/employmentandlabourmarket/peopleinwork/earningsandworkinghours/bulletins/annualsurveyofhoursandearnings/2017provisionaland2016revisedresults. Accessed 3 December 2017.

Office for National Statistics (ONS) (2017i) *Revised GCSE and Equivalent Results in England, 2015 to 2016.* Statistical bulletin, released 19 January 2017. Available at: www.gov.uk/government/uploads/system/uploads/attachment_data/file/584473/SFR03_2017.pdf. Accessed 3 December 2017.

Olsen, T. S., Dehlendorff, C. and Andersen, K. K. (2007) Sex-related time-dependent variations in post-stroke survival – evidence of a female stroke survival advantage. *Neuroepidemiology,* 29(3–4): 218–225.

Orbach, I., Gross, Y., Glaubman, H. and Berman, D. (1986) Children's perception of various determinants of the death concept as a function of intelligence, age, and anxiety. *Journal of Clinical Child Psychology,* 15(2): 120–126.

Parkes, C. M., Stevenson-Hynde, J. and Marris, M. (1991) *Attachment across the Life Cycle.* London: Routledge.

Parliament of Australia (2001) *Child Migrants from the United Kingdom.* Online: www.aph.gov.au/library/intguide/sp/childmigrantuk.htm. Accessed 11 April 2009.

Parry, G., Cleemput, P. V., Peters, J., Walters, S., Thomas, K. and Cooper, C. (2004) *The Health Status of Gypsies and Travellers: Report to Department of Health.* University of Sheffield.

Paul, S. N., Kato, B. S., Hunkin, J. L., Vivekanandan, S. and Spector, T. D. (2006) The big finger: the second to fourth digit ratio is a predictor of sporting ability in women. *British Journal of Sports Medicine*, 40(12): 981–983.

Paus, T., Zijdenbos, A., Worsley, K., Collins, D. L., Blumenthal, J., Giedd, J. N. et al. (1999) Structural maturation of neural pathways in children and adolescents: in vivo study. *Science*, 283: 1908–1911.

Payne, H. and Butler, I. (1998) Improving the health care process and determining health outcomes for children looked after by the local authority. *Ambulatory Child Health*, 4: 165–172.

Payne, M. (2005) *The Origins of Social Work*. Basingstoke and New York: Palgrave.

Pendergast, D. R., Fisher, N. M. and Calkins, E. (1993) Cardiovascular, neuromuscular, and metabolic alterations with age leading to frailty. *Journal of Gerontology*, 48(Spec. No.): 61–67.

Perlman, H. H. (1957) *Social Casework: A Problem-Solving Process*. Chicago: University of Chicago Press.

Phillipson, C. (1982) *Capitalism and the Construction of Old Age*. London: Macmillan.

Phinney, J. S. and Rosenthal, D. A. (1992) Ethnic identity in adolescence: process, context, and outcome. In G. R. Adams, T. P. Gullotta and R. Montemayor (eds) *Adolescent Identity Formation*. Newbury Park, CA: Sage.

Piaget, J. (1950/1997) *The Origin of Intelligence in the Child*. London and New York: Routledge.

Piaget, J., Gruber, H. E. and Vonèche, J. J. (1995) *The Essential Piaget*. Northvale, NJ: J. Aronson.

Pinker, S. (2008) *The Sexual Paradox: Men, Women and the Real Gender Gap*. New York: Scribner.

Piontelli, A. (2002) *Twins: From Fetus to Child*. London and New York: Routledge.

Pollert, A. (1996) Gender and class revisited: or the poverty of patriarchy. *Sociology*, 30(4): 639–659.

Prior, V. and Glaser, D. (2006) *Understanding Attachment and Attachment Disorders: Theory, Evidence and Practice*. London and Philadelphia: Jessica Kingsley.

Prison Reform Trust (2007) *Bromley Briefings Prison Factfile December 2007*. London: Prison Reform Trust. Online: www.prisonreformtrust.org.uk/uploads/documents/factfile5dec.pdf. Accessed 11 December 2017.

Purnine, D. M. and Carey, M. P. (1998) Age and gender differences in sexual behavior preferences: a follow-up report. *Journal of Sex and Marital Therapy*, 24(2): 93–102.

Qualter, P. and Munn, P. (2002) The separateness of social and emotional loneliness in childhood. *Journal of Child Psychology and Psychiatry*, 43(2): 233–244.

Quilgars, D., Johnsen, S. and Pleace, N. (2008) *Youth Homelessness in the UK: A Decade of Progress?* York: Joseph Rowntree Foundation. Online: www.jrf.org.uk/report/youth-homelessness-uk. Accesssed 12 November 2017.

Quinn, P. (1998) *Understanding Disability: A Lifespan Approach*. Thousand Oaks, CA: Sage.

Race, D. G. (2007) *Intellectual Disability: Social Approaches*. Maidenhead and New York: Open University Press/McGraw-Hill Education.

Radford, L., Corral, S., Bradley, C., Fisher, H., Bassett, C., Howat, N. and Collishaw, S. (2011). *Child Abuse and Neglect in the UK Today*. London: NSPCC. Available at: www.nspcc.org.uk/globalassets/documents/research-reports/child-abuse-neglect-uk-today-research-report.pdf. Accessed 12 December 2017.

Raffel, S. (1999) Revisiting role theory: roles and the problem of the self. *Sociological Research Online*, 4(2).

Rainer (2007) *Home Alone: Housing and Support for Young People Leaving Care*. Online: www.crin.org/en/docs/Rainer_home_alone.pdf. Accessed 18 November 2017.

Raphael-Leff, J. (2005) *Psychological Processes of Childbearing*. London: Anna Freud Centre.

Rayner, E., Joyce, A., Rose, J., Twyman, M. and Clulow, C. (2005) *Human Development: An Introduction to the Psychodynamics of Growth, Maturity and Ageing*. Fourth edition. London and New York: Routledge.

Reichard, S., Livson, F. and Petersen, P. G. (1962) *Aging and Personality: A Study of Eighty-Seven Older Men*. New York: Wiley.

Revenson, T. (1982) Predictable loneliness of old age: dispelling the myth. Paper presented at the Annual Convention of the American Psychological Association. Online: www.researchgate.net/publication/234647430_Predictable_Loneliness_of_Old_Age_Dispelling_the_Myth. Accessed 12 December 2017.

Rezmovic, E. L., Sloane, D., Alexander, D., Seltser, B. and Jessor, T. (1996) *Cycle of Sexual Abuse: Research Inconclusive about Whether Child Victims Become Adult Perpetrators*. Washington, DC: United States General Accounting Office.

Ribbens McCarthy, J. and Jessop, J. (2005) *Young People, Bereavement and Loss: Disruptive Transitions?* London: National Children's Bureau/Joseph Rowntree Foundation. Available at: http://oro.open.ac.uk/12980/. Accessed 5 January 2018.

Ridley, M. (1999) *Genome: The Autobiography of a Species in 23 Chapters*. New York: HarperCollins.

Rippon, S. (2004) Interventions in mental health: promoting collaborative working. In T. Ryan and J. Pritchard (eds) *Good Practice in Adult Mental Health*. London and Philadelphia: Jessica Kingsley.

Roberts, V. Z. (1994) The self-assigned impossible task. In A. Obholzer and V. Z. Roberts (eds) *The Unconscious at Work: Individual and Organizational Stress in the Human Services* (pp. 110–120). London and New York: Routledge.

Rogers, A. and Pilgrim, D. (2003) *Mental Health and Inequality*. Basingstoke and New York: Palgrave.

Rogers, C. R. (1959) A theory of therapy, personality, and interpersonal relationships, as developed in the client-centered framework. In S. Koch (ed.) *A Study of a Science: Study 1. Conceptual and Systematic: Vol. 3 Formulations of the Person and the Social Context* (pp. 184–256). New York: McGraw-Hill.

Rogers, C. R. (1961/2004) *On Becoming a Person: A Therapist's View of Psychotherapy*. London: Constable; Boston: Houghton Mifflin.

Roker, D. (1998) *Worth More Than This: Young People Growing Up in Family Poverty*. London: Children's Society.

Ruch, G., Turney, D. and Ward, A. (eds) (2010) *Relationship-Based Social Work: Getting to the Heart of Practice*. London and Philadelphia: Jessica Kingsley.

Rutter, J. (2001) *Supporting Refugee Children in 21st Century Britain*. Staffordshire: Trentham Books.

Rutter, M. (2006) *Genes and Behavior: Nature-Nurture Interplay Explained*. Malden, MA and Oxford: Blackwell

Rutter, M., O Connor, T., Beckett, C., Castle, J., Dunn, J. and Groothues, C. (2000) Recovery and deficit following early profound deprivation. In P. Selman (ed.) *Intercountry Adoption: Developments, Trends and Perspectives*. London: BAAF.

Ryan, T. and Pritchard, J. (eds) (2004) *Good Practice in Adult Mental Health*. London and Philadelphia: Jessica Kingsley.

Scarr, S. (1996) How people make their own environments: implications for parents and policy makers. *Psychology, Public Policy and Law*, 2(2): 204–228.

Scarr, S. and McCartney, K. (1983) How people make their own environments: a theory of genotype-environment effects. *Child Development*, 54(2): 424–435.

Schaffer, H. (1996) *Social Development.* Oxford: Blackwell.

Schonert-Reichl, K. A. (1999) Relations of peer acceptance, friendship adjustment, and social behavior to moral reasoning during early adolescence. *The Journal of Early Adolescence*, 19(2): 249–279.

Schore, A. (1994) *Affect Regulation and the Origin of the Self: The Neurobiology of Emotional Development.* Hillsdale, NJ: Erlbaum.

Schore, A. (1999) Foreword. In J. Bowlby, *Attachment and Loss. Vol. 1, Attachment.* London: Hogarth Press.

Schore, A. (2001a) The effects of a secure attachment relationship on right brain development, affect regulation and infant mental health. *Development and Psychopathology*, 8: 59–87. Online: www.trauma-pages.com/articles.php#Schore. Accessed 6 January 2018.

Schore, A. (2001b) The effects of early relational trauma on right brain development, affect regulation, and infant mental health. *Infant Mental Health Journal*, 22: 201–269. Online: www.trauma-pages.com/articles.php#Schore. Accessed 6 January 2018.

Schore, A. N. (2003) *Affect Dysregulation and Disorders of the Self.* London: Norton.

Schwab, R. (1998) A child's death and divorce: dispelling the myth. *Death Studies*, 22(5): 445–468.

Scott, M. J. and Dryden, W. (2003) The cognitive-behavioural paradigm. In R. Woolfe, W. Dryden and S. Strawbridge (eds) *Handbook of Counselling Psychology.* London and Thousand Oaks, CA: Sage.

Scottish Transgender Alliance (2010) Out of sight, out of mind? Transgender people's experiences of domestic abuse. Available at: www.scottishtrans.org/wp-content/uploads/2013/03/trans_domestic_abuse.pdf. Accessed 17 December 2017.

Seale, C. (1998) *Constructing Death: The Sociology of Dying and Bereavement.* Cambridge: Cambridge University Press.

Sergo, P. (2008) Predicting Alzheimer's: a new technique may give years of advanced warning. *Scientific American Mind*, 19(1).

Shachar, R. (1991) His and her marital satisfaction. *Sex Roles*, 21: 451–467.

Shedler, J. (2010) The efficacy of psychodynamic psychotherapy. *American Psychologist*, 65: 98–109.

Shemmings, D. and Shemmings, Y. (2011) *Understanding Disorganized Attachment: An Evidence-Based Model for Understanding and Supporting Families.* London: Jessica Kingsley.

Shneidman, E. S. (1995) *Voices of Death.* New York: Kodansha International.

Siegenthaler, A. L. and Bigner, J. J. (2000) The value of children to lesbian and non-lesbian mothers. *Journal of Homosexuality*, 39(2): 73–91.

Silverberg, S. B. and Steinberg, L. (1987) Adolescent autonomy, parent-adolescent conflict, and parental wellbeing. *Journal of Youth and Adolescence*, 16: 293–312.

Simon, A., Epstein, L. J. and Association, A. P. (1968) *Aging in Modern Society.* Washington, DC: American Psychiatric Association Committee on Research.

Singh, S., Wulf, D., Samara, R. and Cuca, Y. P. (2000) Gender differences in the timing of first intercourse: data from 14 countries. *International Family Planning Perspectives*, 26(1): 21–28, 43.

Skinner, B. F. (1971) *Beyond Freedom and Dignity.* New York: Knopf.

Slaughter, V. (2005) Young children's understanding of death. *Australian Psychologist*, 40(3): 179–186.

Sloper, T. and Beresford, B. (2006) Families with disabled children. *British Medical Journal*, 333: 928–929.

Small, H. (2007) *The Long Life*. Oxford: Oxford University Press.

Smallwood, S. and Wilson, B. (2007) *Focus on Families*. Basingstoke: Palgrave Macmillan/Office for National Statistics. Online: www.statistics.gov.uk/downloads/theme_compendia/fof2007/FO_Families_2007.pdf.

Smith, M., Edgar, G. and Groom, G. (2008) Health expectancies in the United Kingdom, 2004–06. *Health Statistics Quarterly*, 40. Online: www.statistics.gov.uk.

Smith, P. K., Cowie, H. and Blades, M. (2011) *Understanding Children's Development*. Fifth edition. Chichester: Wiley and Sons.

Smitsman, A. W. (2001) Action in infancy: perspectives, concepts and challenges, development of reaching and grasping. In G. Bremner and F. Fogel (eds) *Blackwell Handbook of Infant Development* (pp. 71–99). Oxford: Blackwell.

Sneed, J. R., Johnson, J. G., Cohen, P., Gilligan, C., Chen, H., Crawford, T. N. et al. (2006) Gender differences in the age-changing relationship between instrumentality and family contact in emerging adulthood. *Developmental Psychology*, 42(5): 787–797.

Soule, A., Baab, P., Evandrou, M., Balchin, S. and Zealey, L., Office for National Statistics (2005) *Focus on Older People*. Basingstoke: Palgrave Macmillan.

Sowell, E. R., Thompson, P. M., Holmes, C. J., Jernigan, T. L. and Toga, A. W. (1999) In vivo evidence for post-adolescent brain maturation in frontal and striatal regions. *Nature Neuroscience*, 2(10): 859–861.

Spencer, M. B. and Dornbusch, S. (1990) Challenges in studying minority youth. In S. S. Feldman and G. R. Elliott (eds) *At the Threshold: The Developing Adolescent*. Cambridge, MA: Harvard University Press.

Sroufe, L. (1988) The role of infant-caregiver attachment in development. In J. Belsky and T. Nezworski (eds) *Clinical Implications of Attachment Theory*. Hillsdale, NJ: Erlbaum.

Steele, M., Hodges, J., Kaniuk, J., Hillman, S. and Henderson, K. (2003) Attachment representations and adoption: associations between maternal states of mind and emotion narratives in previously maltreated children. *Journal of Child Psychotherapy*, 29(2): 187–205.

Sternbach, H. (1998) Age-associated testosterone decline in men: clinical issues for psychiatry. *The American Journal of Psychiatry*, 155(10): 1310–1318.

Stewart, S. and Vaitilingam, R. (eds) (2004) *Seven Ages of Man and Woman*. London: ESRC. Online: www.esrc.ac.uk.

Stonewall (2018) *Domestic Violence: What Does the Law Say?* Available at: www.stonewall.org.uk/help-advice/criminal-law/domestic-violence. Accessed 6 January 2018.

Stroebe, M. S. (2008) *Handbook of Bereavement Research and Practice: Advances in Theory and Intervention*. Washington, DC: American Psychological Association.

Stroebe, M. and Schut, H. (1999) The dual process model of coping with bereavement. *Death Studies*, 23: 197–224.

Stuart-Hamilton, I. (2012) *The Psychology of Ageing: An Introduction*. Fifth edition. London: Jessica Kingsley.

Sudbery, J. (2002) Key features of therapeutic social work: the use of relationship. *Journal of Social Work Practice*, 16(2): 149–162.

Sudbery, J. and Blenkinship, A. (2005) 'Acting as a good parent would'? Psychosocial support for parents in a children's hospital. *Journal of Social Work Practice*, 19(1): 43–57.

Sudbery, J. and Bradley, J. (1996) Staff support in organisations providing therapeutic care. *Journal of Social Work Practice*, 10(1): 51–62.

Sudbery, P. and Sudbery, I. (2009) *Human Molecular Genetics*. Harlow: Pearson Prentice Hall.

Sudbery, J., Hicks, S., Thompson, S., McLaughlin, H. and Bramley, C., with Wilson, K. (2005) *A Bibliography of Family Placement Literature: A Guide to Publications on Children, Parents and Carers*. London: British Association for Adoption and Fostering.

Sugarman, L. (2009) *Lifespan Development: Theories, Concepts and Interventions*. Second edition. Hove: Psychology Press.

Sullivan, A. (2002) Alone again, naturally: the Catholic Church and the homosexual. In E. F. Rogers (ed.) *Theology and Sexuality: Classic and Contemporary Readings*. Oxford and Malden, MA: Blackwell.

Sutherland, N. S. (1998) *Breakdown: A Personal Crisis and a Medical Dilemma*. Oxford and New York: Oxford University Press.

Svanberg, P. O. G. (1998) Attachment, resilience and prevention. *Journal of Mental Health*, 7(6): 543–578.

Tajfel, H. and Turner, J. (1982) Social identity and intergroup relations. In W. G. Austin and S. Worchel (eds) *The Social Psychology of Intergroup Relations*. Cambridge: Cambridge University Press.

Tanner, J. M. (1992) Growth as a measure of the nutritional and hygienic status of a population. *Hormone Research*, 38(Suppl. 1): 106–115.

Taylor, S. E., Klein, L. C., Lewis, B. P., Gruenewald, T. L., Gurung, R. A. R. and Updegraff, J. A. (2000) Biobehavioral responses to stress in females: tend-and-befriend, not fight-or-flight. *Psychological Review*, 107(3): 411–429.

Tharinger, D. and Wells, G. (2000) An attachment perspective on the developmental challenges of gay and lesbian adolescents: the need for continuity of caregiving from family and schools. *School Psychology Review*, 29: 158–172.

Thompson, R. (2005) Multiple relationships multiply considered. *Human Development*, 48: 102–107.

Thompson, S. (1990) Putting a big thing into a little hole: teenage girls' accounts of sexual initiation. *Journal of Sex Research*, 27(3): 341–361.

Tomassini, C. (2005) Demographic profile. In A. Soule, P. Babb, M. Evandrou, S. Balchin and L. Zealey (eds) *Focus on Older People* (pp. 1–10). Basingstoke: Palgrave Macmillan. Online: www.statistics.gov.uk/downloads/theme_compendia/foop05/Olderpeople2005.pdf.

Townsend, P. (1979) *Poverty in the United Kingdom: A Survey of Household Resources and Standards of Living*. Berkeley: University of California Press.

Truax, C. B. and Carkhuff, R. R. (1967) *Toward Effective Counseling and Psychotherapy: Training and Practice*. Chicago: Aldine.

Truckle, S. (2000) Treatment or torture? Working with issues of abuse and torture in the transference. In U. McCluskey and C.-A. Hooper (eds) *Psychodynamic Perpectives on Abuse: The Cost of Fear*. London: Jessica Kingsley.

UK Parliament (2007) *Joint Committee on the Human Tissue and Embryo (Draft) Bill. Session 2006–2007. Volume 1: Report*. London: The Stationery Office. Available at: https://publications.parliament.uk/pa/jt/jtembryos.htm. Accessed 7 January 2018.

UK Parliament (2008) *A Life Like Any Other? Human Rights of Adults with Learning Disabilities*. London: Parliamentary Joint Committee on Human Rights. Available at: https://publications.parliament.uk/pa/jt200708/jtselect/jtrights/40/40i.pdf. Accessed 14 November 2017.

UNHCR (2018) Figures at a glance. Available at: www.unhcr.org/uk/figures-at-a-glance.html. Accessed 2 January 2018.

US Department of Health and Human Services (2007) Re-authorization of Headstart Act. Washington, DC.

van Anders, S. M. and Watson, N. V. (2007) Testosterone levels in women and men who are single, in long-distance relationships, or same-city relationships. *Hormones and Behavior*, 51(2): 286–291.

van Anders, S. M., Hamilton, L. D., Schmidt, N. and Watson, N. V. (2007a) Associations between testosterone secretion and sexual activity in women. *Hormones and Behavior*, 51(4): 477–482.

van Anders, S. M., Hamilton, L. D. and Watson, N. V. (2007b) Multiple partners are associated with higher testosterone in North American men and women. *Hormones and Behavior*, 51(3): 454–459.

van den Akker, O., Andre, J. and Murphy, T. (1999) Adolescent sexual behaviour and knowledge. *British Journal of Midwifery*, 7(12): 765–769.

van der Wal, M. F., van Eijsden, M. and Bonsel, G. J. (2007). Stress and emotional problems during pregnancy and excessive infant crying. *Journal of Developmental and Behavioral Pediatrics*, 28(6).

van IJzendoorn, M. H. and Sagi, A. (1999) Cross-cultural patterns of attachment; universal and contextual dimensions. In J. Cassidy and P. Shaver (eds) *Handbook of Attachment: Theory, Research and Clinical Applications*. New York and London: Guilford Press.

Vincent, J. A. (2003) *Old Age*. London and New York: Routledge.

Vincent, N. (2006) *Self-Made Man: My Year Disguised as a Man*. London: Atlantic.

Von Klitzing, K., Simoni, H. and Bürgin, D. (1999) Child development and early triadic relationships. *International Journal of Psycho-Analysis*, 80: 71–89.

Vygotsky, L. S. and Cole, M. (1978) *L.S. Vygotsky: Mind in Society*. Cambridge, MA: Harvard University Press.

Waddell, M. (2002) *Inside Lives*. London: Duckworth.

Wade, J. and Dixon, J. (2006) Making a home, finding a job: Investigating early housing and employment outcomes for young people leaving care. *Child and Family Social Work*, 11(3): 199–208. Research report online: www.york.ac.uk/inst/spru/research/pdf/leaving.pdf.

Waldfogel, J. (1998) Understanding the gender gap in pay for women with children. *Journal of Economic Perspectives*, 12(1): 137–156.

Walsh, L., Turner, S., Lines, S., Hussey, L., Chen, Y. and Agius, R. (2005) The incidence of work-related illness in the UK health and social work sector: The Health and Occupation Reporting network 2002–2003. *Occupational Medicine*, 55(4): 262–267.

Ward, C. A., Bochner, S. and Furnham, A. (2001) *The Psychology of Culture Shock*. Hove: Routledge.

Warr, P. (2002) *Psychology at Work*. Fifth edition. London: Penguin.

Watson, J. B. (1913). Image and affection in behavior. *Journal of Philosophy, Psychology and Scientific Methods*, 10: 421–428.

Watson, J. B. (1930) *Behaviorism*. Chicago: University of Chicago Press.

Weiner, G. (1994) *Feminisms in Education: An Introduction*. Buckingham: Open University Press.

Weiss, R. S. (1980) *Loneliness: The Experience of Emotional and Social Isolation*. Cambridge, MA: MIT Press.

Wellings, K., Field, J., Johnson, A. M. and Wadsworth, J. (eds) (1994) *Sexual Behavior in Britain: The National Survey of Sexual Attitudes and Lifestyles*. London: Penguin Books.

Wellings, K., Nanchahal, K., Macdowall, W., McManus, S., Erens, B., Mercer, C. et al. (2001) Sexual behaviour in Britain: early heterosexual experience. *Lancet*, 358: 1843–1850.

White, S. (undated) *Death of a Child*. Online: http://support.childbereavement.org.uk/files/Death_of_a_Child_6pp.pdf. Accessed 7 January 2018.

Whiting, R. (2008) 'No room for religion or spirituality or cooking tips': exploring practical atheism as an unspoken consensus in the development of social work values in England. *Ethics and Social Welfare*, 2(1): 67–83.

Whittaker, A. (2011) Social defences and organisational culture in a local authority child protection setting: challenges for the Munro Review? *Journal of Social Work Practice*, 25(4): 481–496.

Whittaker, A. (2012). *Research Skills for Social Work*. Second edition. London: Sage.

Whittaker, A. and Havard, T. (2016) Defensive practice as 'fear-based' practice: social work's open secret? *British Journal of Social Work*, 46(5): 1158–1174.

Whitten, P. L. (1992) Chemical revolution to sexual revolution: historical changes in human reproductive development. In T. Colborn and C. Clement (eds) *Chemically-Induced Alterations in Sexual and Functional Development: The Wildlife/Human Connection* (pp. 311–334). Princeton, NJ: Princeton Scientific Publishing Co.

Wikeley, F., Bullock, K., Muschamp, Y. and Ridge, T. (2007) *Educational Relationships Outside School: Why Access Is Important*. York: Joseph Rowntree Foundation.

Wilkins, D. (2012). Disorganised attachment indicates child maltreatment: how is this link useful for child protection social workers? *Journal of Social Work Practice*, 26(1): 15–30.

Williams, P. and Evans, M. (2013) *Social Work with People with Learning Difficulties*. Third edition. London: Sage.

Wilson, D., Sharp, C. and Patterson, A. (2006) *Young People and Crime: Findings from the 2005 Offending, Crime and Justice Survey (OCJS)*. London: Home Office. Online: www.homeoffice.gov.uk/rds/pdfs06/hosb1706.pdf.

Wilson, K., Ruch, G., Lymbery, M. and Cooper, A. (2011) *Social Work: An Introduction to Contemporary Practice*. Second edition. Harlow: Pearson.

Wine, J. D. (1989/2007) Gynocentric values and feminist psychology. In A. Miles and G. Finn (eds) *Feminism: From Pressure to Politics*. Montreal: Black Rose Books.

Winnicott, D. W. (1952/2007) *Through Paediatrics to Psychoanalysis*. London: Hogarth Press and Institute of Psycho-Analysis.

Winnicott, D. W. (1979) *The Maturational Processes and the Facilitating Environment: Studies in the Theory of Emotional Development*. London: Hogarth Press.

Winterowd, C., Beck, A. T. and Gruener, D. (2003) *Cognitive Therapy with Chronic Pain Patients*. New York: Springer.

Woodmansey, A. C. (1966) The internalization of external conflict. *International Journal of Psychoanalysis*, 47: 349–355.

Woodmansey, C. (1972) The unity of casework. *Social Work Today*, 2(19): 10–12.

Woodmansey, C. (1989) Internal conflict. *British Journal of Psychotherapy*, 6(1): 26–49.

Worden, J. W. (2009) *Grief Counselling and Grief Therapy: A Handbook for the Mental Health Practitioner*. Fourth edition. Philadelphia and Hove: Brunner-Routledge.

World Health Organisation (2017) Female genital mutilation. Online: www.who.int/reproductivehealth/topics/fgm/prevalence/en/. Accessed 2 December 2017.

Xu, X. and Whyte, M. (1990) Love matches and arranged marriages: a Chinese replication. *Journal of Marriage and the Family*, 52(8): 709–722.

Yelsma, P. and Athappilly, K. (1988) Marital satisfaction and communication practices: comparisons among Indian and American couples. *Journal of Comparative Family Studies*, 19(1): 37–54.

Yu, M. and Stiffman, A. R. (2007) Culture and environment as predictors of alcohol abuse/dependence symptoms in American Indian youths. *Addictive Behaviors*, 32(10): 2253–2259.

Zeifman, D. and Hazan, C. (2016) Pair bonds as attachments: mounting evidence in support of Bowlby's hypothesis. In J. Cassidy and P. Shaver (eds) *Handbook of Attachment: Theory, Research and Clinical Applications*. New York and London: Guilford Press.

Zelt, D. (1981) First person account: the Messiah quest. *Schizophrenia Bulletin*, 7(3): 527–531.

Index

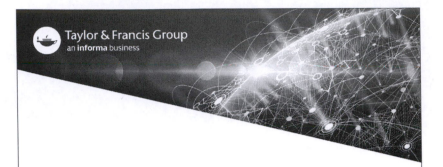